Current Progress in Gastroenterology

Current Progress in Gastroenterology

Edited by Calvin Bush

hayle
medical

New York

Hayle Medical,
750 Third Avenue, 9th Floor,
New York, NY 10017, USA

Visit us on the World Wide Web at:
www.haylemedical.com

© Hayle Medical, 2018

ISBN: 978-1-63241-488-5

Cataloging-in-Publication Data

Current progress in gastroenterology / edited by Calvin Bush.
    p. cm.
Includes bibliographical references and index.
ISBN 978-1-63241-488-5
1. Gastroenterology. 2. Digestive organs--Diseases. I. Bush, Calvin.
RC801 .C87 2018
616.33--dc23

Table of Contents

Preface

In my initial years as a student, I used to run to the library at every possible instance to grab a book and learn something new. Books were my primary source of knowledge and I would not have come such a long way without all that I learnt from them. Thus, when I was approached to edit this book; I became understandably nostalgic. It was an absolute honor to be considered worthy of guiding the current generation as well as those to come. I put all my knowledge and hard work into making this book most beneficial for its readers.

The field of gastroenterology is one of the most important fields in the medicinal science. It deals with the identification, prevention and treatment of disorders and ailments occurring in the digestive system, including alimentary canal. Few of the treatment processes included in this field are endoscopy, liver biopsy, proctology, colonoscopy, etc. This book provides significant information about this discipline to help develop a better understanding of gastroenterology and its sub-fields. Some of the diverse topics covered in the book address the varied branches that fall under this subject. It is a complete source of knowledge on the present status of this important field.

I wish to thank my publisher for supporting me at every step. I would also like to thank all the authors who have contributed their researches in this book. I hope this book will be a valuable contribution to the progress of the field.

Editor

Protective Effect of Daikenchuto on Dextran Sulfate Sodium-Induced Colitis in Mice

Takaharu Matsunaga,[1] **Shinichi Hashimoto,**[1] **Naoki Yamamoto,**[1,2]
Ryo Kawasato,[1] **Tomohiro Shirasawa,**[1] **Atsushi Goto,**[1] **Koichi Fujisawa,**[1,3]
Taro Takami,[1] **Takeshi Okamoto,**[1] **Jun Nishikawa,**[1,4] **and Isao Sakaida**[1]

[1]*Department of Gastroenterology and Hepatology, Yamaguchi University Graduate School of Medicine,
1-1-1 Minami Kogushi, Ube, Yamaguchi 755-8505, Japan*

[2]*Yamaguchi University Health Administration Center, 1677-1 Yoshida, Yamaguchi, Yamaguchi 753-8511, Japan*

[3]*Center of Research and Education for Regenerative Medicine, Yamaguchi University Graduate School of Medicine,
1-1-1 Minami Kogushi, Ube, Yamaguchi 755-8505, Japan*

[4]*Department of Laboratory Science, Yamaguchi University Graduate School of Medicine, 1-1-1 Minami Kogushi,
Ube, Yamaguchi 755-8505, Japan*

Correspondence should be addressed to Shinichi Hashimoto; has-333@yamaguchi-u.ac.jp

Academic Editor: Jean-Francois Beaulieu

Aim. To investigate the effect of daikenchuto (TJ-100; DKT) for ulcerative colitis (UC) model mouse and assess its anti-inflammatory mechanisms. *Methods.* We evaluated the effects of DKT on dextran sulfate sodium- (DSS-) induced experimental colitis. First, we assessed the short-term effects of DKT using two groups: 5% DSS group and 5% DSS with DKT group. Colon length; histological scores; and interleukin- (IL-) 10, IL-1β, and tumor necrosis factor-α mRNA expression profiles were analyzed using real-time PCR. Second, we assessed the long-term effects of DKT, by comparing survival time between 2% DSS and 2% DSS with DKT groups. *Results.* After 7 days, the colon lengths of DSS + DKT group were longer than those of the DSS group (mean values: 6.11 versus 5.69 cm, $p < 0.05$). Furthermore, compared to DSS group, the DSS + DKT group maintained significantly higher levels of serum hemoglobin (13.1 versus 10.7 g/dL, $p < 0.05$) and exhibited significantly higher expression levels of IL-10 ($p < 0.05$). The 2% DSS + DKT group exhibited significantly longer survival time than the 2% DSS group (70 versus 44 days, $p < 0.01$). *Conclusion.* Our results indicate that DKT prevented inflammation in the colon, indicating its potential as a new therapeutic agent for UC.

1. Introduction

Ulcerative colitis (UC) is a chronic, recurrent inflammatory disease of the colon and rectum, characterized by bloody diarrhea, intestinal mucosal ulceration, and infiltration of neutrophils and lymphocytes into the mucous membrane [1]. Although multiple factors such as environmental changes, gene variations, and gut microbiota were thought to be associated with UC, its pathogenesis has not been fully elucidated [2]. In recent years, novel therapeutic agents to treat UC, such as tacrolimus, infliximab, and adalimumab, have become available in Japan, and these new drugs have enabled many patients to avoid surgery [3–5]. However, many of the therapeutic agents used to treat UC are immunosuppressants, and because UC commonly develops in elderly patients, there is a real risk of complications due to infection [6].

Daikenchuto (DKT) is a traditional herbal medicine prepared by mixing Ginseng Radix, Zanthoxyli Fructus, and Zingiberis Processum Rhizoma in a 3 : 2 : 5 ratio, extracting the essence, and then adding Saccharum Granorum. Some studies have reported the clinical efficacy of DKT in treating postoperative paralytic ileus, and recent research has shown that DKT has an inhibitory effect on inflammation in Crohn's disease and prevents colon adhesions in animal models [7–10].

Dextran sulfate sodium (DSS) induces severe mucosal inflammation and colitis, and DSS-induced colitis is considered a type of UC model in terms of morphological and pathophysiological features [11, 12]. DSS-induced colitis model has been generally used to understand the molecular mechanisms of action or to assess the therapeutic effects of test compounds in treatment of UC [13–15].

In this study, we evaluated the effects of DKT on the development of DSS-induced experimental colitis in mice.

2. Materials and Methods

2.1. Mice. Female C57BL/6 mice, eight weeks of age, with an average weight of 18–20 g were purchased from Chiyoda SLC (Tokyo, Japan). They were acclimatized for 1 week before the experiment and were housed individually in a room maintained at 22°C under a 12 h day/night cycle throughout the experiment. The mice were provided with food and drinking water ad libitum. The mice were maintained in specific pathogen-free housing at the Animal Experiment Facility of Yamaguchi University School of Medicine and cared for in accordance with the animal ethics requirements of the Yamaguchi University School of Medicine.

2.2. Assessment of Inflammation in Mouse Model of DSS-Induced Colitis. The mice were divided into three groups ($n = 10$ per group): normal group, DSS group, and DSS + DKT group. Mice in the normal group remained untreated. Mice in the DSS and DSS + DKT groups were both provided with 5% DSS (mol. wt. 5000; Wako Pure Chemical Industries Ltd., Osaka, Japan) through water bottles. Additionally, 6 mg/g body weight of DKT was orally administered using infection tubes in the DSS + DKT group, while 0.2 mL distilled water was orally administered in the same manner in the other two groups. Previous study reported by Case et al. shows that acute oral toxicity study in mice revealed LD50 value 2.64 gm/kg for DSS [16]. Okayasu et al. used 3–10% DSS in their study, and we used 5% DSS for this study [11]. Kono et al. reported anticolitis effect for colitis mouse model using 2.7 mg/g body weight of DKT [10]. According to this study, we used 6 mg/g body weight of DKT which was nearly double to 2.7 mg/g. The intake of both water and food was measured in each group. Serum samples were obtained by eye puncture method on Day 7. In all the experiments, serum hemoglobin (Hb) was measured using an analyzer for clinical chemistry (SPOTCHEM EZ SP-4430; Arkray, Kyoto, Japan). In addition, we recorded the body weight and length of the colon on Day 7.

2.3. Histological Assessment. Mice were anesthetized using halothane (Wako, Japan) and killed by cervical dislocation. Histological examination was performed on samples of the distal colon from each mouse. The samples were fixed in 4% formaldehyde overnight at 4°C. Paraffin sections (4 μm) were stained with hematoxylin and eosin (H&E). All histological evaluations were performed according to the histological score calculation method previously described by Morohoshi

et al. [15]; the histological score was estimated by the combined of inflammatory cell infiltration and tissue damage. The infiltration scoring was as follows: 0, no infiltration; 1, presence of occasional inflammatory cells in the lamina propria; 2, increased numbers of inflammatory cells in the lamina propria; and 3, confluent inflammatory cells extending into the submucosa. The tissue damage scoring was as follows: 0, no mucosal damage; 1, discrete lymphoepithelial lesions; 2, surface mucosal erosion or focal ulceration; and 3, extensive mucosal damage and extension into deeper structures of the bowel wall. The combined histological score was used for examination. The H&E-stained sections were observed using a Keyence BIOREVO BZ9000 microscope (Osaka, Japan).

2.4. Real-Time Quantitative Polymerase Chain Reaction (PCR). Total RNA was isolated from the distal colons of mice. The mRNA expression profiles of interleukin- (IL-) 10, IL-1β, and tumor necrosis factor- (TNF-) α were evaluated using real-time quantitative PCR. Briefly, total RNA was extracted using an RNeasy Mini kit (Qiagen GmbH; Hilden, Germany) according to the manufacturer's instructions. The primers used were as follows: mouse IL-10 primers—sense (5'-CCAGTTTTACCTGGTAGAAGT-GATG-3'), antisense (5'-TGTCTAGGTCCTGGAGTC-CAGCAGACTC-3'); mouse IL-1β primers—sense (5'-CAC-AGCAGCACATCAACAAG-3'), antisense (5'-GTGCTC-ATGTCCTCATCCTG-3'); mouse TNF-α primers—sense (5'-GCCTCTTCTCATTCCTGCTTG-3'), antisense (5'-CTGATGAGAGGGAGGCCATT-3'); and mouse β-actin primers—sense (5'-TGACAGGATGCAGAAGGAGA-3'), antisense (5'-GCTGGAAGGTGGACAGTGAG-3'). PCR amplification was performed in triplicate using the following cycle conditions: 40 cycles at 90°C for 30 s, 55–60°C for 45 s, and 72°C for 1 min. β-Actin was used as the reference gene.

2.5. Survival Time Analysis. To analyze survival time, the mice were divided into two groups: 2% DSS group ($n = 9$) and 2% DSS + DKT ($n = 9$) group, in which the mice were provided 2% DSS or 2% DSS + 3 mg/g body weight DKT, respectively, through water bottles for 100 days.

2.6. Statistical Analysis. All values are expressed as the mean ± standard error of the mean (SEM). Statistical significance was determined using two-tailed Student's t-test. Differences in p values < 0.05 were considered significant. Kaplan–Meier estimator was used for survival time analysis. We used Excel Statistics 2012 (SSRI Co., Ltd.; Tokyo, Japan) for all statistical analyses.

3. Results

3.1. Morphological and Histological Analyses of DKT-Treated Mice. As shown in Figure 1, body weight gain of mice on Day 7 was significantly lower in the DSS group and DSS + DKT group than in the normal group ($p < 0.05$). There was no difference between the DSS and the DSS + DKT group in terms of body weight. Morphology analysis of the colon showed that the colon lengths of mice in the DSS + DKT group were significantly longer than those of DSS

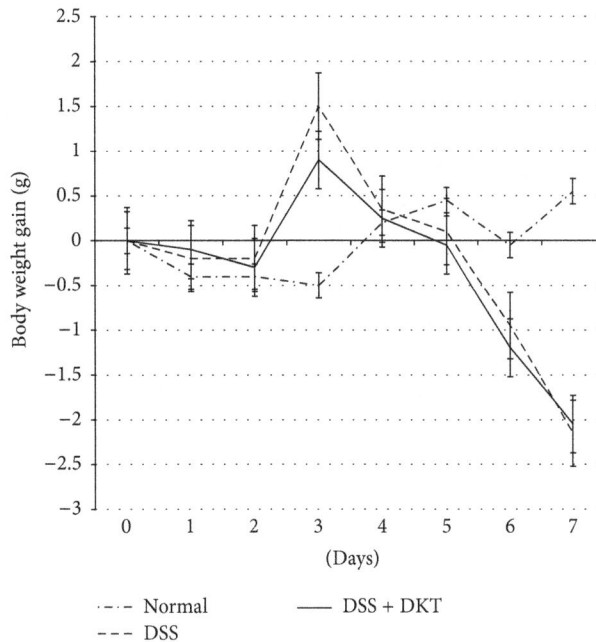

FIGURE 1: Body weight gain of each study group. Normal group, untreated mice. Dextran sulfate sodium (DSS) group, mice provided with 5% DSS for 7 days. DSS + daikenchuto (DKT) group, mice provided with DKT in addition to DSS. $n = 10$ mice (for normal, DSS, and DSS + DKT groups).

group mice ($p < 0.05$). Meanwhile, there was no significant difference between DSS + DKT group and DSS group in colon relative weight (weight/length) (Figure 2). The DSS + DKT group showed significantly higher levels of serum Hb than the DSS group ($p < 0.05$) (Figure 3). DSS-induced colitis is characterized by histological findings such as edema, infiltration of inflammatory cells into the mucosa and submucosa, destruction of epithelial cells, and mucosal thickening (Figures 4(a)–4(f)). The histological score was significantly lower in the DSS + DKT group than that in the DSS group ($p < 0.05$) (Figure 5).

3.2. Gene Expression in the Colon. We analyzed the mRNA expression of IL-10, IL-1β, and TNF-α in the colon after 7 days of the experiment (Figures 6(a), 6(b), and 6(c)). The IL-10 mRNA expression in the DSS + DKT group was significantly higher than that in the DSS group ($p < 0.05$) (Figure 6(a)). The IL-1β and TNF-α mRNA expression levels in the DSS + DKT group were lower than those in the DSS group; however, there was no significant difference in the two groups ($p = 0.06$ and 0.54, resp.) (Figures 6(b) and 6(c)).

3.3. Survival Time Analysis. The survival time in the 2% DSS + DKT group was significantly higher than that in the 2% DSS group (mean value: 70 days versus control 44 days, $p = 0.0038$) (Figure 7).

4. Discussion

The purpose of this study was to elucidate the effects of DKT on DSS-induced colitis, and our results showed that DKT attenuated DSS-induced colitis in mice and prolonged

the survival of DSS-treated mice. In the DSS group, we noted weight loss, shortening of colon length, and significantly higher histological scores compared with the normal group and thus confirmed that DSS did induce colitis. An associated reduction in peripheral blood Hb concentration was also noted. In the DSS + DKT group, although the weight reduction caused by DSS was not inhibited, the shortening of colon length and elevation of the histological score were significantly inhibited, in addition to a milder reduction in the Hb concentration than that in the DSS group. Furthermore, in the molecular biological investigation via real-time PCR analysis, the IL-10 anti-inflammatory cytokine level was significantly elevated in the DSS + DKT group, while although the difference was not significant, the levels of inflammatory cytokines IL-1β and TNF-α decreased. This indicates that DKT also exerts an anti-inflammatory effect at the cytokine level.

Kono et al. [10] evaluated the therapeutic effect of DKT using mouse models of colitis induced by intrarectal instillation of 2,4,6-trinitrobenzenesulfonic acid (TNBS); this TNBS-induced colitis model is widely used as Crohn's disease model. The macroscopic and microscopic evaluation scores in their study were lower in the DKT combination group than in the TNBS-only treatment group. The levels of cytokines TNF-α and interferon- (INF-) γ were lower in the DKT combination group than in the TNBS-only treatment group, and IL-1β levels tended to be lower, though not significantly.

Adrenomedullin (ADM) is attracting attention as a central component of the pathway that drives the anti-inflammatory action of DKT. ADM is a peptide belonging to the calcitonin family and is a potent endogenous vasodilator [17]. It is unevenly distributed in the gastrointestinal tract

(a)

(b)

(c)

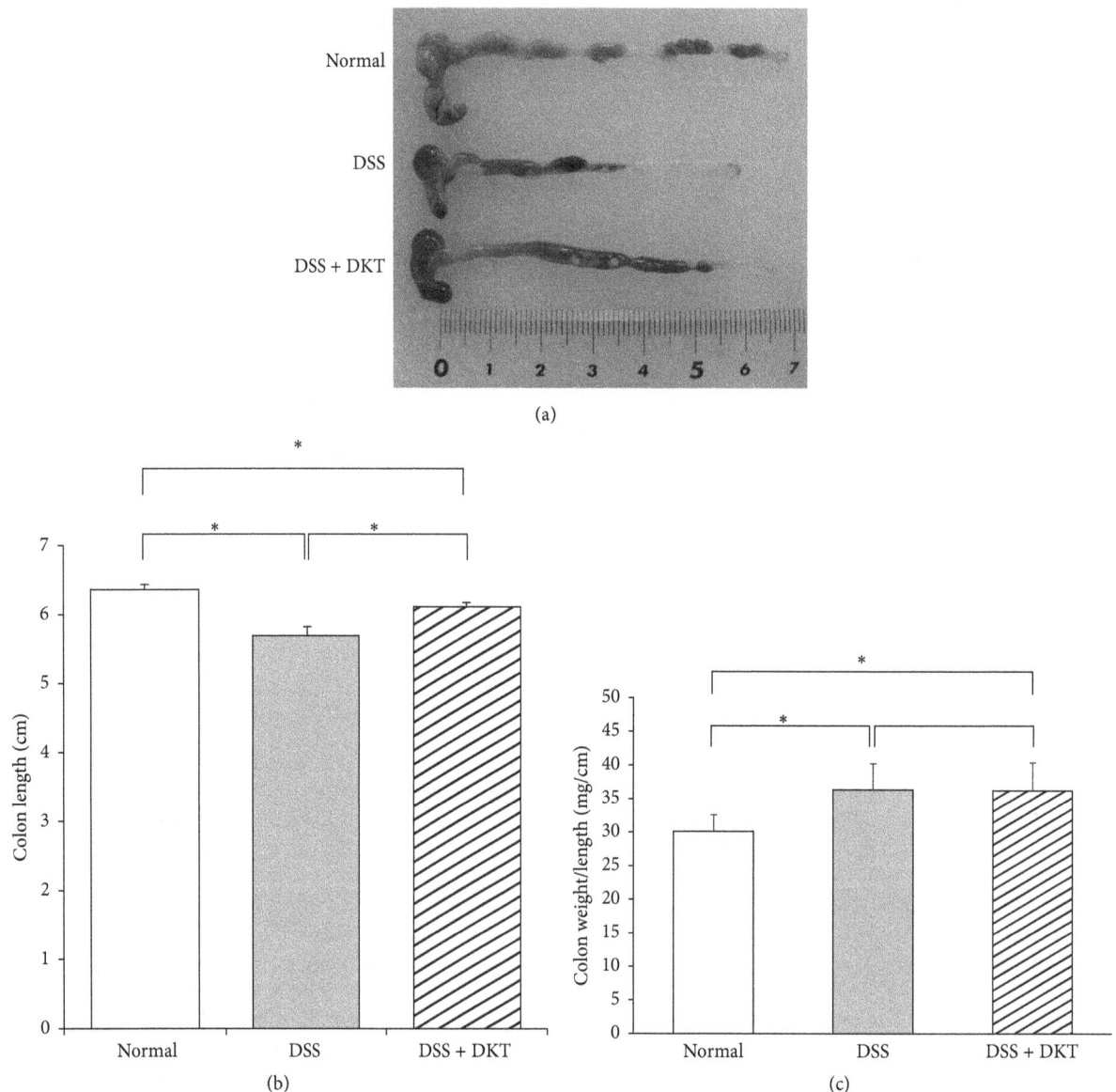

FIGURE 2: (a) Macroscopic appearance and (b) colon length of each study group. Normal group, untreated mice. Dextran sulfate sodium (DSS) group, mice provided with 5% DSS for 7 days. DSS + daikenchuto (DKT) group, mice provided with DKT in addition to DSS. $n = 10$ mice (for normal, DSS, and DSS + DKT groups). (c) Colon relative weight (weight/length) of each study group. $^{*}p < 0.05$.

and plays an important role in regulating microcirculation. ADM also exhibits anti-inflammatory action by inhibiting the production of inflammatory cytokines, particularly TNF-α [18]. TNF-α is an extremely important cytokine in the treatment of Crohn's disease and UC, and investigations have been underway regarding the possibility of using ADM to treat Crohn's disease [19]. In fact, ADM has been found to exert an anti-inflammatory effect in mouse and rat models of Crohn's disease [20, 21]. In a mouse model of DSS-induced colitis, intraperitoneal administration of ADM was shown to inhibit colon inflammation, and research has shown that administration of ADM reduces the levels of cytokines such as TNF-α, IL-1β, and IL-6 [22]. However, exogenous administration of ADM has not yet been put into practical use because of the necessity to verify the effect of ADM on organs other than those of the gastrointestinal tract and also because ADM does not remain for long at the target site owing to metabolism and clearance [23–25]. Conversely, there have been reports that DKT increases endogenous ADM, which manifests as an anti-inflammatory effect in the colon. In addition, DKT is known to have few adverse reactions and hence may be considered as a method to safely induce ADM expression [10]. We additionally found increased expression of IL-10, but the effect of ADM on IL-10 has not yet been investigated. We therefore consider this information vital for elucidating the action mechanisms of both DKT and ADM.

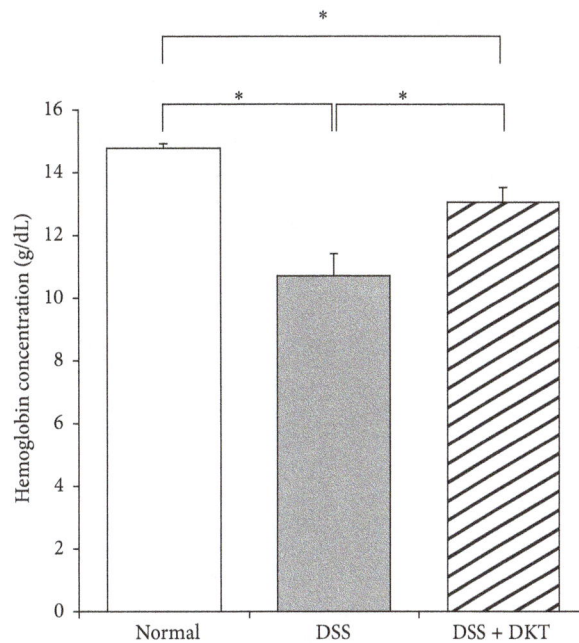

FIGURE 3: Hemoglobin concentration of each study group. Normal group, untreated mice. Dextran sulfate sodium (DSS) group, mice provided with 5% DSS for 7 days. DSS + daikenchuto (DKT) group, mice provided with DKT in addition to DSS. $n = 10$ mice (for normal, DSS, and DSS + DKT groups). $^{*}p < 0.05$.

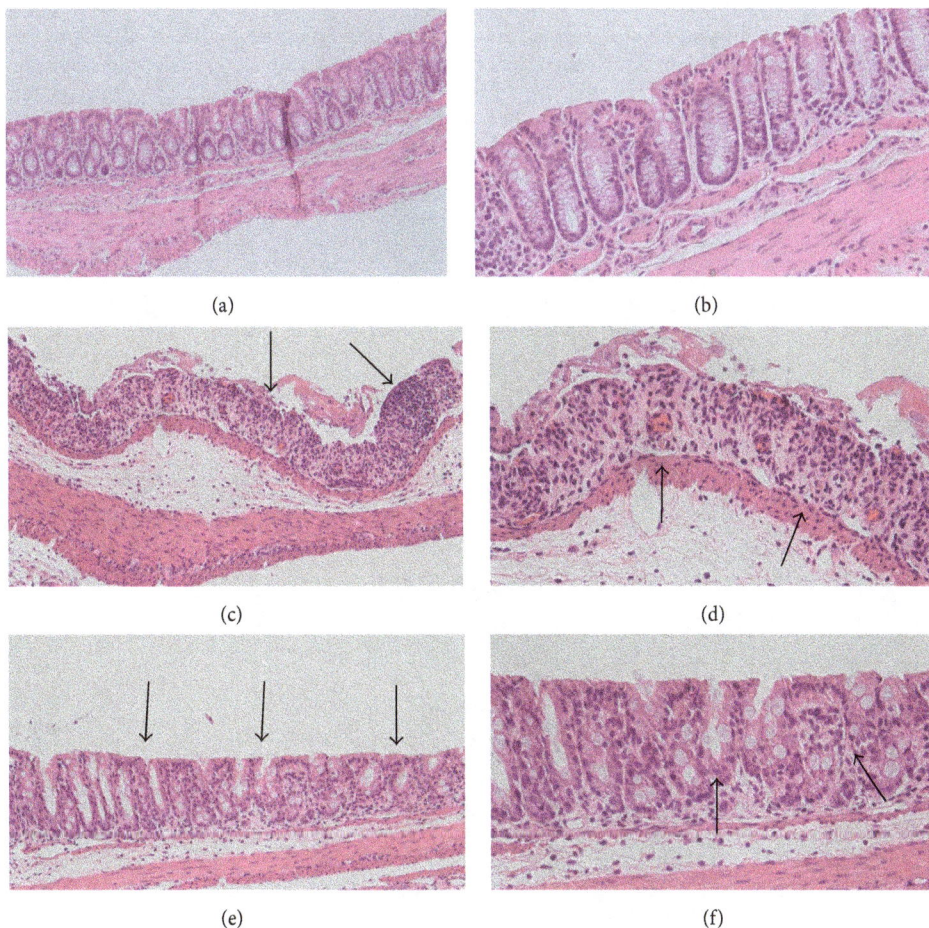

FIGURE 4: Histopathological analysis of hematoxylin and eosin-stained sections of the distal colon. (a, b) Untreated normal mouse: no disturbance of the ductal structure and no thickening of the wall. (c, d) Mouse provided with 5% dextran sulfate sodium (DSS) for 7 days: disturbance in the ductal structure and thickening of the wall *(arrows)*. (e, f) Mouse administered a combination of 5% DSS and daikenchuto: disturbance in the ductal structure and thickening of the wall, but milder than that in mouse provided with DSS alone *(arrows)*. Original magnification (a), (c), and (e): ×20; (b), (d), and (f): ×40.

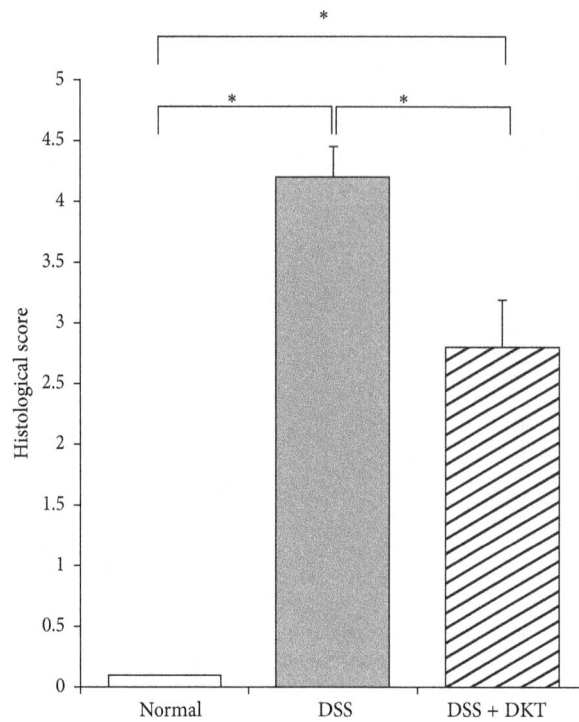

FIGURE 5: Histological score of each study group. Normal group, untreated mice. Dextran sulfate sodium (DSS) group, mice provided with 5% DSS for 7 days. DSS + daikenchuto (DKT) group, mice provided with DKT in addition to DSS. $n = 10$ mice (for normal, DSS, and DSS + DKT groups). $^*p < 0.05$.

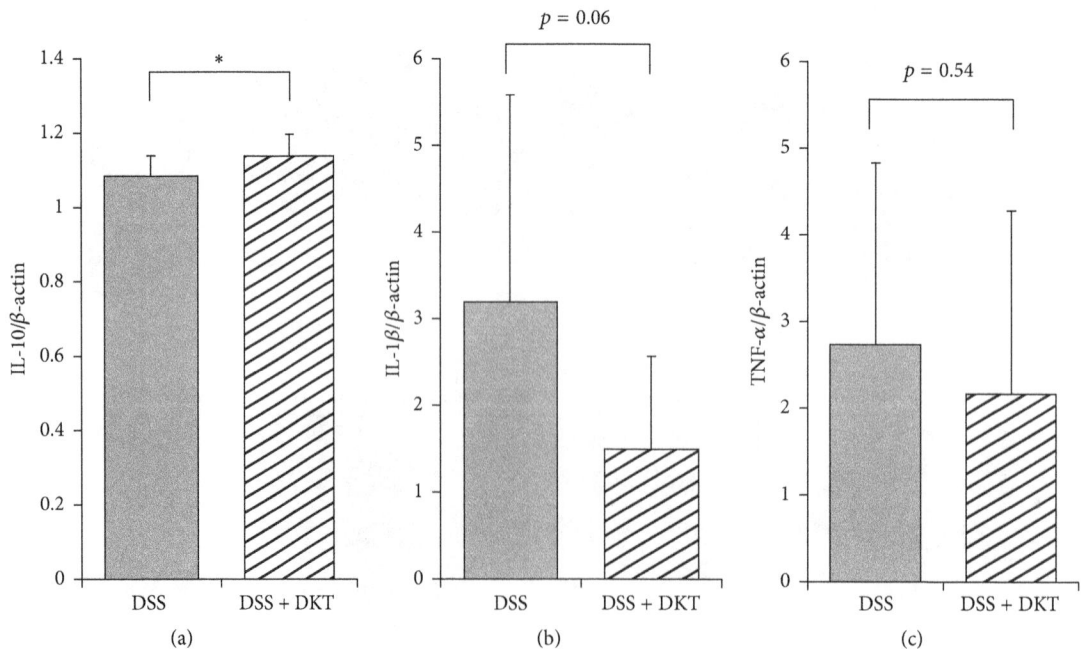

FIGURE 6: Anti-inflammatory and inflammatory cytokine levels of each study group. (a) Interleukin- (IL-) 10. (b) IL-1β. (c) Tumor necrosis factor- (TNF-) α. Normal group, untreated mice. Dextran sulfate sodium (DSS) group, mice administered 5% DSS for 7 days. DSS + daikenchuto (DKT) group, mice provided with DKT in addition to DSS. $n = 10$ mice (for normal, DSS, and DSS + DKT groups). $^*p < 0.05$.

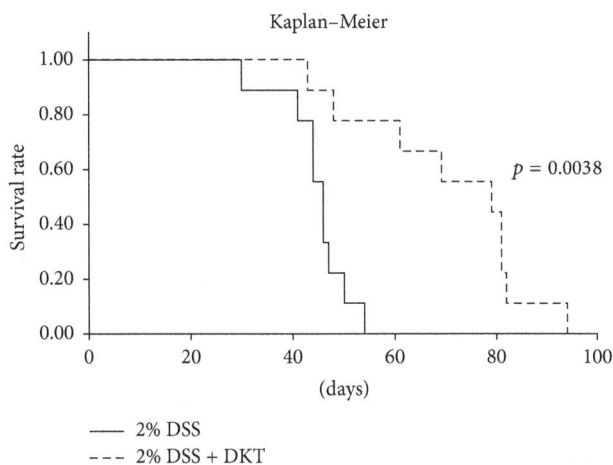

FIGURE 7: Survival time of each study group. 2% dextran sulfate sodium (DSS) group, mice provided with 2% DSS. 2% DSS + daikenchuto (DKT) group, mice provided with DKT in addition to DSS. $n = 9$ mice (for 2% DSS and 2% DSS + DKT groups).

Furthermore, in this study, in mice administered 2% DSS, it was proven that DKT prolonged survival time. In previous studies of the anti-inflammatory effect in DSS-induced colitis, the majority of the evaluations were conducted over a short period, such as 7 days; however, in this study, we clarified that the action of DKT extends over a long period. In actual clinical practice, a variety of treatments can be used to induce UC remission; however, in Japan, options for remission maintenance therapy for UC comprise only 5-aminosalicylic acid, azathioprine, and anti-TNF-α antibodies infliximab and adalimumab. Patients who do not respond adequately to 5-aminosalicylic acid or cannot tolerate azathioprine are administered anti-TNF-α antibodies, which are expensive and not always affordable as therapy. In addition, as these drugs exert an immunosuppressant effect, it is essential to be cautious when administering these drugs to elderly patients. DKT is inexpensive, has no immunosuppressant action, and shows long-term protective effects in DSS-induced colitis model, demonstrating its potential for use in remission maintenance therapy for UC.

Previous studies have shown the efficacy of DKT in maintaining postoperative remission in Crohn's disease; however, to the best of our knowledge, no other studies have yet demonstrated the efficacy of DKT in the treatment of inflammatory bowel disease. We believe that the results of our study will promote further research showing the actual efficacy and safety of DKT in treating patients with UC.

The limitations of this study are as follows: we did not confirm the hypothesized anti-inflammatory action mechanism of DKT. It is essential to verify the actual expression of ADM using real-time PCR and immunohistological tests. Further, DKT is a mixture of Ginseng Radix, Zanthoxyli Fructus, and Zingiberis Processum Rhizoma. Although there are several reports about anti-inflammatory effect of Ginseng Radix (Ginsenoside Rb1) and Zingiberis Processum Rhizoma (6-shoganol), the complementary action of the three components has not been elucidated [26, 27].

5. Conclusion

To the best of our knowledge, this is the first study to demonstrate the anti-inflammatory effect of DKT in DSS-induced colitis mouse model, which serves as a UC disease model. We also reported the involvement of IL-10 and showed that DKT prolonged the survival time of mice with DSS-induced colitis. We believe that these are important findings for the future development of safe and low-cost novel therapeutic agents for the treatment of UC.

Competing Interests

All authors declare no competing financial interests.

Acknowledgments

This study was supported by Grants-in-Aid for Scientific Research from the Japan Society for the Promotion of Science (25460123), the Japan Science and Technology Agency, and the Ministry of Health, Labor, and Welfare. The authors thank Mrs. Mariko Yamada, Mrs. Ihoko Fujimoto, and Mrs. Hiromi Kurose for their technical assistance and support.

References

[1] D. K. Podolsky, "Inflammatory bowel disease," *The New England Journal of Medicine*, vol. 347, no. 6, pp. 417–429, 2002.

[2] H. S. P. De Souza and C. Fiocchi, "Immunopathogenesis of IBD: current state of the art," *Nature Reviews Gastroenterology and Hepatology*, vol. 13, no. 1, pp. 13–27, 2016.

[3] K. Fellermann, D. Ludwig, M. Stahl, T. David-Walek, and E. F. Stange, "Steroid-unresponsive acute attacks of inflammatory bowel disease: immunomodulation by tacrolimus (FK506)," *The American Journal of Gastroenterology*, vol. 93, no. 10, pp. 1860–1866, 1998.

[4] P. Rutgeerts, W. J. Sandborn, B. G. Feagan et al., "Infliximab for induction and maintenance therapy for ulcerative colitis," *The*

New England Journal of Medicine, vol. 353, no. 23, pp. 2462–2476, 2005.

[5] W. Reinisch, W. J. Sandborn, D. W. Hommes et al., "Adalimumab for induction of clinical remission in moderately to severely active ulcerative colitis: results of a randomised controlled trial," *Gut*, vol. 60, no. 6, pp. 780–787, 2011.

[6] A. N. Ananthakrishnan, E. L. McGinley, and D. G. Binion, "Inflammatory bowel disease in the elderly is associated with worse outcomes: a national study of hospitalizations," *Inflammatory Bowel Diseases*, vol. 15, no. 2, pp. 182–189, 2009.

[7] S. Endo, T. Nishida, K. Nishikawa et al., "Dai-kenchu-to, a Chinese herbal medicine, improves stasis of patients with total gastrectomy and jejunal pouch interposition," *American Journal of Surgery*, vol. 192, no. 1, pp. 9–13, 2006.

[8] T. Itoh, J. Yamakawa, M. Mai, N. Yamaguchi, and T. Kanda, "The effect of the herbal medicine dai-kenchu-to on post-operative ileus," *Journal of International Medical Research*, vol. 30, no. 4, pp. 428–432, 2002.

[9] N. Iwai, Y. Kume, O. Kimura, S. Ono, S. Aoi, and T. Tsuda, "Effects of herbal medicine Dai-Kenchu-To on anorectal function in children with severe constipation," *European Journal of Pediatric Surgery*, vol. 17, no. 2, pp. 115–118, 2007.

[10] T. Kono, A. Kaneko, Y. Hira et al., "Anti-colitis and -adhesion effects of daikenchuto via endogenous adrenomedullin enhancement in Crohn's disease mouse model," *Journal of Crohn's and Colitis*, vol. 4, no. 2, pp. 161–170, 2010.

[11] I. Okayasu, S. Hatakeyama, M. Yamada, T. Ohkusa, Y. Inagaki, and R. Nakaya, "A novel method in the induction of reliable experimental acute and chronic ulcerative colitis in mice," *Gastroenterology*, vol. 98, no. 3, pp. 694–702, 1990.

[12] C. G. Whittem, A. D. Williams, and C. S. Williams, "Murine colitis modeling using Dextran Sulfate Sodium (DSS)," *Journal of Visualized Experiments*, no. 35, 2010.

[13] T. Karuppuchamy, E. H. Behrens, P. González-Cabrera et al., "Sphingosine-1-phosphate receptor-1 (S1P$_1$) is expressed by lymphocytes, dendritic cells, and endothelium and modulated during inflammatory bowel disease," *Mucosal Immunology*, 2016.

[14] H. Kim, N. Banerjee, R. C. Barnes et al., "Mango polyphenolics reduce inflammation in intestinal colitis-involvement of the miR-126/PI3K/AKT/mTOR axis in vitro and in vivo," *Molecular Carcinogenesis*, vol. 56, no. 1, pp. 197–207, 2016.

[15] Y. Morohoshi, K. Matsuoka, H. Chinen et al., "Inhibition of neutrophil elastase prevents the development of murine dextran sulfate sodium-induced colitis," *Journal of Gastroenterology*, vol. 41, no. 4, pp. 318–324, 2006.

[16] M. T. Case, J. Knox Smith, and R. A. Nelson, "Acute mouse and chronic dog toxicity studies of danthron, dioctyl sodium sulfosuccinate, poloxalkol and combinations," *Drug and Chemical Toxicology*, vol. 1, no. 1, pp. 89–101, 1978.

[17] K. Kitamura, K. Kangawa, M. Kawamoto et al., "Adrenomedullin: a novel hypotensive peptide isolated from human pheochromocytoma," *Biochemical and Biophysical Research Communications*, vol. 192, no. 2, pp. 553–560, 1993.

[18] R. Wu, M. Zhou, and P. Wang, "Adrenomedullin and adrenomedullin binding protein-1 downregulate TNF-α in macrophage cell line and rat Kupffer cells," *Regulatory Peptides*, vol. 112, no. 1–3, pp. 19–26, 2003.

[19] W. J. Sandborn, "Clinical perspectives in Crohn's disease. Moving forward with anti-TNF-α therapy: current needs and future treatments," *Reviews in gastroenterological disorders*, vol. 7, pp. S23–35, 2007.

[20] E. Gonzalez-Rey, A. Fernandez-Martin, A. Chorny, and M. Delgado, "Therapeutic effect of urocortin and adrenomedullin in a murine model of Crohn's disease," *Gut*, vol. 55, no. 6, pp. 824–832, 2006.

[21] E. Talero, S. Sánchez-Fidalgo, C. A. de la Lastra, M. Illanes, J. R. Calvo, and V. Motilva, "Acute and chronic responses associated with adrenomedullin administration in experimental colitis," *Peptides*, vol. 29, no. 11, pp. 2001–2012, 2008.

[22] Y. Hayashi, K. Narumi, S. Tsuji et al., "Impact of adrenomedullin on dextran sulfate sodium-induced inflammatory colitis in mice: insights from in vitro and in vivo experimental studies," *International Journal of Colorectal Disease*, vol. 26, no. 11, pp. 1453–1462, 2011.

[23] T. Eto, K. Kitamura, and J. Kato, "Biological and clinical roles of adrenomedullin in circulation control and cardiovascular diseases," *Clinical and Experimental Pharmacology and Physiology*, vol. 26, no. 5-6, pp. 371–380, 1999.

[24] K. Meeran, D. O'Shea, P. D. Upton et al., "Circulating adrenomedullin does not regulate systemic blood pressure but increases plasma prolactin after intravenous infusion in humans: a pharmacokinetic study," *The Journal of Clinical Endocrinology & Metabolism*, vol. 82, no. 1, pp. 95–100, 1997.

[25] M. Westphal, M. Booke, and A. T. Dinh-Xuan, "Adrenomedullin: a smart road from pheochromocytoma to treatment of pulmonary hypertension," *European Respiratory Journal*, vol. 24, no. 4, pp. 518–520, 2004.

[26] S. Tan, W. Yu, Z. Lin et al., "Anti-inflammatory effect of ginsenoside Rb1 contributes to the recovery of gastrointestinal motility in the rat model of postoperative ileus," *Biological and Pharmaceutical Bulletin*, vol. 37, no. 11, pp. 1788–1794, 2014.

[27] G. Park, D. Oh, M. G. Lee, C. E. Lee, and Y. Kim, "6-Shogaol, an active compound of ginger, alleviates allergic dermatitis-like skin lesions via cytokine inhibition by activating the Nrf2 pathway," *Toxicology and Applied Pharmacology*, vol. 310, pp. 51–59, 2016.

Feasibility and Safety of Pressurized Intraperitoneal Aerosol Chemotherapy for Peritoneal Carcinomatosis

Martin Hübner,[1] **Hugo Teixeira Farinha,**[1] **Fabian Grass,**[1] **Anita Wolfer,**[2] **Patrice Mathevet,**[3] **Dieter Hahnloser,**[1] **and Nicolas Demartines**[1]

[1]*Department of Visceral Surgery, University Hospital of Lausanne (CHUV), Lausanne, Switzerland*
[2]*Department of Medical Oncology, University Hospital of Lausanne (CHUV), Lausanne, Switzerland*
[3]*Department of Gynecology, University Hospital of Lausanne (CHUV), Lausanne, Switzerland*

Correspondence should be addressed to Martin Hübner; martin.hubner@chuv.ch

Academic Editor: Luis Fernando Moreira

Background. Pressurized intraperitoneal aerosol chemotherapy (PIPAC) has been introduced as a novel repeatable treatment for peritoneal carcinomatosis. The available evidence from the pioneer center suggests good tolerance and high response rates, but independent confirmation is needed. A single-center cohort was analyzed one year after implementation for feasibility and safety. *Methods.* PIPAC was started in January 2015, and every patient was entered into a prospective database. This retrospective analysis included all consecutive patients operated until April 2016 with emphasis on surgical feasibility and early postoperative outcomes. *Results.* Forty-two patients (M : F = 8 : 34, median age 66 (59–73) years) with 91 PIPAC procedures in total (4×: 1, 3×: 17, 2×: 12, and 1×: 12) were analyzed. Abdominal accessibility rate was 95% (42/44); laparoscopic access was not feasible in 2 patients with previous HIPEC. Median initial peritoneal carcinomatosis index (PCI) was 10 (IQR 5–17). Median operation time was 94 min (89–108) with no learning curve observed. One PIPAC application was postponed due to intraoperative intestinal lesion. Overall morbidity was 9% with 7 minor complications (Clavien I-II) and one PIPAC-unrelated postoperative mortality. Median postoperative hospital stay was 3 days (2-3). *Conclusion.* Repetitive PIPAC is feasible in most patients with refractory carcinomatosis of various origins. Intraoperative complications and postoperative morbidity rates were low. This encourages prospective studies assessing oncological efficacy.

1. Introduction

Peritoneal carcinomatosis (PC) remains a condition with limited treatment options and dismal prognosis [1–3]. Outcome appears to be worse for PC compared to other stage IV situations, and response rates to systemic chemotherapy are modest at best, mainly due to limited tissue concentrations [4, 5]. Furthermore, side effects are common, and the use of palliative chemotherapy has therefore been questioned recently [6–8]. Hyperthermic intraperitoneal chemotherapy has been suggested in conjunction with cytoreductive surgery as an alternative in selected patients with encouraging results. However, most patients with PC are not eligible for this major procedure associated with important morbi-mortality [9, 10]. Furthermore, tissue concentrations after HIPEC remain low due to unequal distribution and low penetration [11].

Pressurized intraperitoneal aerosol chemotherapy (PIPAC) has been introduced as a novel treatment for peritoneal carcinomatosis [12, 13]. Pressure application allows for equal distribution and deeper penetration resulting in higher tissue concentrations despite lower doses (low systemic uptake) [14–16]. Minimally invasive access without cytoreduction decreases morbidity and allows for repetitive application. PIPAC is a very new technique, and first human application took place in November 2011 only. So far, all clinical reports but one came from the pioneer center in Herne, Germany [17–20].

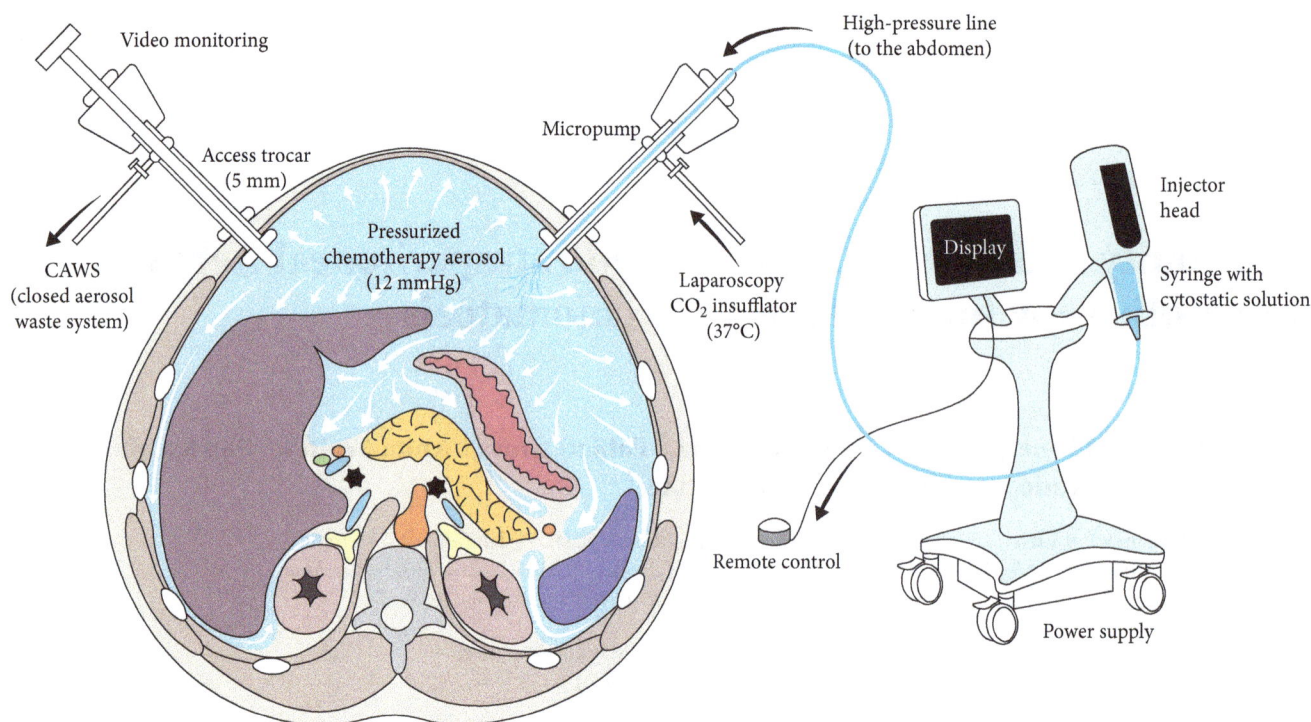

♣ Collapsed splanchnic veins

FIGURE 1: Pressurized intraperitoneal aerosol chemotherapy (PIPAC). The abdominal cavity is accessed with 2 balloon trocars allowing hermetic seal. Liquid chemotherapy is dispersed as aerosol by use of a standard injector and a specific nebulizer. Reprinted from *Rev Med Suisse* [21] with permission from Médicine et Hygiène.

The aim of this study was to analyze and report a consecutive cohort of PIPAC patients in our tertiary center with regard to feasibility and safety of the procedure.

2. Methods

The PIPAC program was started at the Department of Visceral Surgery of the University Hospital of Lausanne, Switzerland (CHUV), in January 2015, and was endorsed by the medical direction. Eligibility criteria for PIPAC treatment were persistent or progressive isolated peritoneal disease under or after at least one line of systemic treatment. Cytoreductive surgery and HIPEC as potentially curative treatment option was always the preferred choice in the absence of contraindications. Exceptionally, patients with predominating symptomatic PC and very limited disease elsewhere were considered. All patients were seen in the outpatient setting by a surgeon together with an oncologist to discuss all available treatment options. All indications were confirmed at the multidisciplinary tumor board. Patients received detailed oral and written information about the nature and risk of this novel procedure, and all patients provided written consent prior to surgery. All patients were treated in a palliative setting since long-term outcomes after PIPAC treatment is not yet available. This important point was explicitly stated in the preoperative information and consenting session. According to Swiss legislation and our institutional directive, all patients were further asked for their

consent for the utilization of their clinical data in anonymous form (general consent).

This retrospective analysis included all consecutive patients scheduled for PIPAC from the beginning of the program (January 2015) until April 2016. Excluded were only those patients refusing to sign the general consent form. The study was approved by the Institutional Review Board (number 2016-00274), conducted and reported in compliance with the STROBE criteria (http://strobe-statement.org/), and registered online (http://www.researchregistry.com; UIN: 1577).

2.1. PIPAC Procedure (Figure 1 [21]). Surgical technique and safety considerations have been described in detail by the Herne group, and our institutional protocol adhered strictly to these empirical standards [13, 16, 22]. Briefly, pneumoperitoneum was established by open placement of one 10 mm and one 5 mm balloon trocar, additional 5 mm trocars only if needed for technical difficulty. The peritoneal carcinomatosis index (PCI) was documented, and representative peritoneal nodules were biopsied. Intraperitoneal chemotherapy was applied by the use of a pressure injector (Accutron HP-D, Medtron®, Saarbrücken, Germany) and a specific nebulizer (MicroPump®, CapnoPen®, Reger, Villingendorf, Germany) at 37°C for 30 min and under standard laparoscopic pressure of 12 mmHg [23]. PIPAC was administered repetitively (3× at least) at an interval of about 6 weeks. In line with current protocols, patients with PC of colorectal origin received oxaliplatin (92 mg/m^2), while a combination of cisplatin ($7.5 \, \text{mg/m}^2$) and doxorubicin ($1.5 \, \text{mg/m}^2$) was applied for the other malignancies [17–19].

2.2. Data Management and Outcome Measures. Demographic information and surgical details were prospectively entered for all patients in a computerized coded database designed specifically for quality control of the PIPAC cohort. Demographic data included age, gender, comorbidities, and nutritional status. American Association of Anesthesiologists (ASA) physical status and Eastern Cooperative Oncology Group (ECOG) performance status were documented as validated tools to describe general condition [24]. Nutritional risk was assessed by the use of the Nutritional Risk Score (NRS 2002) [25].

Surgical information contained operation time, intraoperative complications, need for concomitant adhesiolysis, accessibility of the abdomen, and number of trocars. Extent of peritoneal disease was documented by the use of the peritoneal cancer index (PCI) [26], and volume of ascites was measured. Surgical stress was assessed using the E-PASS (Estimation of Physiologic Ability and Surgical Stress) score [27].

Postoperative morbidity was assessed until 30 days after surgery by use of the Clavien classification, and length of postoperative hospital stay was measured including readmissions. Outpatient appointments were scheduled for all patients at 30 days after each procedure for clinical follow-up and quality control. Moreover, each patient received an emergency phone number and was advised to establish contact if a problem arises.

2.3. Predefined Clinical Questions. Several comparisons and statistical correlations were defined a priori. Univariate analysis was compared between patients with only one PIPAC versus patients with repeated applications. This was done to define conditions rendering repetitive administration difficult.

Gynecological malignancies differ from digestive cancers in many ways including previous surgical and systemic treatments and distribution patterns of peritoneal carcinomatosis. As this has a potential impact on surgical difficulty and approach, surgical aspects between gynecological and digestive patients were compared.

Lastly, increasing peritoneal tumor load might complicate surgery and reflect more advanced disease with consecutive longer hospital stay. In order to test these hypotheses, we correlated PCI to operation time and postoperative hospital stay, respectively.

2.4. Statistical Analysis. Continuous variables were presented as mean with standard deviation (SD) or median value with range or interquartile range (IQR) as appropriate depending on the normality of the distribution and compared using Student's *t*-test and Mann-Whitney *U* test. Categorical variables were given as frequencies with percentages and compared with chi-square test. Spearman's test was used to measure correlations between continuous variables. A *p* value of <0.05 was considered to be statistically significant in all tests. Data analyses were generated using SPSS

v20 statistical software (Chicago, IL, USA); graphics were developed using GraphPad Prism 7 (GraphPad Software Inc., La Jolla, CA, USA).

3. Results

In the study period, 44 patients were scheduled for PIPAC. In 2 patients, no laparoscopic access could be established due to dense adhesions. All remaining patients had signed the general consent form, and no patient was excluded. Final analysis included therefore 42 patients (M : F = 8 : 34, median age 66 (IQR 59–73) years). Overall failure rate (number of nonaccess + aborted procedures/total number of attempted procedures) was 4/95 (4%) (Figure 2). Twenty-one patients (50%) had carcinomatosis of ovarian origin, 14 and 3 from colorectal and gastric cancer, respectively (remainder: 1 small bowel, 1 pseudomyxoma, and 1 mesothelioma). Demographic information is provided in Table 1.

Overall, 91 PIPAC procedures were performed; 18 patients had 3 or more PIPAC procedures, 12 patients had 2 operations, and 12 patients one procedure so far. Reasons for no 2nd PIPAC were progression of systemic disease in 5 patients, patient refusal in 3, absent peritoneal disease during first PIPAC in one, and secondary nonaccess during the 2nd PIPAC in one patient. The 2 remaining patients were awaiting their scheduled 2nd intervention. Patients with higher ASA score, lower BMI, underlying malnutrition, and colorectal origin were less likely to undergo repetitive PIPAC (Table 1).

3.1. Surgical Details (Table 2). In 80 out of the 91 procedures (88%), one 5 mm and one 10 mm trocar were used; 3 trocars were needed in 11 surgeries. Median overall time for all procedures was 94 min (IQR 89–108) showing little variation over time. PIPAC procedures for gynecological peritoneal metastases were significantly shorter as compared with procedures for digestive PC. Surgical stress as measured by the E-PASS was a median of −0.20 (−0.32−−0.11). Median PCI was 10 (5–17), and adhesiolysis was necessary in 16% of cases before applying PIPAC. There was one intraoperative complication: a small bowel lesion occurred during open trocar placement. The enterotomy was recognized and repaired immediately. PIPAC was postponed and successfully performed six weeks later.

In patients with digestive origin, median PCI was significantly higher and operation time significantly longer.

3.2. Postoperative Outcomes. Eight complications occurred after 91 procedures, giving an overall morbidity rate of 8.8%. Seven minor complications were 3 urinary retentions with a need for 24 h catheterization, one ileus treated with nasogastric decompression, one minor scar bleeding, one constipation requiring enema, and one neutropenia with spontaneous resolution. One patient developed cardiogenic shock and arrhythmia 4 days after the 3rd PIPAC procedure with fatal outcome. Autopsy did not find any intra-abdominal complication, and no causative link could be established between PIPAC treatment and death.

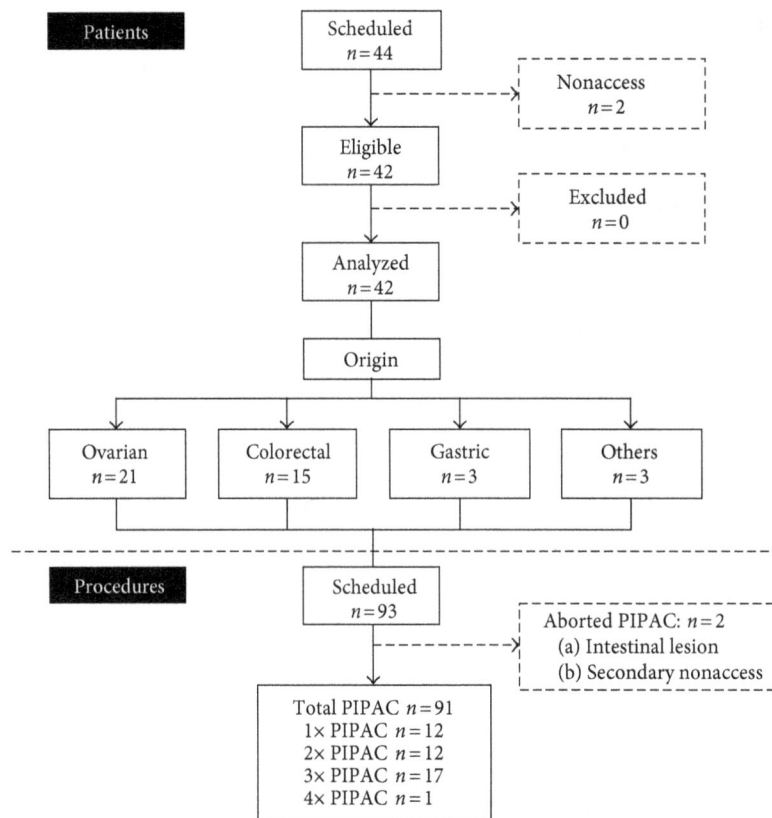

FIGURE 2: Flow of patients treated with pressurized intraperitoneal aerosol chemotherapy (PIPAC).

Median hospital stay was 3 (IQR 2-3) days with 9 and 35 patients, respectively, who left the hospital on the 1st and 2nd postoperative days.

3.3. Correlation of Tumor Load, Operation Time, and Hospital Stay. Higher PCI was significantly associated with shorter OR time ($\rho = -0.291$, $p = 0.005$), while no statistical correlation was found between PCI and hospital stay ($\rho = 0.193$, $p = 0.067$) (Figures 3(a) and 3(b)).

4. Discussion

In the present study, repeated PIPAC was feasible in most patients with peritoneal carcinomatosis. Postprocedure morbidity was low and hospital stay short.

Feasibility of PIPAC includes abdominal access by laparoscopy and repeated application. Minimally invasive surgery in patients with multiple prior surgeries is challenging and associated with higher conversion rates [28, 29]. For PIPAC in particular, the literature is very scarce. Reported primary nonaccess rates vary from 0 to 17%; after at least one PIPAC, secondary nonaccess rate was reported to be 0–35% [17–20]. In our series, we observed primary and secondary nonaccess rates of 4.5% and 2.4%, respectively; of note, both patients with primary nonaccess had prior HIPEC treatment. Repeatability is more complex and depends not only on technical problems but mostly on disease progression and preferences of patients and their care providers. Altogether, 10 out of 42 patients (23.8%) could not

benefit from the 2nd PIPAC mostly due to the development of metastases other than peritoneal ($n = 5$) or for patient's wish to discontinue treatments ($n = 3$). Our findings are in line with the findings from the Herne group reporting repeated application in 64–82% of their patients [17–19].

Intraoperative complications appear to be exceedingly rare, but the risk for small bowel lesions is present in patients with adhesions as also reported by others [18]. Besides the mortality described in this paper, 2 fatal outcomes after PIPAC treatment have been reported in the literature [18]. Mortality was attributed to progressing small bowel disease causing obstruction in one patient and poor general condition with consecutive ascitic decompensation and renal failure in the other patient. Tempfer et al. suggested therefore that impeding small bowel obstruction and refractory ascites should be considered as contraindications to PIPAC treatment. Therefore, proper patient selection is important and challenging as patients tend to accept risks in view of lacking treatment alternatives in most cases. No CTCAE (Common Terminology Criteria for Adverse Events) grade 4 events were reported after PIPAC, while incidence of grade 3 events varied between 23 and 35% [17–20]. Applying the Clavien classification for postoperative complications, we observed an overall morbidity of 9% in our series. Postoperative abdominal pain, which was present in the Herne experience in up to 100% [17], required rarely other analgesics than those routinely used after other laparoscopic procedures like cholecystectomy. The median hospital stay was 3 days, similar as reported by an Italian group [20]. Reporting

TABLE 1: Baseline demographics of patients treated with pressurized intraperitoneal aerosol chemotherapy (PIPAC).

	All patients ($n = 42$)	1 PIPAC ($n = 12$)	2 or >3 PIPAC ($n = 30$)	p value
Demographics				
Median age (years)	66 (59–73)	62 (52–88)	67 (61–63)	0.185
Age ≥ 70 years	16 (38%)	4 (33%)	12 (40%)	0.687
Gender (male)	8 (19%)	4 (33%)	4 (13%)	0.135
Median BMI (kg/m^2)	22.5 (20–25)	19 (19–23)	22.7 (21.3–26)	*0.018*
BMI < 18.5 kg/m^2	2 (5%)	1	1	0.491
Comorbidities				
ASA (I-II)	28 (66%)	5 (42%)	23 (77%)	*0.029*
ECOG (0-1)	36 (86%)	9 (75%)	27 (90%)	0.209
Diabetes	1 (2%)	1	0	0.109
Malnutrition	14 (33%)	7 (58%)	7 (23%)	*0.029*
NRS < 3	29 (69%)	6 (50%)	23 (77%)	0.091
Previous laparotomy	1 (0–4)	1 (0–3)	1 (0–4)	*0.040*
≥2	15 (36%)	2 (16%)	13 (43%)	0.103
Disease				
Origin				*0.007*
Colorectal	15 (33%)	8 (66%)	6 (20%)	
Gastric	3 (7%)	0	3 (10%)	
Gynecological	21 (50%)	2 (17%)	19 (63%)	
Other	3	1	2	
Prior chemotherapy				0.229
No chemo	2	1	1	
1 line	9 (21%)	5 (42%)	4 (13%)	
2 lines	13 (31%)	2 (17%)	11 (36%)	
3 lines	9 (21%)	1	8 (26%)	
More than 3	9 (21%)	3 (25%)	6 (20%)	
Prior HIPEC	4 (10%)	2 (17%)	2 (7%)	0.318
Diagnosis—1st PIPAC (mo)	16 (1–104)	18 (1–73)	16 (1–104)	0.928

Median (range) for previous laparotomy and diagnosis—1st PIPAC, otherwise median (IQR) or number (%) as appropriate. Statistical significance ($p < 0.05$) is highlighted in italics.
BMI: body mass index; ASA: American Association of Anesthesiologists physical status classification system; ECOG: Eastern Cooperative Oncology Group performance status; HIPEC: hyperthermic intraperitoneal chemotherapy.

TABLE 2: Surgical details of pressurized intraperitoneal aerosol chemotherapy (PIPAC).

	Overall ($n = 91$)	GYN ($n = 51$)	Digestive ($n = 40$)	p value
Surgical feasibility				
Number of trocars	2 (2-3)	2 (2-3)	2 (2-3)	0.668
Operation time	94 (89–108)	91 (87–97)	100 (92–117)	*0.002*
Intra-OP findings				
PCI	10 (5–17)	9 (4–14)	15 (7–19)	*0.002*
Ascites (mL)	50 (0–4000)	0 (0–300)	50 (0–4000)	0.982
Adhesiolysis	15 (16%)	9 (18%)	6 (15%)	0.735
Median E-PASS	−0.20 (−0.32−−0.11)	−0.20 (−0.31−−0.10)	−0.20 (−0.31−−0.09)	0.733

Median (range) for number of trocars and ascites and median (IQR) for operation time, PCI, and E-PASS. Statistical significance ($p < 0.05$) is highlighted in italics.
PCI: peritoneal cancer index; E-PASS: Modified Estimation of Physiologic Ability and Surgical Stress.

a considerable number of patients leaving hospital already 1-2 days after surgery, even outpatient surgery might be considered in the future for well-selected patients in good general condition. However, it must be underlined that the usual PIPAC patient is frail and in reduced general condition due to the disease and previous treatments. Caution is

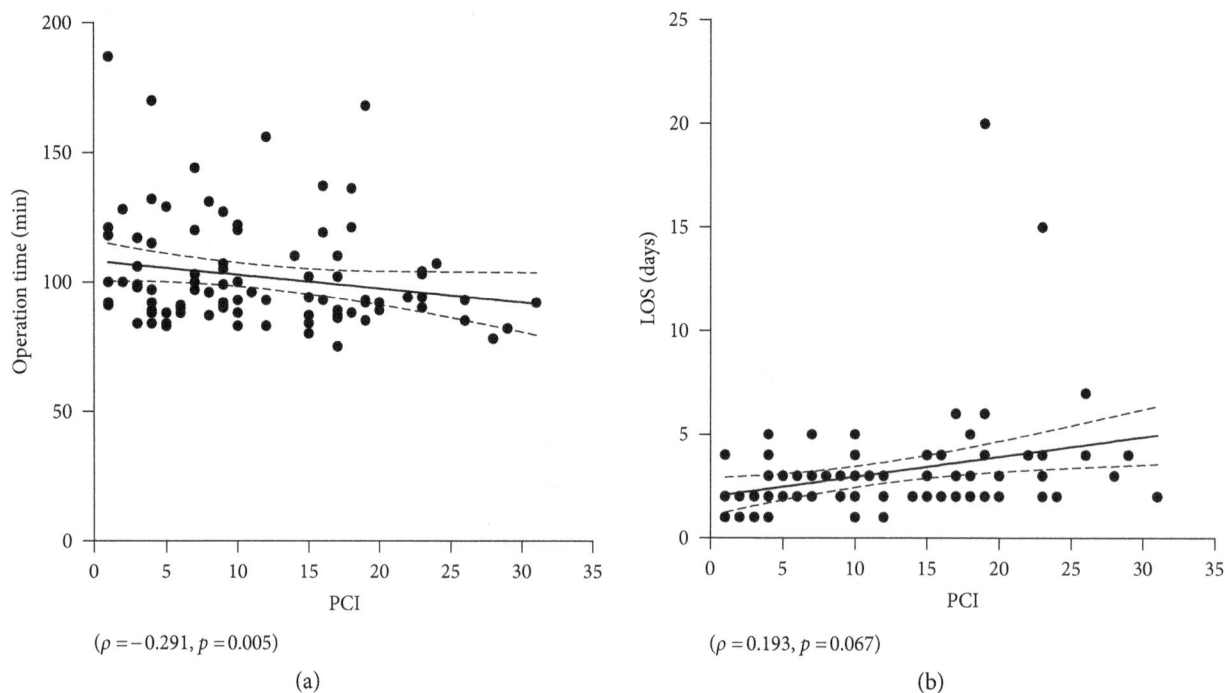

$(\rho = -0.291, p = 0.005)$

(a)

$(\rho = 0.193, p = 0.067)$

(b)

FIGURE 3: Correlation of tumor load with operation time and hospital stay. The extent of peritoneal disease (measured by the peritoneal cancer index: PCI) was plotted against operation time (a) and length of hospital stay (LOS) (b).

advocated especially for malnourished patients presenting with ascites as postoperative fluid shifts can be important entailing consecutive electrolyte disturbances and renal failure. But even those negatively selected patients required rarely more than 3 days after surgery before being fit for discharge.

Extent of peritoneal disease (as measured by the PCI) was in the present experience not associated with increased operation time, rather the contrary. Most patients with advanced peritoneal disease had considerable amounts of ascites facilitating abdominal access and also choice of appropriate location for biopsies. To our knowledge, impact of PCI on operation time has not been investigated by other groups. The present study did not observe any significant correlation between PCI and postoperative stay; these findings confirm that PIPAC treatment is feasible and safe within short hospital stay even for patients with very advanced disease [20].

Selection and reporting bias are important limitations of retrospective studies. The present analysis included all consecutive patients without any exclusion. All reported endpoints were defined a priori and documented online in a prospectively maintained database designed for quality control. The study sample however was modest and heterogeneous. Heterogeneity concerns especially prior surgical and systemic chemotherapy treatments which is a methodological problem in studies on peritoneal carcinomatosis in general. Comparisons with other cohorts treated intraperitoneally or systemically are hence problematic. Therefore, further data is certainly needed to confirm the present findings even if they are in line with data published so far.

In conclusion, the present study suggests that repetitive PIPAC is feasible in most patients with refractory carcinomatosis of various origins. Intraoperative events and postoperative complications are low. These findings encourage designing prospective studies assessing oncological efficacy.

Abbreviations

IQR: Interquartile range
PC: Peritoneal carcinomatosis
PCI: Peritoneal cancer index
PIPAC: Pressurized intraperitoneal aerosol chemotherapy.

Disclosure

This study was included as a poster presentation at the ESCP congress, September 28–30, 2016, in Milano, Italy.

Competing Interests

The authors declare that there is no conflict of interest regarding the publication of this paper.

Authors' Contributions

Martin Hübner and Hugo Teixeira Farinha contributed equally to this work.

References

[1] L. C. Hanker, S. Loibl, N. Burchardi et al., "The impact of second to sixth line therapy on survival of relapsed ovarian cancer after primary taxane/platinum-based therapy," *Annals of Oncology*, vol. 23, no. 10, pp. 2605–2612, 2012.

[2] Y. L. Klaver, V. E. Lemmens, G. J. Creemers, H. J. Rutten, S. W. Nienhuijs, and I. H. de Hingh, "Population-based survival of patients with peritoneal carcinomatosis from colorectal origin in the era of increasing use of palliative chemotherapy," *Annals of Oncology*, vol. 22, no. 10, pp. 2250–2256, 2011.

[3] V. E. Lemmens, Y. L. Klaver, V. J. Verwaal, H. J. Rutten, J. W. Coebergh, and I. H. de Hingh, "Predictors and survival of synchronous peritoneal carcinomatosis of colorectal origin: a population-based study," *International Journal of Cancer*, vol. 128, no. 11, pp. 2717–2725, 2011.

[4] J. Franko, Q. Shi, C. D. Goldman et al., "Treatment of colorectal peritoneal carcinomatosis with systemic chemotherapy: a pooled analysis of north central cancer treatment group phase III trials N9741 and N9841," *Journal of Clinical Oncology*, vol. 30, no. 3, pp. 263–267, 2012.

[5] A. I. Minchinton and I. F. Tannock, "Drug penetration in solid tumours," *Nature Reviews Cancer*, vol. 6, no. 8, pp. 583–592, 2006.

[6] H. G. Prigerson, Y. Bao, M. A. Shah et al., "Chemotherapy use, performance status, and quality of life at the end of life," *JAMA Oncology*, vol. 1, no. 6, pp. 778–784, 2015.

[7] M. M. Garrido, H. G. Prigerson, Y. Bao, and P. K. Maciejewski, "Chemotherapy use in the months before death and estimated costs of care in the last week of life," *Journal of Pain and Symptom Management*, vol. 51, no. 5, pp. 875–881, 2016.

[8] A. A. Wright, B. Zhang, N. L. Keating, J. C. Weeks, and H. G. Prigerson, "Associations between palliative chemotherapy and adult cancer patients' end of life care and place of death: prospective cohort study," *BMJ*, vol. 348, p. g1219, 2014.

[9] O. Glehen, F. N. Gilly, F. Boutitie et al., "Toward curative treatment of peritoneal carcinomatosis from nonovarian origin by cytoreductive surgery combined with perioperative intraperitoneal chemotherapy: a multi-institutional study of 1,290 patients," *Cancer*, vol. 116, no. 24, pp. 5608–5618, 2010.

[10] V. J. Verwaal, "Long-term results of cytoreduction and HIPEC followed by systemic chemotherapy," *Cancer Journal*, vol. 15, no. 3, pp. 212–215, 2009.

[11] W. P. Ceelen, L. Pahlman, and H. Mahteme, "Pharmacodynamic aspects of intraperitoneal cytotoxic therapy," *Cancer Treatment and Research*, vol. 134, pp. 195–214, 2007.

[12] W. Solass, R. Kerb, T. Mürdter et al., "Intraperitoneal chemotherapy of peritoneal carcinomatosis using pressurized aerosol as an alternative to liquid solution: first evidence for efficacy," *Annals of Surgical Oncology*, vol. 21, no. 2, pp. 553–559, 2014.

[13] W. Solass, A. Hetzel, G. Nadiradze, E. Sagynaliev, and M. A. Reymond, "Description of a novel approach for intraperitoneal drug delivery and the related device," *Surgical Endoscopy*, vol. 26, no. 7, pp. 1849–1855, 2012.

[14] P. Esquis, D. Consolo, G. Magnin et al., "High intra-abdominal pressure enhances the penetration and antitumor effect of intraperitoneal cisplatin on experimental peritoneal carcinomatosis," *Annals of Surgery*, vol. 244, no. 1, pp. 106–112, 2006.

[15] O. Facy, S. Al Samman, G. Magnin et al., "High pressure enhances the effect of hyperthermia in intraperitoneal chemotherapy with oxaliplatin: an experimental study," *Annals of Surgery*, vol. 256, no. 6, pp. 1084–1088, 2012.

[16] W. Solass, A. Herbette, T. Schwarz et al., "Therapeutic approach of human peritoneal carcinomatosis with Dbait in combination with capnoperitoneum: proof of concept," *Surgical Endoscopy*, vol. 26, no. 3, pp. 847–852, 2012.

[17] C. B. Tempfer, G. Winnekendonk, W. Solass et al., "Pressurized intraperitoneal aerosol chemotherapy in women with recurrent ovarian cancer: a phase 2 study," *Gynecologic Oncology*, vol. 137, no. 2, pp. 223–228, 2015.

[18] G. Nadiradze, U. Giger-Pabst, J. Zieren, D. Strumberg, W. Solass, and M. A. Reymond, "Pressurized intraperitoneal aerosol chemotherapy (PIPAC) with low-dose cisplatin and doxorubicin in gastric peritoneal metastasis," *Journal of Gastrointestinal Surgery*, vol. 20, no. 2, pp. 367–373, 2015.

[19] C. Demtroder, W. Solass, J. Zieren, D. Strumberg, U. Giger-Pabst, and M. A. Reymond, "Pressurized intraperitoneal aerosol chemotherapy (PIPAC) with oxaliplatin in colorectal peritoneal metastasis," *Colorectal Disease*, vol. 18, no. 4, pp. 364–371, 2015.

[20] M. Robella, M. Vaira, and M. De Simone, "Safety and feasibility of pressurized intraperitoneal aerosol chemotherapy (PIPAC) associated with systemic chemotherapy: an innovative approach to treat peritoneal carcinomatosis," *World Journal of Surgical Oncology*, vol. 14, no. 1, p. 128, 2016.

[21] M. Hubner, H. Teixeira, T. Boussaha, M. Cachemaille, K. Lehmann, and N. Demartines, "PIPAC–pressurized intraperitoneal aerosol chemotherapy. A novel treatment for peritoneal carcinomatosis," *Revue Médicale Suisse*, vol. 11, no. 479, pp. 1325–1330, 2015.

[22] W. Solass, U. Giger-Pabst, J. Zieren, and M. A. Reymond, "Pressurized intraperitoneal aerosol chemotherapy (PIPAC): occupational health and safety aspects," *Annals of Surgical Oncology*, vol. 20, no. 11, pp. 3504–3511, 2013.

[23] H. Jung do, S. Y. Son, A. M. Oo et al., "Feasibility of hyperthermic pressurized intraperitoneal aerosol chemotherapy in a porcine model," *Surgical Endoscopy*, vol. 30, no. 10, pp. 4258–4264, 2016.

[24] M. M. Oken, R. H. Creech, D. C. Tormey et al., "Toxicity and response criteria of the Eastern Cooperative Oncology Group," *American Journal of Clinical Oncology*, vol. 5, no. 6, pp. 649–655, 1982.

[25] J. Kondrup, H. H. Rasmussen, O. Hamberg, Z. Stanga, and Ad Hoc ESPEN Working Group, "Nutritional risk screening (NRS 2002): a new method based on an analysis of controlled clinical trials," *Clinical Nutrition*, vol. 22, no. 3, pp. 321–336, 2003.

[26] A. G. Portilla, K. Shigeki, B. Dario, and D. Marcello, "The intraoperative staging systems in the management of peritoneal surface malignancy," *Journal of Surgical Oncology*, vol. 98, no. 4, pp. 228–231, 2008.

[27] Y. Haga, K. Ikejiri, Y. Wada et al., "A multicenter prospective study of surgical audit systems," *Annals of Surgery*, vol. 253, no. 1, pp. 194–201, 2011.

[28] D. S. Chi, N. R. Abu-Rustum, Y. Sonoda et al., "Ten-year experience with laparoscopy on a gynecologic oncology service: analysis of risk factors for complications and conversion to laparotomy," *American Journal of Obstetrics and Gynecology*, vol. 191, no. 4, pp. 1138–1145, 2004.

[29] S. Palomba, F. Ghezzi, A. Falbo et al., "Conversion in endometrial cancer patients scheduled for laparoscopic staging: a large multicenter analysis: conversions and endometrial cancer," *Surgical Endoscopy*, vol. 28, no. 11, pp. 3200–3209, 2014.

3

Survival after Abdominoperineal and Sphincter-Preserving Resection in Nonmetastatic Rectal Cancer: A Population-Based Time-Trend and Propensity Score-Matched SEER Analysis

Rene Warschkow,[1,2] Sabrina M. Ebinger,[1,3] Walter Brunner,[1] Bruno M. Schmied,[1] and Lukas Marti[1,4]

[1]Department of Surgery, Cantonal Hospital of St. Gallen, 9007 St. Gallen, Switzerland
[2]Institute of Medical Biometry and Informatics, University of Heidelberg, 69120 Heidelberg, Germany
[3]Department of Surgery, Hospital of Thun, 3600 Thun, Switzerland
[4]Department of Surgery, Universitätsmedizin Mannheim, Medical Faculty Mannheim, University of Heidelberg, 68167 Mannheim, Germany

Correspondence should be addressed to Lukas Marti; lukas.marti@kssg.ch

Academic Editor: Francesco Selvaggi

Background. Abdominoperineal resection (APR) has been associated with impaired survival in nonmetastatic rectal cancer patients. It is unclear whether this adverse outcome is due to the surgical procedure itself or is a consequence of tumor-related characteristics. *Study Design.* Patients were identified from the Surveillance, Epidemiology, and End Results database. The impact of APR compared to coloanal anastomosis (CAA) on survival was assessed by Cox regression and propensity-score matching. *Results.* In 36,488 patients with rectal cancer resection, the APR rate declined from 31.8% in 1998 to 19.2% in 2011, with a significant trend change in 2004 at 21.6% ($P < 0.001$). To minimize a potential time-trend bias, survival analysis was limited to patients diagnosed after 2004. APR was associated with an increased risk of cancer-specific mortality after unadjusted analysis (HR = 1.61, 95% CI: 1.28–2.03, $P < 0.01$) and multivariable adjustment (HR = 1.39, 95% CI: 1.10–1.76, $P < 0.01$). After optimal adjustment of highly biased patient characteristics by propensity-score matching, APR was not identified as a risk factor for cancer-specific mortality (HR = 0.85, 95% CI: 0.56–1.29, $P = 0.456$). *Conclusions.* The current propensity score-adjusted analysis provides evidence that worse oncological outcomes in patients undergoing APR compared to CAA are caused by different patient characteristics and not by the surgical procedure itself.

1. Introduction

Abdominoperineal resection (APR) has long been considered the standard of care for curative treatment of distal rectal cancer. Recently, this dogma has been increasingly questioned [1–3]. Besides the fact that APR defines the sphincter's fortune by creating a permanent colostomy, it has also been associated with an impaired oncological outcome and survival compared to restorative operations [4–6], even if performed for distal rectal cancer with coloanal anastomosis (CAA) [7].

Decision-making for sphincter preservation versus sphincter resection is related to numerous tumor- and patient-related characteristics. Whether an adverse outcome is due to one or a combination of these factors or to the surgical procedure of APR itself is a matter of debate [8]. A prominent factor is a tumor's distance to the anal sphincters. Because a wide distal margin has formerly been considered to be of particular importance, tumors less than 5 cm from the anal verge could not be operated on except by APR. Because local recurrence and overall survival were then proved not to be impaired by a limited margin, the recommended distal resection margin was incrementally reduced from 5 cm to 1 cm [9–11] and even to 0.5 cm in special cases of tumors that were downstaged after neoadjuvant chemoradiotherapy [12]. However, in patients with higher tumor grades, a broader distal margin is recommended [13]. Other factors that might lead to performing an APR and not a sphincter-preserving procedure are higher T-stage [14, 15], male gender with a narrow pelvis [14, 16], higher age [17], and impaired preoperative sphincter function to avoid postoperative incontinence [16].

In the literature, there are contradictions about the impact of APR on oncological outcome and survival [1, 6, 17–19]. Of note, some of the factors favoring APR over restorative operations (e.g., T-stage, age, and distance to the anal verge) are independent risk factors for poor oncologic outcome after APR [5]. Additionally, the rate of APR has decreased significantly during the last two decades [20]. Hence, a comparison of APR versus CAA should consider such a selection and time-trend bias.

Therefore, the aims of the current population-based investigation were to first define the optimal study period by time-trend analysis and then to assess the putative impact of APR versus CAA on survival in unadjusted and multivariable Cox proportional hazard regression analyses. Finally, a statistically optimal adjustment for imbalances in patient characteristics was undertaken by propensity score matching to further elaborate the prognostic impact of APR.

2. Materials and Methods

2.1. Cohort Definition: Surveillance, Epidemiology, and End Results. Data from the Surveillance, Epidemiology, and End Results (SEER) Program of the National Cancer Institute in the United States, covering approximately 28% of cancer cases in the United States, were the source of the present population-based analysis [21]. The SEER data were collected and reported using data items and codes as documented by the North American Association of Central Cancer Registries (NAACCR) [22]. Primary cancer site and histology were coded according to the criteria in the third edition of the International Classification of Diseases for Oncology (ICD-O-3) [23]. Rectal cancer patients were identified by the ICD-O-3 site code C20.9 and behavior code 3 (NAACCR Items 522 and 523). Patients diagnosed at autopsy or only by death certificate were excluded, as well as patients without histologically confirmed cancer (NAACCR Items 490 and 2180) and patients with occurrence of another malignancy preceding rectal cancer (NAACCR Item 380). The analysis was further restricted to patients with adenocarcinoma identified by the ICD-O-3 histology codes 8140, 8144, 8210, 8211, 8220, 8221, 8261, 8262, and 8263 (NAACCR Item 522), patients without distant metastases (NAACCR Item 790 in 1998 to 2003 and Item 3000 in 2004 to 2011), and patients without intraoperative radiation (NAACCR Item 1360). For trend analysis, patients with any rectal cancer resection were included (NAACCR Item 1290, codes 30 to 80). To analyze the impact of APR on prognosis, the cohort was further limited to patients diagnosed between 2005 and 2011 and undergoing either APR or rectal cancer resection with sphincter preservation and CAA (NAACCR Item 1290, codes 50 and 40). Patients undergoing rectal cancer resection with colorectal anastomosis were not included in the survival analysis because they were mixed with patients undergoing

anterior resection without complete mesorectal excision and patients treated with Hartmann's procedure (NAACCR Item 1290, code 30).

2.2. Statistical Analysis. Statistical analyses were performed using R statistical software (https://www.r-project.org/). A two-sided P value < 0.05 was considered statistically significant. Continuous data are expressed as medians (interquartile range). Chi-square statistics and Mann–Whitney U tests were used to compare proportions and continuous variables. In regression analysis, all P values were computed by likelihood-ratio tests. Wald-type confidence intervals were estimated.

To analyze the time trend in the APR rate, logistic regression and Davis tests [24] were applied to test for points in time at which a significant change in APR rate had occurred. Joinpoint regression analysis [25] was applied to define the best fitting point for a change in the time trend of the APR rate. The trends in the two segments defined by the joinpoint were characterized by the annual percentage change [25]. For sensitivity analysis, the time trend was finally assessed by LOESS regression analysis [26].

After comparing patients with APR and CAA in descriptive analysis, APR was assessed as a prognostic factor for overall and cancer-specific survival in Kaplan-Meier analysis and in Cox regression analyses with and without risk adjustment for tumor stage according to the American Joint Committee on Cancer (AJCC, 6th edition) for retrieved regional lymph nodes, grading, year of diagnosis, age, gender, ethnicity, and marital status (risk set). The full model Cox regression was further elucidated by a backward variable selection procedure from the full model based on Akaike's information criterion. The proportional hazard assumption was tested by scaled Schoenfeld residuals and by inspection of the hazard ratio (HR) plots [27]. Thereafter, predictors of APR in the risk set were assessed in multivariable logistic regression to assess the bias concerning APR. Moreover, a propensity score analysis was performed as a superior and more refined statistical method to adjust for all potential baseline-confounding variables in the risk set [28–30]. Propensity score matching was performed as exact matching. In this procedure, each patient undergoing APR was matched to all possible patients undergoing CAA with exactly the same values on all the covariates, forming subclasses such that within each subclass both groups had exactly the same covariate values after assigning weights to each individual. Patients undergoing APR who did not have a counterpart among the patients undergoing CAA and vice versa were excluded from this analysis. Finally, overall and cancer-specific survival in patients undergoing APR was assessed in a Cox regression analysis using the weights obtained by the matching propensity score analysis.

3. Results

3.1. Trend Analysis. The trend analysis was based on 36,488 patients who underwent resection of nonmetastatic rectal adenocarcinoma. The rate of APR declined significantly from 31.8% in 1998 to 19.2% in 2011 ($P < 0.001$). Further analyzing this trend (Figure 1), joinpoint regression analysis identified

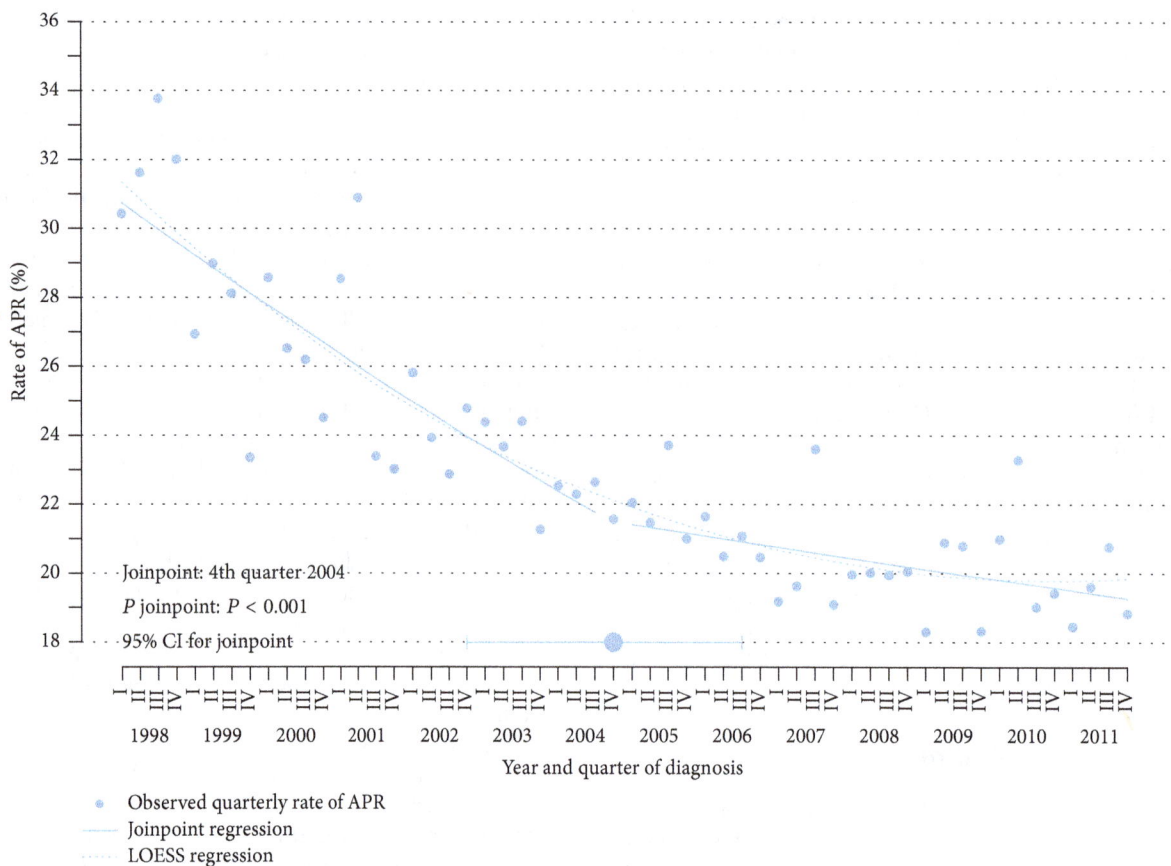

FIGURE 1: Trend analysis for abdominoperineal resection, 1998 to 2011.

one notable change in the APR rate at the 4th quarter of 2004 ($P < 0.001$). The 95% confidence interval for this break in the time trend was estimated to be between the 4th quarter of 2002 and the 3rd quarter of 2006. There was no evidence for additional relevant changes in the trend ($P = 0.716$). From the 1st quarter of 1998 until the 4th quarter of 2004, the observed rate of APR declined from 30.4% to 21.6%, corresponding to an annual percent change of −7.1% (95% CI: −9.1% to −5.2%, $P < 0.001$). Thereafter, the rate of APR declined further to 18.8% at the 4th quarter of 2011 ($P = 0.018$), but to a much lower extent. The annual percent change after 2004 was −2.0% (95% CI: −3.6% to −0.3%). A LOESS regression was performed for sensitivity analysis and confirmed a lower decline after 2004 (Figure 1).

3.2. Patient Characteristics for Abdominoperineal Resection. The comparative analysis of oncologic outcomes after APR versus CAA was limited to patients diagnosed after 2004 to minimize a potential time-trend bias, leaving 4,700 patients eligible for this part of the analysis. Of these, 3,898 patients (82.9%) underwent APR and 802 (17.1%) underwent rectal resection with CAA. Table 1 summarizes the patient characteristics for both groups. Patients with APR had more advanced cancer stages, less regional lymph nodes retrieved, more advanced grading, and more applications of radiotherapy, were significantly older, were less often African-Americans, and were less often married.

3.3. Abdominoperineal Resection as a Prognostic Factor for Survival. Panels (a) and (b) in Figure 2 display the Kaplan-Meier curves for overall and cancer-specific survival in patients with APR and CAA. In unadjusted Cox proportional hazards regression analysis, patients undergoing APR had a 58% increased risk of overall mortality (HR = 1.58, 95% CI: 1.31 to 1.91, $P < 0.001$) and a 61% increased risk of cancer-specific mortality (HR = 1.61, 95% CI: 1.28 to 2.03, $P < 0.001$). The 5-year overall survival for patients with APR was 65.6% (95% CI: 63.6 to 67.7%) compared with 76.7% (95% CI: 72.5 to 81.0%) for patients undergoing CAA ($P < 0.001$). The 5-year cancer-specific survival for patients with APR was 74.3% (95% CI: 72.4 to 76.2%) compared with 83.3% (95% CI: 79.5 to 87.3%) for patients undergoing CAA. After multivariable risk adjustment in the Cox regression analysis (Table 2), APR was persistently associated with an increased risk of overall mortality (hazard ratio of death = 1.37, 95% CI: 1.13 to 1.67, $P = 0.001$) and cancer-specific mortality (hazard ratio of death = 1.39, 95% CI: 1.10 to 1.76, $P = 0.004$). These results were additionally confirmed after variable selection (Table 2).

3.4. Adjusting for Patient Characteristics with Propensity Score Matching. To further corroborate the bias for APR in the patient characteristics and its potential influence on survival, logistic regression analysis with multivariable adjustment was performed (Table 3). Patients undergoing APR had more advanced cancer stages and more radiotherapy treatments,

TABLE 1: Patient characteristics.

	Total N = 4,700	APR N = 3,898	CAA N = 802	P^A
Patient characteristics				
Tumor stage (AJCC 6th ed.)				
Stage I	1106 (23.5%)	859 (22.0%)	247 (30.8%)	
Stage IIA	1417 (30.1%)	1185 (30.4%)	232 (28.9%)	
Stage IIB	160 (3.4%)	150 (3.8%)	10 (1.2%)	<0.001^A
Stage IIIA	283 (6.0%)	219 (5.6%)	64 (8.0%)	
Stage IIIB	1159 (24.7%)	993 (25.5%)	166 (20.7%)	
Stage IIIC	575 (12.2%)	492 (12.6%)	83 (10.3%)	
Retrieved regional lymph nodes				
<12	2180 (46.4%)	1845 (47.3%)	335 (41.8%)	0.004^A
12+	2520 (53.6%)	2053 (52.7%)	467 (58.2%)	
Grading				
G1	338 (7.2%)	264 (6.8%)	74 (9.2%)	
G2	3307 (70.4%)	2731 (70.1%)	576 (71.8%)	0.007^A
G3/4	686 (14.6%)	581 (14.9%)	105 (13.1%)	
Unknown	369 (7.9%)	322 (8.3%)	47 (5.9%)	
Radiation				
None	1165 (24.8%)	897 (23.0%)	268 (33.4%)	
Before surgery	2953 (62.8%)	2512 (64.4%)	441 (55.0%)	<0.001^A
After surgery	582 (12.4%)	489 (12.5%)	93 (11.6%)	
Year of diagnosis				
2005	744 (15.8%)	620 (15.9%)	124 (15.5%)	
2006	671 (14.3%)	566 (14.5%)	105 (13.1%)	
2007	688 (14.6%)	568 (14.6%)	120 (15.0%)	
2008	636 (13.5%)	547 (14.0%)	89 (11.1%)	0.070^A
2009	653 (13.9%)	526 (13.5%)	127 (15.8%)	
2010	685 (14.6%)	572 (14.7%)	113 (14.1%)	
2011	623 (13.3%)	499 (12.8%)	124 (15.5%)	
Age				
<50	799 (17.0%)	629 (16.1%)	170 (21.2%)	
50–64	1854 (39.4%)	1497 (38.4%)	357 (44.5%)	<0.001^A
65–79	1564 (33.3%)	1342 (34.4%)	222 (27.7%)	
80+	483 (10.3%)	430 (11.0%)	53 (6.6%)	
Gender				
Male	2972 (63.2%)	2477 (63.5%)	495 (61.7%)	0.329^A
Female	1728 (36.8%)	1421 (36.5%)	307 (38.3%)	
Ethnicity				
Caucasian	3940 (83.8%)	3275 (84.0%)	665 (82.9%)	
African-American	366 (7.8%)	285 (7.3%)	81 (10.1%)	0.011^A
Other/unknown	394 (8.4%)	338 (8.7%)	56 (7.0%)	
Marital status				
Married	2822 (60.0%)	2296 (58.9%)	526 (65.6%)	
Single/widowed	1174 (25.0%)	1003 (25.7%)	171 (21.3%)	0.002^A
Other/unknown	704 (15.0%)	599 (15.4%)	105 (13.1%)	
Outcome variables				
Cause of death				
Alive	3668 (78.0%)	2988 (76.7%)	680 (84.8%)	
Dead from cancer	714 (15.2%)	631 (16.2%)	83 (10.3%)	<0.001^A
Dead not from cancer	318 (6.8%)	279 (7.2%)	39 (4.9%)	
Follow-up				
Months	35.5 (23.4)	35.4 (23.4)	36.3 (23.8)	0.353^B

n (%) and mean (SD).
[A]Chi-square test [B]Mann–Whitney *U* test.

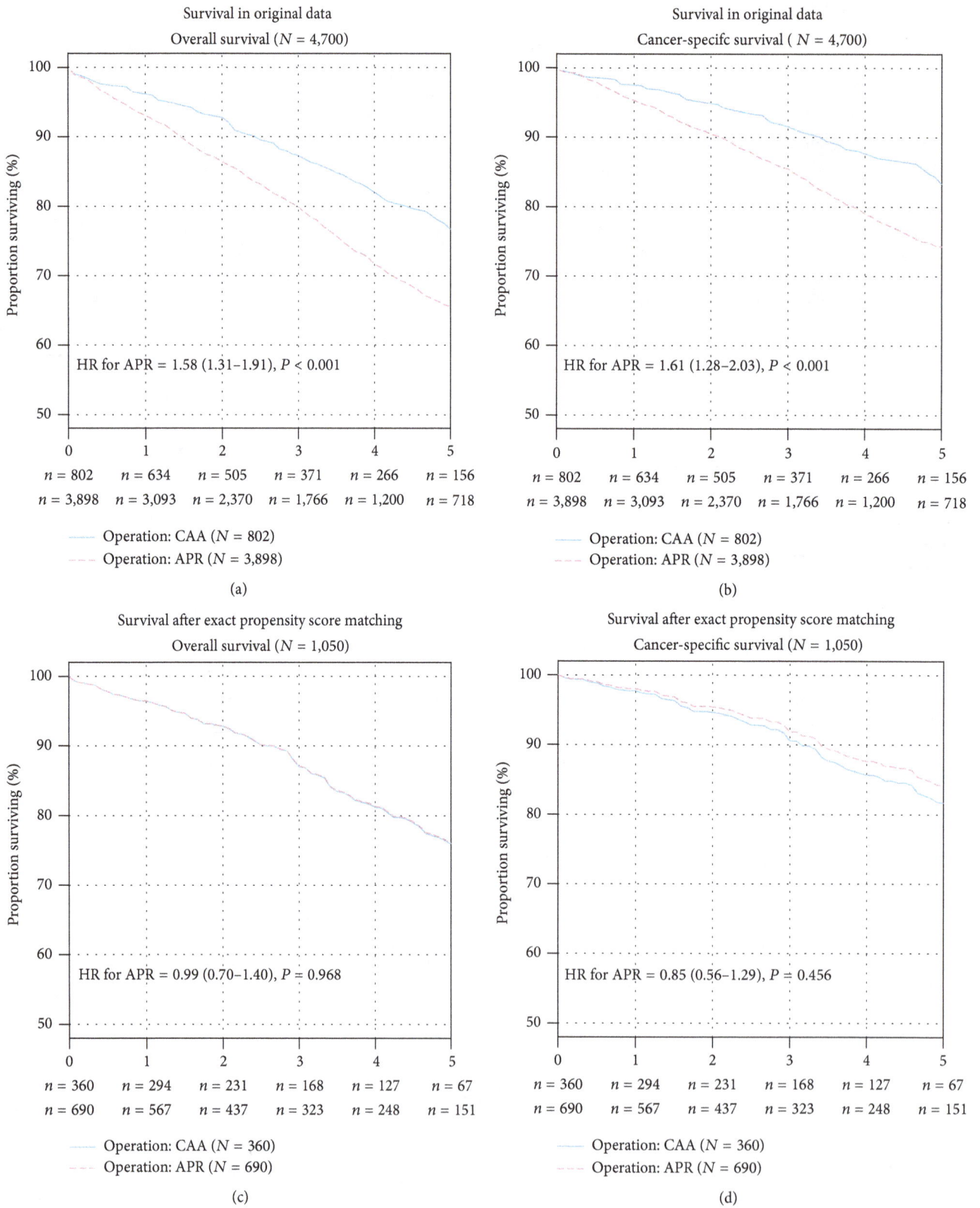

FIGURE 2: Kaplan-Meier curves for overall (panels a, c) and cancer-specific (panels b, d) survival in unadjusted and propensity score adjusted analysis. The overall survival (panels a, c) and cancer-specific survival (panels b, d) in unadjusted and propensity score adjusted analysis are depicted. The number of rectal cancer patients at risk in the two groups is given below each plot. HR: hazard ratio for APR compared with CAA with P value from likelihood-ratio test.

Table 2: Prognostic factors for overall and cancer-specific mortality.

| | Overall mortality | | | | | | Cancer-specific mortality | | | | | |
| | Unadjusted[A] | | Cox regression, full model[B] | | Cox regression, variable selection[C] | | Unadjusted[A] | | Cox regression, full model[B] | | Cox regression, variable selection[C] | |
	HR (95% CI)	P^D	HR (95% CI)	P^D	HR (95% CI)	P^D	HR (95% CI)	P^D	HR (95% CI)	P^D	HR (95% CI)	P^D
Operation												
CAA	Reference		Reference		Reference		Reference		Reference		Reference	
APR	1.58 (1.31–1.91)	<0.001	1.37 (1.13–1.67)	0.001	1.36 (1.12–1.64)	0.001	1.61 (1.28–2.03)	<0.001	1.39 (1.10–1.76)	0.004	1.39 (1.11–1.76)	0.004
Tumor stage (AJCC 6th ed.)												
Stage I	Reference		Reference		Reference		Reference		Reference		Reference	
Stage IIA	1.23 (1.02–1.50)		1.47 (1.20–1.80)		1.49 (1.22–1.82)		1.67 (1.28–2.18)		1.90 (1.44–2.50)		1.91 (1.45–2.51)	
Stage IIB	2.17 (1.58–2.99)		2.71 (1.96–3.76)		2.67 (1.93–3.70)		3.83 (2.63–5.59)		4.51 (3.06–6.65)		4.45 (3.02–6.55)	
Stage IIIA	1.50 (1.11–2.01)	<0.001	1.82 (1.34–2.46)	<0.001	1.82 (1.34–2.46)	<0.001	2.13 (1.45–3.11)	<0.001	2.50 (1.69–3.69)	<0.001	2.47 (1.67–3.64)	<0.001
Stage IIIB	1.76 (1.46–2.13)		2.28 (1.87–2.80)		2.29 (1.87–2.81)		2.81 (2.18–3.63)		3.39 (2.59–4.43)		3.38 (2.58–4.42)	
Stage IIIC	3.42 (2.81–4.17)		4.11 (3.33–5.08)		4.09 (3.31–5.06)		5.90 (4.56–7.65)		6.57 (4.99–8.65)		6.54 (4.97–8.61)	
Retrieved regional lymph nodes												
<12	Reference		Reference		Reference		Reference		Reference		Reference	
12+	0.95 (0.84–1.07)	0.391	0.79 (0.69–0.90)	<0.001	0.78 (0.69–0.88)	<0.001	0.96 (0.83–1.11)	0.576	0.77 (0.66–0.90)	0.001	0.76 (0.65–0.89)	0.001
Grading												
G1	Reference		Reference		Reference		Reference		Reference		Reference	
G2	1.43 (1.08–1.89)		1.26 (0.95–1.68)		1.28 (0.96–1.70)		2.29 (1.50–3.52)		1.92 (1.25–2.95)		1.95 (1.27–3.00)	
G3/4	2.15 (1.59–2.92)	<0.001	1.59 (1.17–2.16)	0.006	1.61 (1.19–2.19)	0.004	4.15 (2.66–6.46)	<0.001	2.80 (1.79–4.38)	<0.001	2.84 (1.82–4.45)	<0.001
Unknown	1.07 (0.74–1.55)		1.15 (0.79–1.66)		1.16 (0.80–1.68)		1.63 (0.97–2.75)		1.55 (0.92–2.61)		1.59 (0.94–2.68)	
Radiation												
None	Reference		Reference		Reference		Reference		Reference		Reference	
Before surgery	0.58 (0.51–0.67)		0.56 (0.48–0.66)		0.56 (0.48–0.66)		0.74 (0.62–0.87)		0.62 (0.51–0.75)		0.61 (0.51–0.74)	
After surgery	0.82 (0.68–0.99)	<0.001	0.62 (0.51–0.76)	<0.001	0.63 (0.51–0.77)	<0.001	1.00 (0.80–1.25)	<0.001	0.63 (0.49–0.80)	<0.001	0.64 (0.50–0.81)	<0.001
Year												
2005	Reference		Reference		—		Reference		Reference		—	
2006	0.94 (0.79–1.12)		0.99 (0.83–1.18)		—		0.97 (0.79–1.20)		1.02 (0.83–1.25)		—	
2007	0.85 (0.71–1.03)		0.85 (0.71–1.03)		—		0.86 (0.69–1.08)		0.86 (0.69–1.09)		—	
2008	0.95 (0.77–1.17)		0.99 (0.80–1.22)		—		1.00 (0.78–1.28)		1.02 (0.80–1.31)		—	
2009	0.88 (0.69–1.12)	0.068	1.06 (0.83–1.35)	0.141	—		0.83 (0.62–1.11)	0.029	0.96 (0.71–1.30)	0.072	—	
2010	0.76 (0.56–1.03)		0.84 (0.62–1.15)		—		0.60 (0.40–0.90)		0.65 (0.44–0.98)		—	
2011	0.43 (0.22–0.82)		0.51 (0.26–0.97)		—		0.36 (0.15–0.89)		0.40 (0.16–0.99)		—	
Age												
<50	Reference		Reference		Reference		Reference		Reference		Reference	
50–64	1.07 (0.86–1.32)		1.10 (0.89–1.37)		1.09 (0.88–1.35)		0.96 (0.76–1.21)		1.01 (0.80–1.27)		1.00 (0.79–1.27)	
65–79	1.80 (1.47–2.21)	<0.001	1.76 (1.43–2.16)	<0.001	1.74 (1.42–2.15)	<0.001	1.37 (1.09–1.72)	<0.001	1.37 (1.09–1.73)	<0.001	1.38 (1.09–1.74)	<0.001
80+	3.88 (3.10–4.86)		3.25 (2.56–4.12)		3.14 (2.47–3.98)		2.49 (1.92–3.25)		2.23 (1.68–2.96)		2.21 (1.67–2.93)	

TABLE 2: Continued.

	Overall mortality						Cancer-specific mortality					
	Unadjusted[A]		Cox regression, full model[B]		Cox regression, variable selection[C]		Unadjusted[A]		Cox regression, full model[B]		Cox regression, variable selection[C]	
	HR (95% CI)	P^D	HR (95% CI)	P^D	HR (95% CI)	P^D	HR (95% CI)	P^D	HR (95% CI)	P^D	HR (95% CI)	P^D
Gender												
Male	Reference		Reference		—	—	Reference		Reference		—	—
Female	1.18 (1.04–1.33)	0.012	0.93 (0.81–1.06)	0.282	—	—	1.15 (0.99–1.34)	0.066	0.96 (0.82–1.13)	0.641	—	—
Ethnicity												
Caucasian	Reference		Reference		—	—	Reference		Reference		Reference	
African-American	1.24 (1.00–1.54)	0.122	1.25 (1.00–1.55)	0.152	—	—	1.34 (1.04–1.72)	0.061	1.30 (1.00–1.67)	0.145	1.30 (1.01–1.68)	0.135
Other/unknown	0.95 (0.75–1.19)		1.02 (0.80–1.28)		—		0.91 (0.68–1.21)		0.97 (0.73–1.30)		0.96 (0.72–1.28)	
Marital status												
Married	Reference		Reference		Reference		Reference		Reference		Reference	
Single/widowed	1.81 (1.57–2.07)	<0.001	1.42 (1.22–1.65)	<0.001	1.41 (1.22–1.62)	<0.001	1.66 (1.41–1.97)	<0.001	1.34 (1.12–1.60)	0.001	1.31 (1.10–1.56)	0.001
Other/unknown	1.41 (1.19–1.67)		1.41 (1.18–1.68)		1.41 (1.19–1.68)		1.44 (1.17–1.76)		1.37 (1.11–1.69)		1.35 (1.10–1.66)	

Hazard ratios (HR) with 95% confidence intervals; [A] univariate Cox regression analysis; [B] multivariable Cox regression analysis full model; [C] backward variable selection from full model multivariable Cox regression analysis full model; [D] likelihood ratio tests.

TABLE 3: Bias for abdominoperineal resection.

	Logistic regression in raw data ($N = 4,700$)[A]		Patient characteristics after exact propensity score matching ($N = 1,050$)[C]		
	OR (95% CI)	P[B]	Total $N = 1,050$	APR $N = 690$	CAA $N = 360$
Tumor stage (AJCC 6th ed.)					
Stage I	Reference		295.2 (28.1%)	194 (28.1%)	101.2 (28.1%)
Stage IIA	1.21 (0.98–1.51)		398.7 (38.0%)	262 (38.0%)	136.7 (38.0%)
Stage IIB	3.53 (1.91–7.31)		1.5 (0.1%)	1 (0.1%)	0.5 (0.1%)
Stage IIIA	0.90 (0.65–1.25)	<0.001	36.5 (3.5%)	24 (3.5%)	12.5 (3.5%)
Stage IIIB	1.42 (1.12–1.80)		261.7 (24.9%)	172 (24.9%)	89.7 (24.9%)
Stage IIIC	1.52 (1.14–2.04)		56.3 (5.4%)	37 (5.4%)	19.3 (5.4%)
Retrieved regional lymph nodes					
<12	Reference	0.155	503.7 (48.0%)	331 (48.0%)	172.7 (48.0%)
12+	0.89 (0.75–1.05)		546.3 (52.0%)	359 (52.0%)	187.3 (52.0%)
Grading					
G1	Reference		22.8 (2.2%)	15 (2.2%)	7.8 (2.2%)
G2	1.22 (0.92–1.61)	0.072	969.3 (92.3%)	637 (92.3%)	332.3 (92.3%)
G3/4	1.34 (0.95–1.88)		41.1 (3.9%)	27 (3.9%)	14.1 (3.9%)
Unknown	1.69 (1.12–2.57)		16.7 (1.6%)	11 (1.6%)	5.7 (1.6%)
Radiation					
None	Reference		228.3 (21.7%)	150 (21.7%)	78.3 (21.7%)
Before surgery	1.75 (1.43–2.13)	<0.001	768.5 (73.2%)	505 (73.2%)	263.5 (73.2%)
After surgery	1.58 (1.20–2.10)		53.3 (5.1%)	35 (5.1%)	18.3 (5.1%)
Year					
2005	Reference		176.5 (16.8%)	116 (16.8%)	60.5 (16.8%)
2006	1.05 (0.79–1.41)		152.2 (14.5%)	100 (14.5%)	52.2 (14.5%)
2007	0.92 (0.69–1.23)		149.1 (14.2%)	98 (14.2%)	51.1 (14.2%)
2008	1.19 (0.88–1.62)	0.155	94.3 (9.0%)	62 (9.0%)	32.3 (9.0%)
2009	0.82 (0.62–1.09)		172 (16.4%)	113 (16.4%)	59 (16.4%)
2010	0.98 (0.73–1.31)		172 (16.4%)	113 (16.4%)	59 (16.4%)
2011	0.81 (0.61–1.08)		133.9 (12.8%)	88 (12.8%)	45.9 (12.8%)
Age					
<50	Reference		132.4 (12.6%)	87 (12.6%)	45.4 (12.6%)
50–64	1.20 (0.97–1.48)	<0.001	544.8 (51.9%)	358 (51.9%)	186.8 (51.9%)
65–79	1.86 (1.48–2.33)		343.9 (32.8%)	226 (32.8%)	117.9 (32.8%)
80+	2.76 (1.96–3.94)		28.9 (2.8%)	19 (2.8%)	9.9 (2.8%)
Gender					
Male	Reference	0.066	833.9 (79.4%)	548 (79.4%)	285.9 (79.4%)
Female	0.86 (0.73–1.01)		216.1 (20.6%)	142 (20.6%)	74.1 (20.6%)
Ethnicity					
Caucasian	Reference		1033.3 (98.4%)	679 (98.4%)	354.3 (98.4%)
African-American	0.71 (0.55–0.94)	0.008	7.6 (0.7%)	5 (0.7%)	2.6 (0.7%)
Other/unknown	1.30 (0.97–1.77)		9.1 (0.9%)	6 (0.9%)	3.1 (0.9%)
Marital status					
Married	Reference		897.8 (85.5%)	590 (85.5%)	307.8 (85.5%)
Single/widowed	1.29 (1.06–1.58)	0.006	106.5 (10.1%)	70 (10.1%)	36.5 (10.1%)
Other/unknown	1.33 (1.06–1.69)		45.7 (4.3%)	30 (4.3%)	15.7 (4.3%)

After exclusion of 3,650 patients for the exact propensity score matching, no bias was observed in the remaining 1,050 patients for APR versus CAA (all $P = 1$).
[A]Multivariable logistic regression with the odds ratio (OR) for APR in the original raw data set ($N = 4,700$).
[B]Likelihood ratio tests.
[C]All $P = 1$ for comparison of APR versus CAA in weighted Chi-square tests after exact weighted propensity score matching ($N = 1,050$).
Weighted matching causes decimals for the number of patients in the group with CAA.

were significantly older, were less often African-Americans, and were less often married.

For exact propensity score matching, 3,650 patients were excluded because they did not have a counterpart in the other group who had exactly the same values for all baseline covariates. In the remaining 1,050 patients, no differences between patients undergoing APR and CAA were observed (for all covariates, $P = 1.0$), demonstrating a perfect matching. In Cox regression analyses after propensity score matching, the risk of overall mortality (HR of death = 0.99, 95% CI: 0.70 to 1.40, $P = 0.968$) and cancer-specific mortality (HR of death = 0.85, 95% CI: 0.56 to 1.29, $P = 0.456$) was not increased in patients undergoing APR. In the propensity score-matched analysis, the 5-year overall survival for patients undergoing APR was 76.1% (95% CI: 71.9 to 80.5%) compared with 76.0% (95% CI: 70.4 to 81.9%) for patients undergoing CAA (Figure 2). The 5-year cancer-specific survival in patients undergoing APR was 84.1% (95% CI: 80.5 to 88.0%) compared with 81.7% (95% CI: 76.5 to 87.2%) in patients undergoing CAA (Figure 2).

4. Discussion and Conclusions

The present study is, to the best of our knowledge, the first SEER analysis applying propensity score matching to determine the prognostic relevance of APR versus CAA. Based on the assessed cohort of nonmetastatic rectal cancer patients, the current study revealed the following two central results.

First, the rate of APR declined from 31.8% in 1998 to 19.2% in 2011, with a significant change in this trend at the end of 2004. Second, APR was associated with a significant survival disadvantage in univariate analysis and after conventional multivariable adjustment. This finding was in contrast to the lack of influence of APR on survival when optimally adjusting by exact propensity score matching. Consequently, the association between APR and worse survival observed in conventional analysis is not due to the APR itself but caused by highly biased patient characteristics.

The decline in the APR rate confirms previous research that has indicated a rate of 23% decrease in nonrestorative rectal resections between 2005 and 2010 in the regions covered by the SEER registry [15, 20]. In England, analysis of the national administrative database between 1996 and 2004 demonstrated that the APR rate significantly decreased from 29% to 21% [20]. Besides the declining trend of APR, the rates of APR vary immensely within the literature. In their retrospective analysis of discharge data from 21 states in the US from 2002 to 2004, Ricciardi et al. documented an APR rate of 50% [31].

The trend change in 2004 observed in the present investigation might be explained by the increasing implementation of preoperative chemoradiotherapy at that time. In 2004, Sauer et al. demonstrated better local control and a decreased rate of APR in patients with preoperative compared to postoperative chemoradiotherapy [32]. Another reason for the trend change in 2004 might be the increased use of phased array coil MRI [33], which proved to be a more accurate diagnostic technique in the prediction of a positive

circumferential resection margin and sphincter infiltration and might thus have minimized potential overtreatment by APR. Furthermore, the more prevalent use of stapling devices might have contributed to the declining rate of APR [34, 35]. Inevitably, for a portion of patients, that is, those with sphincter-infiltrating tumors, APR is still the only curative treatment. In the future, the application of preoperative, targeted therapy to nonmetastatic rectal cancer could further reduce the nearly stagnating rate [36].

The risk of mortality for APR compared to CAA was exclusively analyzed in patients diagnosed after 2005, a time period with only moderate changes in APR rate. Thus, the time-trend bias was minimized. In this analysis, APR was associated with a significantly increased risk of mortality, which was approximately 60% after univariate analysis and approximately 38% after conventional multivariable adjustment. In contrast, after exact propensity score matching, no increased risk of mortality was observed after APR. To elaborate this discrepancy, patient and tumor characteristics were considered.

Of note, conventional multivariable analysis cannot fully adjust for confounders; for example, it cannot take into account the combined effect of two confounders (e.g., age and gender). Furthermore, effects such as collinearity cannot be ruled out. In contrast, the exact weighted propensity score matching that was applied in the present study is a modern, superior statistical method of building two identical groups, thus simulating randomization and precluding selection bias [28–30]. There was a statistically significant and clinically relevant bias in patient and tumor characteristics between the APR and CAA groups that strongly favored CAA against APR. Independent risk factors for a poor oncologic outcome after APR [5] occurred more often in the APR group. Patients undergoing APR were older, had more advanced cancer stages, and had fewer regional lymph nodes retrieved. The risk of mortality after APR versus CAA decreased with a higher degree of adjustment and was zero when an optimal adjustment was performed by exact propensity score matching. Hence, the association between APR and worse overall and cancer-specific survival is not caused by APR itself but rather reflects disadvantageous patient and tumor characteristics.

The relationship between the level of adjustment for patient and tumor characteristics and the oncologic outcome explains some of the contradictory findings in the literature [1, 3, 5, 6, 17–19, 37, 38]. A SEER-based analysis from 1998 to 2007 found a 35% increased risk of mortality for APR after conventional multivariable-adjusted Cox regression [37]. A Swedish population-based analysis from 1995 to 2003 [17] and two single center analyses from 1989 to 2002 and from 1990 to 2006 did not find such a negative impact [18, 19]. In contrast, in a pooled analysis of five European trials between 1987 and 2003 published by den Dulk et al., APR was associated with a higher rate of a positive circumferential margin and of local recurrences as well as decreased survival, although the likelihood of undergoing APR was included in the multivariable analysis [5]. Another investigation of the data in the Dutch Surgical Colorectal Audit conducted between 2010 and 2011 by the same research group did not find an increased rate of positive circumferential margin after APR [38].

The recent introduction of a more radical operative technique might explain potential improvement in oncological outcome after APR. In 2005, Marr and coauthors showed that in standard APR the specimen has a smaller diameter at the location of the tumor compared to anterior resection with total mesorectal excision (TME). The consequences of a smaller diameter were a smaller median distance from the tumor to the circumferential resection margin (CRM) and more CRM positive specimens [2]. At the beginning of the 21st century, Holm et al. started to perform more extensive APR, stopping the abdominal dissection above the beginning of the levators and dissecting more radically from beneath to completely remove these muscles [39]. West et al. demonstrated in 2010 that this cylindrical or extralevator APR approach led to reduced rates of positive CRM and intraoperative perforations [40]. Recent systematic reviews and meta-analyses showed significantly fewer local recurrences after the more extensive procedure [41, 42]. Data on the effect on survival is still scarce; some studies show an improvement [43], whereas smaller analyses have not yielded significantly better oncological outcomes compared with standard APR [34, 44]. The partial or complete adaption of this new form of APR in the last years, which is not referred to in most studies, might add to the contradictory results regarding oncologic outcome.

We would like to acknowledge the limitations of the present investigation. First, data corresponding to tumor height, adjuvant therapy, comorbidities, quality of TME, and CRM involvement are not available in the SEER registry. Therefore, the extent to which these parameters might have influenced prognosis remains unclear. Although we performed risk adjustment for known confounders, potential bias due to unknown confounding cannot be excluded. Additionally, survival is not the only oncological outcome in cancer patient care. Continence, genitourinary function and the superordinate criterion of quality of life are essential for deciding what type of operation to perform. Unfortunately, the SEER database does not provide data about quality of life. According to a recent Cochrane meta-analysis, reliable conclusions concerning quality of life after APR versus CAA have not been possible to date [45]. Additionally, data about postoperative morbidity after APR and CAA are sparse, with some evidence for a similar rate after both procedures [19].

The main strength of the present investigation comes from the great power associated with its large sample size. Because randomized controlled trials directly comparing results after APR and CAA are lacking and difficult to perform due to ethical reasons, the present analysis is probably the most appropriate study design.

5. Conclusion

In summary, the present population-based investigation on nonmetastatic rectal cancer patients provides evidence that APR itself is not associated with worse overall or cancer-specific survival. APR is performed in the presence of poor prognostic factors, such as age and tumor stage. Hence,

overall and cancer-specific survival should not be an issue when deciding whether to perform APR.

Competing Interests

The authors declare that they have no competing interests.

Authors' Contributions

Rene Warschkow and Sabrina M. Ebinger contributed equally to this work.

References

[1] R. J. Heald, R. K. Smedh, A. Kald, R. Sexton, and B. J. Moran, "Abdominoperineal excision of the rectum—an endangered operation. Norman Nigro Lectureship," *Diseases of the Colon and Rectum*, vol. 40, no. 7, pp. 747–751, 1997.

[2] R. Marr, K. Birbeck, J. Garvican et al., "The modern abdominoperineal excision: the next challenge after total mesorectal excision," *Annals of Surgery*, vol. 242, no. 1, pp. 74–82, 2005.

[3] I. D. Nagtegaal, C. J. H. Van De Velde, C. A. M. Marijnen, J. H. J. M. Van Krieken, and P. Quirke, "Low rectal cancer: a call for a change of approach in abdominoperineal resection," *Journal of Clinical Oncology*, vol. 23, no. 36, pp. 9257–9264, 2005.

[4] P. P. Tekkis, A. G. Heriot, J. Smith, M. R. Thompson, P. Finan, and J. D. Stamatakis, "Comparison of circumferential margin involvement between restrorative and nonrestorative resections for rectal cancer," *Colorectal Disease*, vol. 7, no. 4, pp. 369–374, 2005.

[5] M. den Dulk, H. Putter, L. Collette et al., "The abdominoperineal resection itself is associated with an adverse outcome: the European experience based on a pooled analysis of five European randomised clinical trials on rectal cancer," *European Journal of Cancer*, vol. 45, no. 7, pp. 1175–1183, 2009.

[6] W. L. Law and K. W. Chu, "Abdominoperineal resection is associated with poor oncological outcome," *British Journal of Surgery*, vol. 91, no. 11, pp. 1493–1499, 2004.

[7] E. J. Silberfein, K. M. Kattepogu, C.-Y. Hu et al., "Long-term survival and recurrence outcomes following surgery for distal rectal cancer," *Annals of Surgical Oncology*, vol. 17, no. 11, pp. 2863–2869, 2010.

[8] A. B. Benson III, T. Bekaii-Saab, E. Chan et al., "Rectal cancer," *JNCCN Journal of the National Comprehensive Cancer Network*, vol. 10, no. 12, pp. 1528–1564, 2012.

[9] K. Bujko, A. Rutkowski, G. J. Chang, W. Michalski, E. Chmielik, and J. Kusnierz, "Is the 1-cm rule of distal bowel resection margin in rectal cancer based on clinical evidence? A systematic review," *Annals of Surgical Oncology*, vol. 19, no. 3, pp. 801–808, 2012.

[10] F. Rullier, C. Laurent, F. Bretagnol, A. Rullier, V. Vendrely, and F. Zerbib, "Sphincter-saving resection for all rectal carcinomas: the end of the 2-cm distal rule," *Annals of Surgery*, vol. 241, no. 3, pp. 465–469, 2005.

[11] N. S. Williams, M. F. Dixon, and D. Johnston, "Reappraisal of the 5 centimetre rule of distal excision for carcinoma of the rectum: a study of distal intramural spread and of patients' survival," *The British Journal of Surgery*, vol. 70, no. 3, pp. 150–154, 1983.

[12] K. M. Madbouly and A. M. Hussein, "Changing operative strategy from abdominoperineal resection to sphincter preservation in T3 low rectal cancer after downstaging by neoadjuvant chemoradiation: a preliminary report," *World Journal of Surgery*, vol. 39, no. 5, pp. 1248–1256, 2015.

[13] E. L. Bokey, B. Öjerskog, P. H. Chapuis, O. F. Dent, R. C. Newland, and G. Sinclair, "Local recurrence after curative excision of the rectum for cancer without adjuvant therapy: role of total anatomical dissection," *British Journal of Surgery*, vol. 86, no. 9, pp. 1164–1170, 1999.

[14] M. den Dulk, C. A. M. Marijnen, H. Putter et al., "Risk factors for adverse outcome in patients with rectal cancer treated with an abdominoperineal resection in the total mesorectal excision trial," *Annals of Surgery*, vol. 246, no. 1, pp. 83–90, 2007.

[15] S. Mohammed, D. A. Anaya, S. S. Awad, D. Albo, D. H. Berger, and A. Artinyan, "Sphincter preservation rates after radical resection for rectal cancer in the United States veteran population: opportunity for improvement in early disease," *Annals of Surgical Oncology*, vol. 22, no. 1, pp. 216–223, 2015.

[16] J. G. Guillem, "Ultra-low anterior resection and coloanal pouch reconstruction for carcinoma of the distal rectum," *World Journal of Surgery*, vol. 21, no. 7, pp. 721–727, 1997.

[17] C. Anderin, A. Martling, H. Hellborg, and T. Holm, "A population-based study on outcome in relation to the type of resection in low rectal cancer," *Diseases of the Colon and Rectum*, vol. 53, no. 5, pp. 753–760, 2010.

[18] K. L. Mathis, D. W. Larson, E. J. Dozois et al., "Outcomes following surgery without radiotherapy for rectal cancer," *The British Journal of Surgery*, vol. 99, no. 1, pp. 137–143, 2012.

[19] E. W. L. Chuwa and F. Seow-Choen, "Outcomes for abdominoperineal resections are not worse than those of anterior resections," *Diseases of the Colon and Rectum*, vol. 49, no. 1, pp. 41–49, 2006.

[20] H. S. Tilney, A. G. Heriot, S. Purkayastha et al., "A national perspective on the decline of abdominoperineal resection for rectal cancer," *Annals of Surgery*, vol. 247, no. 1, pp. 77–84, 2008.

[21] Surveillance, Epidemiology and End Results (SEER) Program, Research Data (1973–2011), National Cancer Institute, DCCPS, Surveillance Research Program, Surveillance Systems Branch, April 2014, https://seer.cancer.gov/.

[22] P. A. Wingo, P. M. Jamison, R. A. Hiatt et al., "Building the infrastructure for nationwide cancer surveillance and control— a comparison between The National Program of Cancer Registries (NPCR) and The Surveillance, Epidemiology, and End Results (SEER) Program (United States)," *Cancer Causes & Control*, vol. 14, no. 2, pp. 175–193, 2003.

[23] A. Fritz, C. Percy, A. Jack et al., *International Classification of Diseases for Oncology*, World Health Organization, Geneva, Switzerland, 3rd edition, 2000.

[24] R. B. Davies, "Hypothesis testing when a nuisance parameter is present only under the alternative," *Biometrika*, vol. 74, no. 1, pp. 33–43, 1987.

[25] V. M. R. Muggeo, "Estimating regression models with unknown break-points," *Statistics in Medicine*, vol. 22, no. 19, pp. 3055–3071, 2003.

[26] W. S. Cleveland and S. J. Devlin, "Locally weighted regression: an approach to regression analysis by local fitting," *Journal of the American Statistical Association*, vol. 83, no. 403, pp. 596–610, 1988.

[27] P. M. Grambsch and T. M. Therneau, "Proportional hazards tests and diagnostics based on weighted residuals," *Biometrika*, vol. 81, no. 3, pp. 515–526, 1994.

[28] D. B. Rubin, "Estimating causal effects from large data sets using propensity scores," *Annals of Internal Medicine*, vol. 127, no. 8, pp. 757–763, 1997.

[29] M. M. Joffe and P. R. Rosenbaum, "Invited commentary: propensity scores," *American Journal of Epidemiology*, vol. 150, no. 4, pp. 327–333, 1999.

[30] P. R. Rosenbaum, "Model-based direct adjustment," *Journal of the American Statistical Association*, vol. 82, no. 398, pp. 387–394, 1987.

[31] R. Ricciardi, P. L. Roberts, T. E. Read, P. W. Marcello, D. J. Schoetz, and N. N. Baxter, "Variability in reconstructive procedures following rectal cancer surgery in the United States," *Diseases of the Colon and Rectum*, vol. 53, no. 6, pp. 874–880, 2010.

[32] R. Sauer, H. Becker, W. Hohenberger et al., "Preoperative versus postoperative chemoradiotherapy for rectal cancer," *The New England Journal of Medicine*, vol. 351, no. 17, pp. 1731–1810, 2004.

[33] R. G. H. Beets-Tan, G. L. Beets, R. F. A. Vliegen et al., "Accuracy of magnetic resonance imaging in prediction of tumour-free resection margin in rectal cancer surgery," *The Lancet*, vol. 357, no. 9255, pp. 497–504, 2001.

[34] A. Krishna, M. J. F. X. Rickard, A. Keshava, O. F. Dent, and P. H. Chapuis, "A comparison of published rates of resection margin involvement and intra-operative perforation between standard and 'cylindrical' abdominoperineal excision for low rectal cancer," *Colorectal Disease*, vol. 15, no. 1, pp. 57–65, 2013.

[35] N. S. Williams, J. Murphy, and C. H. Knowles, "Anterior Perineal PlanE for ultra-low Anterior Resection of the rectum (the APPEAR technique): a prospective clinical trial of a new procedure," *Annals of Surgery*, vol. 247, no. 5, pp. 750–758, 2008.

[36] L. Fornaro, C. Caparello, C. Vivaldi et al., "Bevacizumab in the pre-operative treatment of locally advanced rectal cancer: a systematic review," *World Journal of Gastroenterology*, vol. 20, no. 20, pp. 6081–6091, 2014.

[37] D. A. Etzioni, T. M. Young-Fadok, R. R. Cima et al., "Patient survival after surgical treatment of rectal cancer: impact of surgeon and hospital characteristics," *Cancer*, vol. 120, no. 16, pp. 2472–2481, 2014.

[38] N. van Leersum, I. Martijnse, M. den Dulk et al., "Differences in circumferential resection margin involvement after abdominoperineal excision and low anterior resection no longer significant," *Annals of Surgery*, vol. 259, no. 6, pp. 1150–1155, 2014.

[39] T. Holm, A. Ljung, T. Häggmark, G. Jurell, and J. Lagergren, "Extended abdominoperineal resection with gluteus maximus flap reconstruction of the pelvic floor for rectal cancer," *The British Journal of Surgery*, vol. 94, no. 2, pp. 232–238, 2007.

[40] N. P. West, C. Anderin, K. J. E. Smith, T. Holm, and P. Quirke, "Multicentre experience with extralevator abdominoperineal excision for low rectal cancer," *British Journal of Surgery*, vol. 97, no. 4, pp. 588–599, 2010.

[41] H.-C. Yu, H. Peng, X.-S. He, and R.-S. Zhao, "Comparison of short- and long-term outcomes after extralevator abdominoperineal excision and standard abdominoperineal excision for rectal cancer: a systematic review and meta-analysis," *International Journal of Colorectal Disease*, vol. 29, no. 2, pp. 183–191, 2014.

[42] S. Stelzner, C. Koehler, J. Stelzer, A. Sims, and H. Witzigmann, "Extended abdominoperineal excision vs. standard abdominoperineal excision in rectal cancer—a systematic overview," *International Journal of Colorectal Disease*, vol. 26, no. 10, pp. 1227–1240, 2011.

[43] P. G. Vaughan-Shaw, T. Cheung, J. S. Knight, P. H. Nichols, S. A. Pilkington, and A. H. Mirnezami, "A prospective case-control study of extralevator abdominoperineal excision (ELAPE) of the rectum versus conventional laparoscopic and open abdominoperineal excision: comparative analysis of short-term outcomes and quality of life," *Techniques in Coloproctology*, vol. 16, no. 5, pp. 355–362, 2012.

[44] D. Asplund, E. Haglind, and E. Angenete, "Outcome of extralevator abdominoperineal excision compared with standard surgery: results from a single centre," *Colorectal Disease*, vol. 14, no. 10, pp. 1191–1196, 2012.

[45] J. Pachler and P. Wille-Jørgensen, "Quality of life after rectal resection for cancer, with or without permanent colostomy," *Cochrane database of systematic reviews*, vol. 12, Article ID Cd004323, 2012.

4

Cost-Effectiveness Analysis of *Helicobacter pylori* Diagnostic Methods in Patients with Atrophic Gastritis

Fumio Omata,[1,2] **Takuro Shimbo,**[3] **Sachiko Ohde,**[2] **Gautam A. Deshpande,**[2] **and Tsuguya Fukui**[1,2]

[1]*Department of Internal Medicine, St. Luke's International Hospital, Chuo-Ku, Japan*
[2]*Center for Clinical Epidemiology, St. Luke's International University, Chuo-Ku, Japan*
[3]*Ohta Nishinouchi Hospital, Koriyama, Japan*

Correspondence should be addressed to Fumio Omata; omataf@icloud.com

Academic Editor: Tatsuya Toyokawa

Background. There are several diagnostic methods for *Helicobacter pylori (H. pylori)* infection. A cost-effective analysis is needed to decide on the optimal diagnostic method. The aim of this study was to determine a cost-effective diagnostic method in patients with atrophic gastritis (AG). *Methods.* A decision-analysis model including seven diagnostic methods was constructed for patients with AG diagnosed by esophagogastroduodenoscopy. Expected values of cost and effectiveness were calculated for each test. *Results.* If the prevalence of *H. pylori* in the patients with AG is 85% and CAM-resistant *H. pylori* is 30%, histology, stool *H. pylori* antigen (SHPAg), bacterial culture (BC), and urine *H. pylori* antibody (UHPAb) were dominated by serum *H. pylori* IgG antibody (SHPAb), rapid urease test (RUT), and urea breath test (UBT). Among three undominated methods, the incremental cost-effective ratios (ICER) of RUT versus SHPAb and UBT versus RUT were $214 and $1914, respectively. If the prevalence of CAM-sensitive *H. pylori* was less than 55%, BC was not dominated, but its *H. pylori* eradication success rate was 0.86. *Conclusions.* RUT was the most cost-effective at the current prevalence of CAM-resistant *H. pylori*. BC could not be selected due to its poor effectiveness even if CAM-resistant *H. pylori* was more than 45%.

1. Introduction

While the prevalence of *Helicobacter pylori (H. pylori)* has been decreasing [1, 2], it remains a critical public health issue. Recently, increasing prevalence of CAM-resistant *H. pylori* is an emerging problem of public health all over the world as CAM is included in most first-line empiric *H. pylori* eradication regimens [3, 4].

Since the discovery of *H. pylori*, its association with peptic ulcer disease (PUD) [5], atrophic gastritis (AG) [6], gastric cancer [7], mucosa-associated lymphoid tissue (MALT) lymphoma [8], and immune thrombocytopenia [9] has been elucidated. Accordingly, the indication of *H. pylori* eradication therapy has been broadened from only PUD to some of the above diseases.

Among these *H. pylori*-related diseases, AG is more common than PUD or early gastric cancer; in Japan, its prevalence is reported to be approximately 27.9% even in healthy individuals [10]. 85% of AG patients were reported to have *H. pylori* infection [11]. It is a common situation that, during either diagnostic or screening esophagogastro-duodenoscopy (EGD), physicians must choose between one of several *H. pylori* diagnostic methods.

There are three invasive methods to diagnose *H. pylori* infection during EGD, including rapid urease test (RUT), histology, and bacterial culture (BC) from biopsy specimens. Other noninvasive options to diagnose *H. pylori* are serum *H. pylori* IgG antibody (SHPAb), urea breath test (UBT), stool *H. pylori* antigen (SHPAg), and urine *H. pylori* IgG antibody (UHPAb).

The diagnostic performance of these tests differs. Using BC for diagnosing *H. pylori* infection allows us to perform antibiotic- (typically macrolide-) sensitivity testing. The results of the sensitivity testing are useful to make appropriate decisions when choosing the correct first regimen for treatment, a strategy called antimicrobial susceptibility-guided therapy (AMSGT). AMSGT is assumed to be more cost-effective when the prevalence of CAM-resistant *H. pylori* has been increasing. However, there have been no prior reports mainly focusing on the impact of the prevalence of CAM-resistant *H. pylori* infection. The aim of this study was to determine a cost-effective diagnostic method for *H. pylori* infection in patients with AG.

2. Methods

This study was conducted from a social perspective. A decision-analysis model was constructed for patients in Japan diagnosed with AG suggesting *H. pylori* infection, using screening or diagnostic EGD. Time horizon was until successful *H. pylori* eradication or the end of the third regimen. We assumed that this time horizon would fall within 1 year and did not discount either effectiveness or cost.

Undergoing one of seven diagnostic tests (RUT, histology, BC, SHPAb, UBT, SHPAg, and UHPAb), patients' *H. pylori* infection status was unknown. Excluding BC which can be applied for AMSGT, if one of six tests (RUT, histology, SHPAb, UBT, SHPAg, and UHPAb) was selected and was positive, the patient underwent empiric antibiotic treatment, as none of these six tests provided any information on CAM-sensitivity. If the first standard regimen failed, patients followed the second and third regimens without additional CAM-sensitivity testing. If BC was initially selected as the diagnostic test and was positive, subsequent antibiotic susceptibility testing results were used to decide on the treatment regimen. If detected *H. pylori* was sensitive to CAM, these patients were treated with CAM-included regimen. If not, these patients were treated with metronidazole-included regimen. In the decision tree, all eradication failure was measured by UBT after the previous diagnostic step. We did not include the strategy of initial six diagnostic tests followed by AMSGT as BC required repeat EGD and we considered it unaffordable to perform repeat EGD only for the purpose of BC.

Diagnostic performance, including sensitivity and specificity of invasive and noninvasive diagnostic tests, was obtained from past English literatures, searched manually through MEDLINE and EMBASE. If there was a literature of meta-analysis, we adopted pooled values of sensitivity and specificity. Otherwise, we conducted a meta-analysis (bivariate random effects model) to calculate pooled values of sensitivity and specificity. Effectiveness was measured by rate of successful *H. pylori* eradication.

We used the success rate of *H. pylori* eradication by the first regimen (lansoprazole 30 mg bid, amoxicillin 750 mg or 1000 mg bid, and CAM 200 mg or 500 mg bid for one week) including CAM in the patients with CAM-sensitive or CAM-resistant *H. pylori* [12–15]. We also used success rate of metronidazole included triple therapy (omeprazole 20 mg bid or lansoprazole 30 mg bid, amoxicillin 500 or 750 mg bid, metronidazole 500 mg in the morning and 250 mg in the evening or 250 mg tid for one week) in the

patients with CAM-sensitive or CAM-resistant *H. pylori* [16]. In case of AMSGT, the *H. pylori* eradication rate of the 2nd regimen for the patients with CAM-resistant *H. pylori* was used [15]. The success rate of the third regimen (lansoprazole 30 mg bid, amoxicillin 750 mg bid, and sitafloxacin 100 mg bid for one week) for the patients who failed metronidazole-based triple therapy was also used [17].

Costs of each diagnostic procedure and *H. pylori* eradication regimens were derived from reimbursement of the Japanese governmental health insurance [18], and costs of gastric cancer treatments were derived from diagnosis procedure combination (DPC) by the Japanese government [19].

Our main outcome was a success rate of *H. pylori* eradication. Cost-effective thresholds, in other words willingness to pay (WTP), were estimated by treatment costs of preventable gastric cancer divided by the number needed to eradicate *H. pylori* infection.

Ford et al. [20] reported a pooled relative risk of 0.66 (95% confidence interval 0.46 to 0.95), and a number needed to eradicate *H. pylori* to prevent one patient of gastric cancer was as low as 15 for Chinese men, compared to 245 for US women.

Early gastric cancer is treated by endoscopic mucosal resection (EMR) or endoscopic submucosal dissection (ESD), and advanced gastric cancer is treated by laparoscopic or open gastrectomy. These DPC costs ranged from \$2500 to \$16000 [19].

At least, we may save \$167 (\$2500 × (1/15)) in high-prevalence areas or \$10 (\$2500 × (1/245)) in low-prevalence areas by successfully eradicating *H. pylori* infection in one patient. This means that WTP is at least \$10 in low-prevalence areas and \$167 in high-prevalence areas.

Expected values of cost and effectiveness were calculated for BC potentially for AMSGT and other six diagnostic strategies (RUT, histology, SHPAb, UBT, SHPAg, and UHPAb). Costs of each diagnostic method and each *H. pylori* eradication regimen were estimated from National Health Insurance data in Japan and expressed in US dollars at the exchange rate of 100 yen/US dollar (Table 1) [18, 19, 21]. We did not include cost of EGD as all patients in our model underwent EGD.

We first performed cost-effective analysis of base-case and calculated incremental cost-effective ratio (ICER) for comparing pairs of undominated diagnostic methods. Then, we conducted a one-way sensitivity analysis, focusing on the prevalence of CAM-resistant *H. pylori*, prevalence of *H. pylori* in the patients with AG, and the success rate of the 1st regimen for *H. pylori* to determine its threshold (Table 1).

We also performed a Monte Carlo simulation using range of uncertain probability in two scenarios of 0.4 or 0.45 of CAM-resistant *H. pylori* prevalence. All variables were assumed to follow a triangular distribution (Table 1). Ten thousand trials were conducted for simulation. We reported acceptability curve by a simulation of 10000 trials.

We used STATA® version14.1 (StataCorp, College Station, TX) for meta-analysis and TreeAge Pro® version 2016 (TreeAge Software, Inc., Williamstown, MA) for cost-effective analysis.

TABLE 1: Probabilities and costs.

Variable	Base case	References	Range for one-way sensitivity analysis	Range in Monte Carlo analysis
Probabilities				
Prevalence of *H. pylori* in AG	0.85	[11]	0.2–0.9	0.2–0.9
Proportion of CAM-resistant *H. pylori*	0.3	[37]	0.1–0.7	n. a.
Sensitivity				
Bacterial culture	0.87	[22]	n. a.	0.77–0.97
Rapid urease test	0.94	[22]	n. a.	0.84–1
Histology	0.96	[22]	n. a.	0.86–1
UBT	0.96	[23]	n. a.	0.86–1
Serum *H. pylori* IgG antibody	0.85	[24]	n. a.	0.75–0.95
Stool *H. pylori* antigen	0.93	[25]	n. a.	0.83–1
Urine *H. pylori* antibody	0.87	[26–36]	n. a.	0.77–0.97
Specificity				
Bacterial culture	0.96	[22]	n. a.	0.86–1
Rapid urease test	0.91	[22]	n. a.	0.81–1
Histology	0.77	[22]	n. a.	0.67–0.87
UBT	0.93	[23]	n. a.	0.83–1
Serum *H. pylori* IgG antibody	0.79	[24]	n. a.	0.69–0.89
Stool *H. pylori* antigen	0.96	[25]	n. a.	0.86–1
Urine *H. pylori* antibody	0.94	[26–36]	n. a.	0.84–1
Success rate of eradication regimens				
Success rate of 1st regimen for all	0.76	[12]	0.6–0.9	0.66–0.86
Success rate of 1st regimen for CAM-sensitive *H. pylori*	0.92	[13]	n. a.	0.82–1
Success rate of 1st regimen for CAM-resistant *H. pylori*	0.2	[14, 15]	n. a.	0.1–0.3
Success rate of 2nd regimen for CAM-resistant *H. pylori*	1	[15]	n. a.	0.9–1
Success rate of 2nd regimen for CAM-sensitive *H. pylori* after 1st regimen failure	0.9	[16]	n. a.	0.8–1
Success rate of 2nd regimen for CAM-resistant *H. pylori* after 1st regimen failure	0.9	[16]	n. a.	0.8–1
Success rate of 3rd regimen for CAM-sensitive *H. pylori* after 1st and 2nd regimen	0.67	[17]	n. a.	0.57–0.77
Success rate of 3rd regimen for CAM-resistant *H. pylori* after 1st and 2nd regimen	0.73	[17]	n. a.	0.63–0.83
Costs				
Diagnostics costs				
Bacterial culture with antibiotics sensitivity during EGD	$62	[18]	n. a.	n. a.
Bacterial culture only during EGD	$45	[18]	n. a.	n. a.
Rapid urease test during EGD	$20	[18]	n. a.	n. a.
Histology including immunohistochemistry during EGD	$234	[18]	n. a.	n. a.
UBT	$53	[18]	n. a.	n. a.
Serum *H. pylori* IgG antibody	$14	[18]	n. a.	n. a.
Stool *H. pylori* antigen	$33	[18]	n. a.	n. a.
Urine *H. pylori* antibody	$25	[18]	n. a.	n. a.

Variable	Base case	References	Range for one-way sensitivity analysis	Range in Monte Carlo analysis
Antibiotics and administration costs				
LAC for one week (1st line)	$45	[21]	n. a.	n. a.
LAM for one week (2nd line)	$35	[21]	n. a.	n. a.
LAS for one week (3rd line)	$92	[21]	n. a.	n. a.

H. pylori, Helicobacter pylori; AG, atrophic gastritis; CAM, clarithromycin, UBT, urea breath test; EGD, esophagogastroduodenoscopy; LAC, lansoprazole 30 mg bid, amoxicillin 750 mg bid, and clarithromycin 200 mg bid; LAM, lansoprazole 30 mg bid, amoxicillin 750 mg bid, and metronidazole 500 mg bid; LAS, lansoprazole 30 mg bid, amoxicillin 500 mg bid, and sitafloxacin 100 mg bid; EMR, endoscopic mucosal resection; ESD, endoscopic submucosal dissection; n. a., not applicable.
*This range was not used in Monte Carlo analysis but in one-way sensitivity analysis.

3. Results and Discussion

A decision-analysis model starting at the point of diagnosing *H. pylori* infection during or just after EGD was constructed (Figure 1). Costs and probabilities used in the decision model are presented in Table 1.

Regarding diagnostic performance of BC, RUT, histology, UBT, SHPAb, and SHPAg, pooled values reported in past meta-analyses [22–25] were used. Our meta-analysis of 11 studies [26–36] about UHPAb showed that pooled sensitivity and specificity [95% CI] of UHPAb was 0.87 [0.72–0.94] (I^2, 96%) and 0.94 [0.88–0.97] (I^2, 84%), respectively. The publication bias was not significant ($P = 0.62$).

With the current prevalence of CAM-resistant *H. pylori* of 30% [37], the most effective test for *H. pylori* diagnosis was UBT or histology, while the least effective test was SHPAb. Additionally, the most expensive test was histology, while the least expensive test was SHPAb. Histology, SHPAg, and BC were absolutely and UHPAb was weakly dominated by SHPAb, RUT, and UBT. Among the three undominated methods, the ICER of RUT versus SHPAb and UBT versus RUT was $214 and $1914, respectively. The *H. pylori* eradication success rate of SHPAb, RUT, and UBT was 0.87, 0.94, and 0.96, respectively (Figure 2).

One-way sensitivity analysis with change of prevalence of CAM-resistant *H. pylori* was showed in Figures 3 and 4. In cost-effective plane, BC was dominated if the proportion of CAM-resistant *H. pylori* was less than or equal to 44%. However, if the proportion of CAM-resistant *H. pylori* was 45%, BC was not dominated. The *H. pylori* eradication success rate of SHPAb, UHPAb, BC, RUT, and UBT was 0.86, 0.88, 0.89, 0.94, and 0.96, respectively. The ICER of UHPAb versus SHPAb, BC versus UHPAb, RUT versus BC, and UBT versus RUT was $657, $932, $8, and $1853, respectively (Figure 4).

One-way sensitivity analyses using other two variables the prevalence of *H. pylori* in the patients with AG and *H. pylori* eradication success rate by the 1st regimen suggested that our results were insensitive for these two variables (Table 2).

In acceptability curves using Monte Carlo simulation with current (0.3) and increased (0.45) prevalence of CAM-resistant *H. pylori*, the optimal strategy was either SHPAb, RUT, or UBT (Figures 5(a) and 5(b)).

This is the first cost-effective analysis of *H. pylori* diagnostic methods mainly taking into account increasing prevalence of CAM-resistant *H. pylori*. First, our study showed that SHPAb, RUT, and UBT were undominated and RUT was the most cost-effective at the current prevalence of CAM-resistant *H. pylori* considering both their effectiveness and WTP. Second, although BC for AMSGT can be a suitable option if the proportion of CAM-resistant *H. pylori* increases to more than 45%, RUT was the most cost-effective as the effectiveness of BC was remarkably poorer than RUT and UBT. Third, although SHPAg was dominated in the base-case analysis, Monte-Carlo analyses showed that SHPAg was cost-effective in about 20% of trials if WTP was more than $1000. This would be caused by uncertainty of diagnostic performance of UBT and SHPAg.

Elwyn et al. [38] performed cost-effective analysis including three methods (SHPAb, SHPAg, and UBT) and concluded that UBT was dominated by SHPAg and the ICER of SHPAg versus SHPAb was €10. This study disregarded the three invasive tests, as well as UHPAb, all of which were included in our decision model. The cost of SHPAg ($33) is relatively more expensive than other diagnostic tests in Japan, and the above study used higher sensitivity and specificity data for SHPAg than those used in our model. The outcome of this study by Elwyn et al. was not the *H. pylori* eradication rate but the number of true outcomes. Additionally, authors did not discuss about WTP. These might be some of the reasons why SHPAg was not found to be cost-effective in our study. They followed "test and treat" policy without considering a referral to EGD, common in general practitioners' practice outside of Japan. In our decision model, we assumed that EGD would be performed prior to *H. pylori* testing in patients with or without dyspepsia.

According to the most recent guidelines for gastric cancer screening in Japan, EGD can be used not only as an opportunistic screening but also as a population-based screening tool [39]. It is anticipated that the number of asymptomatic individuals with the diagnosis of AG will increase and a cost-effective diagnostic tool for *H. pylori* infection is therefore needed. As such, the results of our study can be applied to choosing a diagnostic method for *H. pylori* infection mainly in the context of a screening population undergoing EGD.

Considering poor effectiveness of SHPAb and ICER of UBT versus RUT, RUT was the optimal choice for diagnosing *H. pylori* infection at the current CAM-resistant *H. pylori* prevalence.

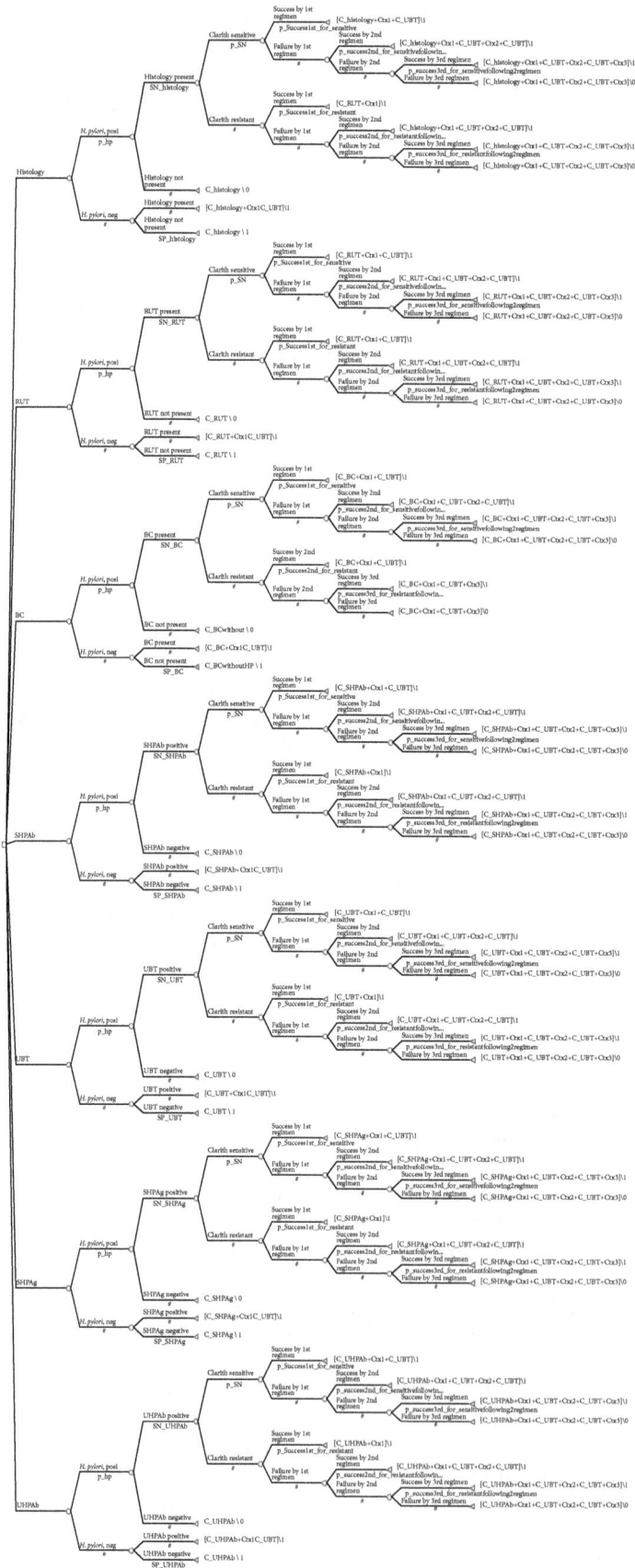

FIGURE 1: Decision tree. Decision tree was constructed on the assumption that treatment was selected after performing esophagogastroduodenoscopy in all patients.

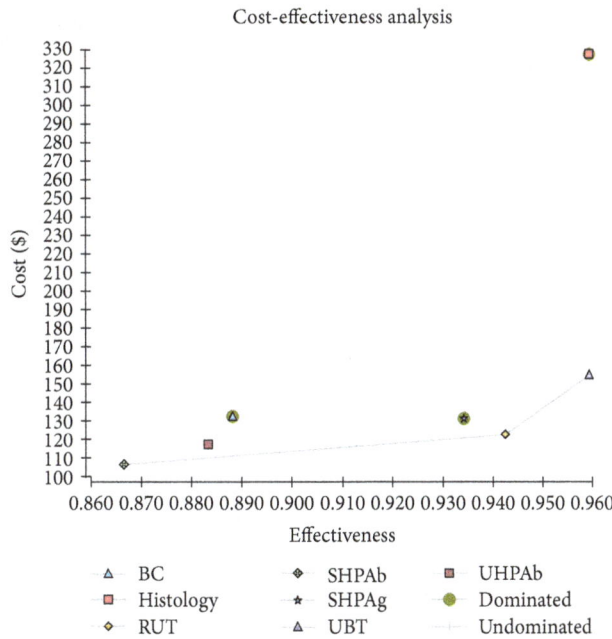

FIGURE 2: Cost-effectiveness graph. Cost-effectiveness analysis showed that histology, stool *H. pylori* antigen, and bacterial culture were absolutely and urine *H. pylori* antibody was weakly dominated by serum *H. pylori* IgG antibody, rapid urease test, and urea breath test.

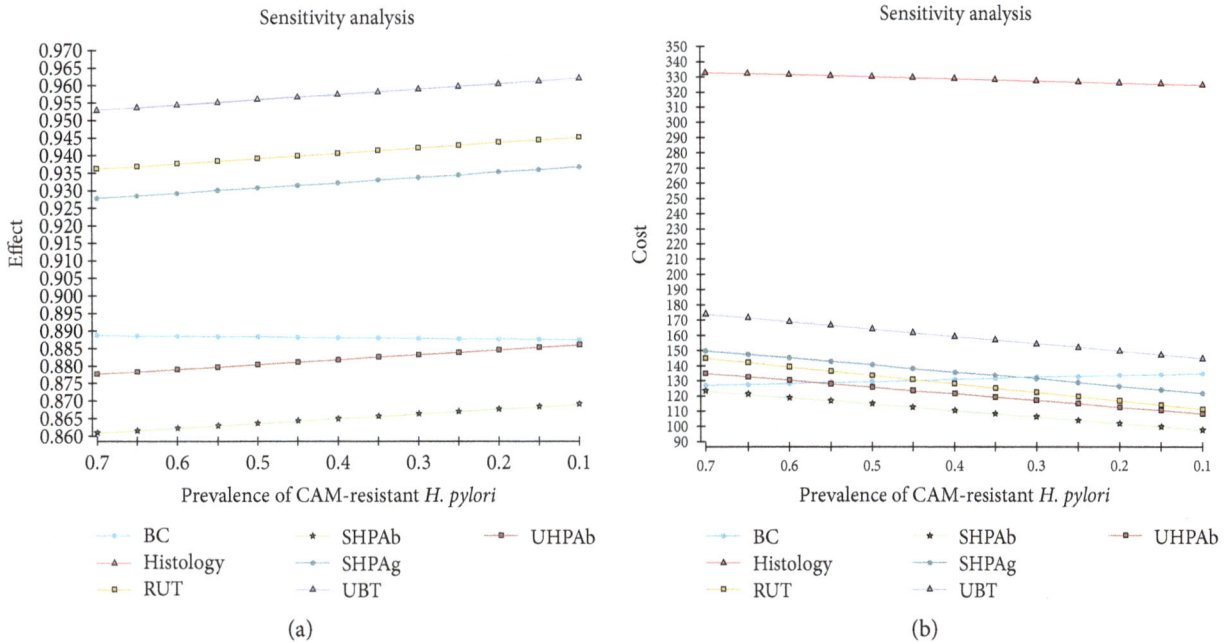

FIGURE 3: One-way sensitivity analysis. Sensitivity analysis using prevalence of clarithromycin- (CAM-) resistant *Helicobacter pylori* (*H. pylori*) showed that the order of effectiveness of seven diagnostic methods did not change between a CAM-resistant *H. pylori* prevalence of 0.1 and 0.7. The lines of histology and urea breath test were overlapped (a). In contrast, the cost of bacterial culture became equal to urine *H. pylori* antibody or rapid urease test or stool *H. pylori* antigen at between a CAM-resistant *H. pylori* prevalence of 0.3 and 0.58 (b).

If the prevalence of CAM-resistant *H. pylori* infection increases to 45%, BC becomes one of the options. Considering not only ICERs of UHPAb versus SHPAb ($657), BC versus UHPAb ($932), RUT versus BC ($8), and UBT versus RUT ($1853) but also poor effectiveness of SHPAb (0.86), UHPAb (0.88), and BC (0.89), RUT was again a preferred diagnostic method.

The CAM resistance of *H. pylori* was reported to be caused by mutations at two positions within 23S rRNA [40]. Okamura et al. [41] reported that the proportion of CAM-resistant *H. pylori* was significantly higher in younger groups. They also reported that the proportion of CAM-resistant *H. pylori* increased between 2000 and 2013, while the proportion of metronidazole-resistant *H. pylori* did

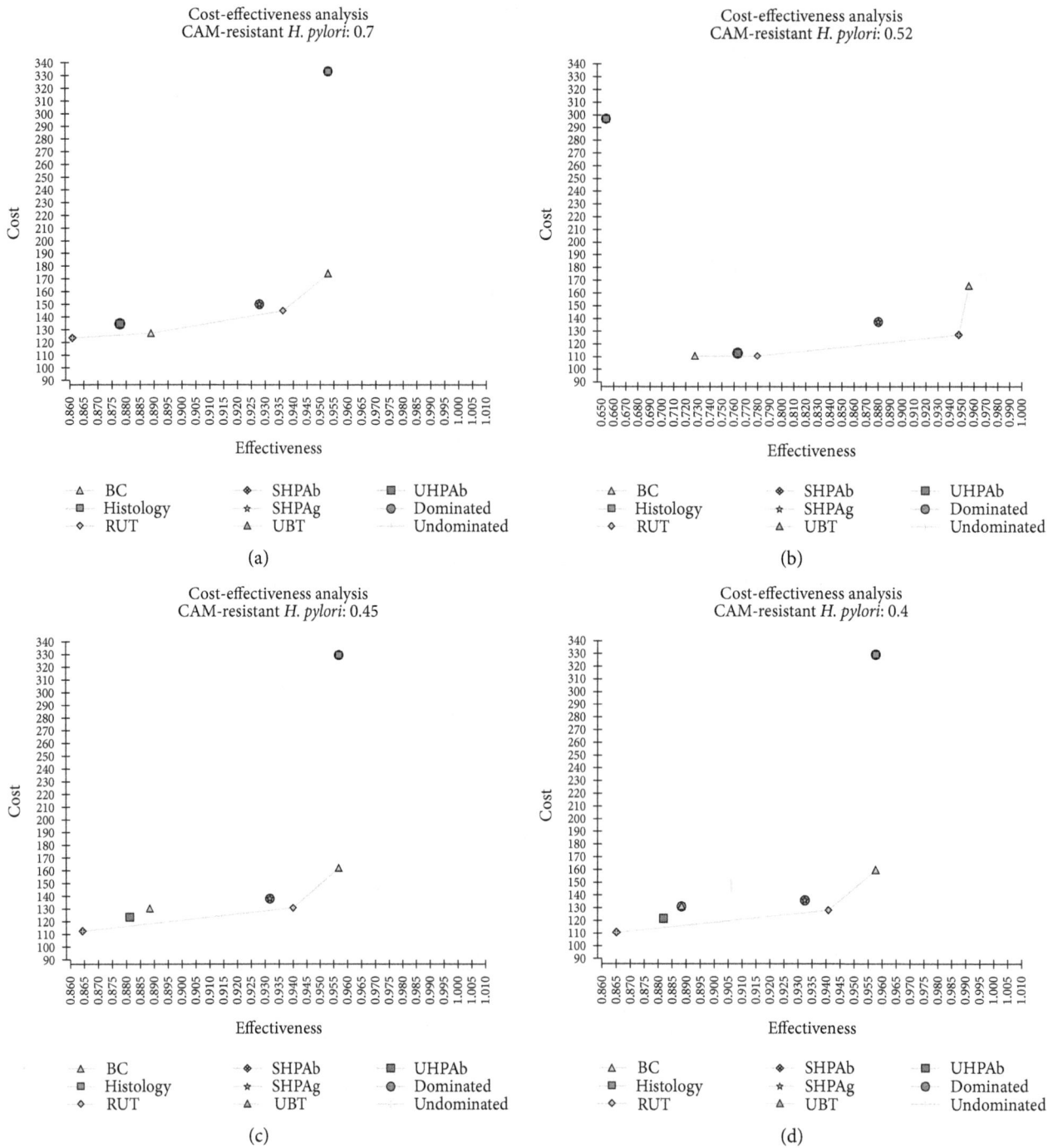

Figure 4: Cost-effectiveness plane of sensitivity analysis. If the prevalence of clarithromycin- (CAM-) resistant *H. pylori* was ≥0.45 (a), bacterial culture (BC) with antibiotics susceptibility testing was not dominated. However, if the prevalence of CAM-resistant *H. pylori* was ≤0.44, BC was dominated by serum *H. pylori* IgG antibody, rapid urease test, and urea breath test (b–d).

TABLE 2: Results of one-way sensitivity analysis.

Variable	Base case	Threshold	Results of sensitivity analysis
Proportion of CAM-resistant *H. pylori*	0.3	0.45	BC was not dominated if CAM-resistant *H. pylori* ≥ 0.45.
Prevalence of *H. pylori* in AG	0.85	—	BC was dominated. RUT was the most cost-effective.
Success rate of 1st regimen for all	0.76	—	BC was dominated. RUT was the most cost-effective.

CAM, clarithromycin; *H. pylori, Helicobacter pylori*; AG, atrophic gastritis; BC, bacterial culture; RUT, rapid urease test.

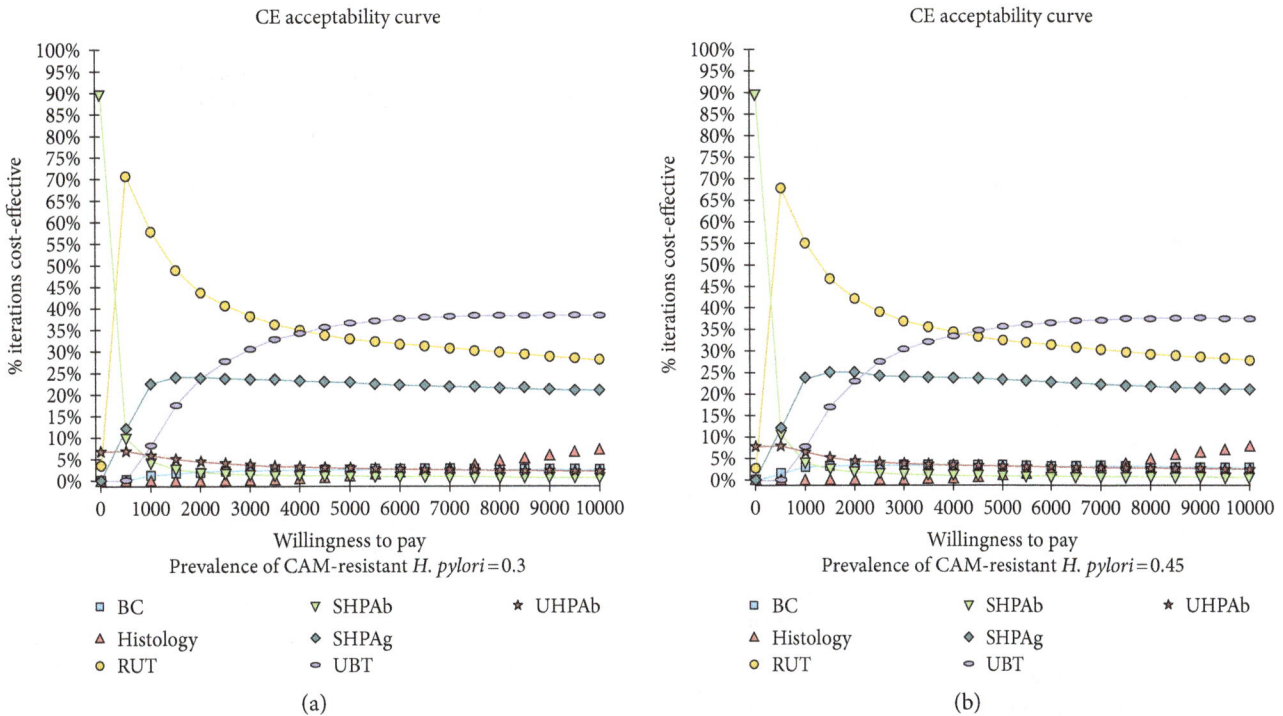

FIGURE 5: Acceptability curves using Monte Carlo simulation analysis with 0.3 (a) and 0.45 (b) of clarithromycin- (CAM-) resistant *Helicobacter pylori* (H. pylori). Acceptability curve showed that serum H. pylori antibody or rapid urease test or urea breath test was an optimal diagnostic method depending on willingness to pay (WTP). Even if the prevalence of CAM-resistant H. pylori increased to 0.45, the probability that bacterial culture becomes an optimal method was low regardless of WTP.

not. We should clarify cost-effective diagnostic methods, anticipating future trends of increasing CAM-resistant *H. pylori* infections.

With recent understanding about pharmacokinetics of PPI, it has been reported that the efficacy of PPI included triple therapy is associated not only with antibiotics susceptibility but also with polymorphism of S-mephenytoin 4'-hydroxylase (CYP2C19) [42], a marker of rapid PPI metabolizers. We did not make our decision model considering this factor as the CYP2C19 test is not commercially available.

Our analysis has some limitations and strengths. First, we did not take into account possible adverse events from taking antibiotics or taking biopsy specimen for invasive tests, which we anticipate are very rare and not severe. Second, as treatment completion was assumed to be within 1 year, we did not consider the time needed until *H. pylori* eradication. Third, we did not take into account costs of several *H. pylori*-associated diseases except gastric cancer in estimating WTP. Fourth, our results can apply only for medical practice in Japan as our model assumes AG prevalence and standard *H. pylori* eradication regimen in Japan, both of which are different from western countries.

However, this is the first study to investigate the impact of increasing prevalence of CAM-resistant *H. pylori* infection from a cost-effectiveness perspective. In addition, we used the results of meta-analyses for all diagnostic methods' performance, which should be valid.

In conclusion, RUT was the most cost-effective diagnostic procedure given the present prevalence of CAM-resistant *H. pylori*. Although BC can be a cost-effective diagnostic method if the proportion of CAM-resistant *H. pylori* continues to increase to ≥45%, BC potentially for AMSGT will not be cost-effective due to its poor effectiveness.

Competing Interests

The authors declare that there is no conflict of interest regarding the publication of this paper.

Acknowledgments

The authors thank Rie Ozeki, Shuji Nakamura, and Masato Ichikawa for providing the cost of the procedure and medicine and Atsuko Tomita for the excellent secretarial support.

References

[1] Y. Hirayama, T. Kawai, J. Otaki, K. Kawakami, and Y. Harada, "Prevalence of *Helicobacter pylori* infection with healthy subjects in Japan," *Journal of Gastroenterology and Hepatology*, vol. 29, Supplement 4, pp. 16–19, 2014.

[2] T. Kamada, K. Haruma, M. Ito et al., "Time trends in *Helicobacter pylori* infection and atrophic gastritis over 40 years in Japan," *Helicobacter*, vol. 20, no. 3, pp. 192–198, 2015.

[3] V. De Francesco, F. Giorgio, C. Hassan et al., "Worldwide *H. pylori* antibiotic resistance: a systematic review," *Journal of*

Gastrointestinal and Liver Diseases, vol. 19, no. 4, pp. 409–414, 2010.

[4] S. Shiota, R. Reddy, A. Alsarraj, H. B. El-Serag, and D. Y. Graham, "Antibiotic resistance of *Helicobacter pylori* among male United States veterans," *Clinical Gastroenterology and Hepatology*, vol. 13, no. 9, pp. 1616–1624, 2015.

[5] T. T. Schubert, S. D. Bologna, Y. Nensey, A. B. Schubert, E. J. Mascha, and C. K. Ma, "Ulcer risk factors: interactions between *Helicobacter pylori* infection, nonsteroidal use, and age," *The American Journal of Medicine*, vol. 94, no. 4, pp. 413–418, 1993.

[6] A. Fukao, S. Komatsu, Y. Tsubono et al., "*Helicobacter pylori* infection and chronic atrophic gastritis among Japanese blood donors: a cross-sectional study," *Cancer Causes & Control: CCC*, vol. 4, no. 4, pp. 307–312, 1993.

[7] D. Forman, D. G. Newell, F. Fullerton et al., "Association between infection with *Helicobacter pylori* and risk of gastric cancer: evidence from a prospective investigation," *BMJ*, vol. 302, no. 6788, pp. 1302–1305, 1991.

[8] Y. S. Kim, J. S. Kim, H. C. Jung et al., "Regression of low-grade gastric mucosa-associated lymphoid tissue lymphoma after eradication of *Helicobacter pylori*: possible association with p16 hypermethylation," *Journal of Gastroenterology*, vol. 37, no. 1, pp. 17–22, 2002.

[9] T. Suzuki, M. Matsushima, A. Masui et al., "Effect of *Helicobacter pylori* eradication in patients with chronic idiopathic thrombocytopenic purpura-a randomized controlled trial," *The American Journal of Gastroenterology*, vol. 100, no. 6, pp. 1265–1270, 2005.

[10] H. Watabe, T. Mitsushima, M. H. Derakhshan et al., "Study of association between atrophic gastritis and body mass index: a cross-sectional study in 10,197 Japanese subjects," *Digestive Diseases and Sciences*, vol. 54, no. 5, pp. 988–995, 2009.

[11] S. Eun Bae, J. Hoon Lee, Y. Soo Park et al., "Decrease of serum total ghrelin in extensive atrophic gastritis: comparison with pepsinogens in histological reference," *Scandinavian Journal of Gastroenterology*, vol. 51, no. 2, pp. 137–144, 2016.

[12] K. Murakami, Y. Sakurai, M. Shiino, N. Funao, A. Nishimura, and M. Asaka, "Vonoprazan, a novel potassium-competitive acid blocker, as a component of first-line and second-line triple therapy for *Helicobacter pylori* eradication: a phase III, randomised, double-blind study," *Gut*, vol. 65, no. 9, pp. 1439–1446, 2016.

[13] M. Asaka, T. Sugiyama, M. Kato et al., "A multicenter, double-blind study on triple therapy with lansoprazole, amoxicillin and clarithromycin for eradication of *Helicobacter pylori* in Japanese peptic ulcer patients," *Helicobacter*, vol. 6, no. 3, pp. 254–261, 2001.

[14] J. A. Ducons, S. Santolaria, R. Guirao, M. Ferrero, M. Montoro, and F. Gomollón, "Impact of clarithromycin resistance on the effectiveness of a regimen for *Helicobacter pylori*: a prospective study of 1-week lansoprazole, amoxycillin and clarithromycin in active peptic ulcer," *Alimentary Pharmacology & Therapeutics*, vol. 13, no. 6, pp. 775–780, 1999.

[15] C. S. Park, S. M. Lee, C. H. Park et al., "Pretreatment antimicrobial susceptibility-guided vs. clarithromycin-based triple therapy for *Helicobacter pylori* eradication in a region with high rates of multiple drug resistance," *The American Journal of Gastroenterology*, vol. 109, no. 10, pp. 1595–1602, 2014.

[16] T. Matsuhisa, T. Kawai, T. Masaoka et al., "Efficacy of metronidazole as second-line drug for the treatment of *Helicobacter pylori* infection in the Japanese population: a multicenter study

in the Tokyo metropolitan area," *Helicobacter*, vol. 11, no. 3, pp. 152–158, 2006.

[17] K. Murakami, T. Furuta, T. Ando et al., "Multi-center randomized controlled study to establish the standard third-line regimen for *Helicobacter pylori* eradication in Japan," *Journal of Gastroenterology*, vol. 48, no. 10, pp. 1128–1135, 2013.

[18] Igakutsushinsha, *Quick Manual for Reimbursement, April 2015 Version: Igakutsushinsha*, 2015.

[19] Igakutsushinsha, *Quick Manual for DPC Score, April 2015 Version: Igakutsushinsha*, 2015.

[20] A. C. Ford, D. Forman, R. H. Hunt, Y. Yuan, and P. Moayyedi, "*Helicobacter pylori* eradication therapy to prevent gastric cancer in healthy asymptomatic infected individuals: systematic review and meta-analysis of randomised controlled trials," *BMJ*, vol. 348, article g3174, 2014.

[21] Yakugyokenkyukai, *Insured Drug Dictionary*, Jihosha, Plus, 2015.

[22] F. Omata, S. Ohde, G. A. Deshpande et al., "Diagnostic performance of three endoscopic tests for *Helicobacter pylori* infection: systematic review and meta-analysis," *The American Journal of Gastroenterology*, vol. 110, 2015.

[23] M. Ferwana, I. Abdulmajeed, A. Alhajiahmed et al., "Accuracy of urea breath test in *Helicobacter pylori* infection: meta-analysis," *World Journal of Gastroenterology*, vol. 21, no. 4, pp. 1305–1314, 2015.

[24] C. T. Loy, L. M. Irwig, P. H. Katelaris, and N. J. Talley, "Do commercial serological kits for *Helicobacter pylori* infection differ in accuracy? A meta-analysis," *The American Journal of Gastroenterology*, vol. 91, no. 6, pp. 1138–1144, 1996.

[25] J. P. Gisbert, F. de la Morena, and V. Abraira, "Accuracy of monoclonal stool antigen test for the diagnosis of *H. pylori* infection: a systematic review and meta-analysis," *The American Journal of Gastroenterology*, vol. 101, no. 8, pp. 1921–1930, 2006.

[26] S. Yamamoto, N. Uemura, S. Okamoto, S. Yamaguchi, H. Mashiba, and T. Tachikawa, "A new rapid test for detecting anti-*Helicobacter pylori* antibody excreted into urine," *Helicobacter*, vol. 5, no. 3, pp. 160–164, 2000.

[27] D. Y. Graham and S. Reddy, "Rapid detection of anti-*Helicobacter pylori* IgG in urine using immunochromatography," *Alimentary Pharmacology & Therapeutics*, vol. 15, no. 5, pp. 699–702, 2001.

[28] T. Fujisawa, T. Kaneko, T. Kumagai et al., "Evaluation of urinary rapid test for *Helicobacter pylori* in general practice," *Journal of Clinical Laboratory Analysis*, vol. 15, no. 3, pp. 154–159, 2001.

[29] W. M. Wong, B. C. Wong, H. H. Xia et al., "An evaluation of a rapid urine test for the diagnosis of *Helicobacter pylori* infection in the Chinese population," *Alimentary Pharmacology & Therapeutics*, vol. 16, no. 4, pp. 813–817, 2002.

[30] K. Adachi, A. Kawamura, M. Ono et al., "Comparative evaluation of urine-based and other minimally invasive methods for the diagnosis of *Helicobacter pylori* infection," *Journal of Gastroenterology*, vol. 37, no. 9, pp. 703–708, 2002.

[31] A. Leodolter, D. Vaira, F. Bazzoli et al., "European multicentre validation trial of two new non-invasive tests for the detection of *Helicobacter pylori* antibodies: urine-based ELISA and rapid urine test," *Alimentary Pharmacology & Therapeutics*, vol. 18, no. 9, pp. 927–931, 2003.

[32] C. Y. Lu, F. C. Kuo, S. W. Wang et al., "The clinical applications and accuracy of 2 rapid near-patient tests in detecting

Helicobacter pylori infection," *Diagnostic Microbiology and Infectious Disease*, vol. 56, no. 3, pp. 241–246, 2006.

[33] A. R. Opekun, P. Luu, A. B. Gotschall et al., "Point-of-care *Helicobacter pylori* urine antibody detection in a multi-ethnic adult population in the United States," *Translational Research*, vol. 148, no. 1, pp. 13–18, 2006.

[34] E. Demiray Gurbuz, C. Gonen, N. Bekmen et al., "The diagnostic accuracy of urine IgG antibody tests for the detection of *Helicobacter pylori* infection in Turkish dyspeptic patients," *The Turkish Journal of Gastroenterology*, vol. 23, no. 6, pp. 753–758, 2012.

[35] D. T. Quach, T. Hiyama, F. Shimamoto et al., "Value of a new stick-type rapid urine test for the diagnosis of *Helicobacter pylori* infection in the Vietnamese population," *World Journal of Gastroenterology*, vol. 20, no. 17, pp. 5087–5091, 2014.

[36] A. F. Syam, M. Miftahussurur, W. B. Uwan, D. Simanjuntak, T. Uchida, and Y. Yamaoka, "Validation of urine test for detection of *Helicobacter pylori* infection in Indonesian population," *BioMed Research International*, vol. 2015, Article ID 152823, 6 pages, 2015.

[37] N. Horiki, F. Omata, M. Uemura et al., "Annual change of primary resistance to clarithromycin among *Helicobacter pylori* isolates from 1996 through 2008 in Japan," *Helicobacter*, vol. 14, no. 5, pp. 86–90, 2009.

[38] G. Elwyn, M. Taubert, S. Davies, G. Brown, M. Allison, and C. Phillips, "Which test is best for *Helicobacter pylori*? A cost-effectiveness model using decision analysis," *The British Journal of General Practice*, vol. 57, no. 538, pp. 401–403, 2007.

[39] *Research Center of Cancer Prevention and Screening NCI. Gastric Cancer Screening Guideline Based on Effectiveness, 2014 Version*, National cancer institute, USA, 2014.

[40] D. E. Taylor, "Pathophysiology of antibiotic resistance: clarithromycin," *Canadian Journal of Gastroenterology*, vol. 14, no. 10, pp. 891–894, 2000.

[41] T. Okamura, T. Suga, T. Nagaya et al., "Antimicrobial resistance and characteristics of eradication therapy of *Helicobacter pylori* in Japan: a multi-generational comparison," *Helicobacter*, vol. 19, no. 3, pp. 214–220, 2014.

[42] H. Kawabata, Y. Habu, H. Tomioka et al., "Effect of different proton pump inhibitors, differences in CYP2C19 genotype and antibiotic resistance on the eradication rate of *Helicobacter pylori* infection by a 1-week regimen of proton pump inhibitor, amoxicillin and clarithromycin," *Alimentary Pharmacology & Therapeutics*, vol. 17, no. 2, pp. 259–264, 2003.

5

Effects of Combined Simultaneous and Sequential Endostar and Cisplatin Treatment in a Mice Model of Gastric Cancer Peritoneal Metastases

Lin Jia,[1] Shuguang Ren,[2] Tao Li,[3] Jianing Wu,[4] Xinliang Zhou,[5] Yan Zhang,[4] Jianhua Wu,[2] and Wei Liu[6]

[1]*Department of Medical Oncology, The Affiliated Hospital of Hebei University, Baoding 071000, China*
[2]*Department of Animal Center, The Fourth Hospital, Hebei Medical University, Shijiazhuang 050017, China*
[3]*Department of Epidemiology and Health Statistics, School of Public Health, Hebei Medical University, Shijiazhuang 050011, China*
[4]*Hebei Province China-Japan Friendship Center for Cancer Detection, Shijiazhuang 050017, China*
[5]*Department of Medical Oncology, The Fourth Hospital, Hebei Medical University, Shijiazhuang 050017, China*
[6]*Department of Palliative Care Center, Beijing Cancer Hospital, Beijing 100000, China*

Correspondence should be addressed to Wei Liu; liuweihebei1026@163.com

Academic Editor: Charles Honore

Objective. Aimed to study the effects of endostar and cisplatin using an in vivo imaging system (IVIS) in a model of peritoneal metastasis of gastric cancer. *Methods.* NUGC-4 gastric cancer cells transfected with luciferase gene (NUGC-4-Luc) were injected i.p. into nude mice. One week later, mice were randomly injected i.p.: group 1, cisplatin (d1–3) + endostar (d4–7); group 2, endostar (d1–4) + cisplatin (d5–7); group 3, endostar + cisplatin d1, 4, and 7; group 4, saline for two weeks. One week after the final administration, mice were sacrificed. Bioluminescent data, microvessel density (MVD), and lymphatic vessel density (LVD) were analyzed. *Results.* Among the four groups, there were no significant differences in the weights and in the number of cancer cell photons on days 1 and 8 ($P > 0.05$). On day 15, the numbers in groups 3 and 1 were less than that in group 2 ($P < 0.05$). On day 21, group 3 was significantly less than group 2 ($P < 0.05$). MVD of group 4 was less than that of groups 1 and 2 ($P < 0.01$). There was no significant difference between groups 2 and 3 ($P > 0.05$) or in LVD number among the four groups ($P > 0.05$). *Conclusions.* IVIS® was more useful than weight, volume of ascites, and number of peritoneal nodules. The simultaneous group was superior to sequential groups in killing cancer cells and inhibiting vascular endothelium. Cisplatin-endostar was superior to endostar-cisplatin in killing cancer cells, while the latter in inhibiting peritoneal vascular endothelium.

1. Introduction

Malignant ascites is common in gastrointestinal and gynecological cancers and has been associated with a median survival of less than 20 weeks [1]. Patients with malignant ascites caused by gastrointestinal cancers have especially poor prognosis, and their survival times are only 12–20 weeks [2]. The treatment of malignant effusions is often a challenge for physicians. Currently, the conventional treatment of malignant effusions is mainly composed of diuresis, salt restriction, serous cavity paracentesis, intracavitary chemotherapy, biological response modifiers, traditional Chinese medicine, or thermotherapy. However, these therapies are not all satisfactory. After treatment with these methods, there is no significant decrease in effusions, and relapses often occur. Furthermore, almost all of these treatment methods have toxic side effects to various degrees [3].

Thus, it is important to understand the underlying molecular mechanisms associated with malignant effusion. Previous studies have shown that elevated levels of vascular endothelial growth factor (VEGF), tumor angiogenesis, and increased vascular permeability after tumor invasion or metastasis to the pleuroperitoneum are important mechanisms of serous cavity effusions [4, 5]. VEGF has attracted attention due to its presence in the pleural fluid and its potential use as a therapeutic target [6–8]. Many clinical studies have also demonstrated the potential benefit of inhibition of VEGF-A in patients with malignant effusions [4]. Antiangiogenic therapy (such as bevacizumab, a monoclonal antibody targeting VEGF-A) adjuvant to chemotherapy was found to have a potential role in management of pleural effusion in advanced nonsquamous non-small-cell lung cancer [8].

Recombinant human endostatin (rh-endostatin, endostar) is a Chinese broad spectrum humanized antiangiogenic drug that targets vascular endothelial cells, but not tumor cells. Furthermore, this drug has been shown to downregulate the protecting effect of a variety of proangiogenic factors on the vascular endothelium. In addition, it has direct and indirect antiangiogenic effects. Endostar was approved by the State Food and Drug Administration of China (SFDA) for the treatment of non-small-cell lung cancer in 2005 [9]. A number of researchers have explored the application of endostar alone or in combination with chemotherapy for treatment of malignant serous effusion showing high efficiency and low toxicity. It has been shown that the control of effusions is stronger than other agents and that this can significantly improve quality of life of patients. Using a malignant pleural effusion (MPE) model, it has been demonstrated that endostar had an efficient anticancer activity in MPE through its suppressive effect on angiogenesis and lymphangiogenesis. However, bevacizumab does not inhibit lymphangiogenesis. This provided a theoretical basis for the use of endostar for MPE treatment [10]. However, the efficacy of endostar when administered simultaneously and sequentially with chemotherapy remains to be determined.

In mice subcutaneous tumor models, tumor growth can be easily monitored by caliper measurements. However, in pleural metastasis models, it is difficult to continuously measure tumor growth and evaluate the response to a treatment. Surrogate markers such as weight loss may be employed to monitor toxicity. However, the real treatment efficacy can usually be evaluated only after mice are sacrificed. In addition to computed tomography (CT), magnetic resonance imaging (MRI), and positron emission tomography (PET), an in vivo noninvasive bioluminescent imaging (BLI) system has recently been developed using the adenosine triphosphate- (ATP-) dependent light-emitting reaction of the firefly (*Photinus pyralis*) luciferase and its substrate, D-luciferin [D-(−)-2-(6-hydroxy-2-benzothiazolyl) thiazone-4-carboxylic acid] [11, 12]. Using this system, the temporal and spatial monitoring of the pathophysiological processes can be performed in vivo, thus, reducing the number of animals needed to achieve statistical power [11–18].

We established a stably expressing luciferase gastric NUGC-4-Luc cell line. On the basis of this cell line, we established a gastric cancer ascites tumor model in nude mice for the first time and demonstrated the therapeutic effects of the simultaneous and sequential administration of endostar with cisplatin on the intraperitoneal disseminated foci using an in vivo imaging system (IVIS) and detected the peritoneal nodules with microvessel density (MVD) and lymphatic vessel density (LVD).

2. Materials and Methods

2.1. Cell Line and Animals. Human gastric adenocarcinoma cell line NUGC-4 was obtained from Japan RIKEN BioResource (Tokyo, Japan). A luciferase-expressing human gastric cancer cell line, NUGC-4-Luc, was established by GenScript Co., Ltd. (Nanjing, China). Cells were maintained at 37°C in RPMI-1640 medium (Gibco, Grand Island, NY) supplemented with 10% fetal bovine serum at 37°C in a humidified atmosphere containing 5% CO_2. Five- to six-week old female nude mice (BALB/c nu/nu) were purchased from the Institute of Laboratory Animal Science, the Chinese Academy of Medical Sciences, Beijing, China, and were housed in environmentally controlled conditions (22°C, 12-hour light/dark cycles, with the light cycle from 6:00 to 18:00 and the dark cycle from 18:00 to 6:00) with ad libitum access to standard laboratory chow. The study protocol was approved by the local Institutional Review Board, and animal experiments were conducted in accordance with the guideline of the local Institutional Animal Care and Use Committee, which has been accredited by the Association for Assessment and Accreditation of Laboratory Animal Care International.

2.2. Ascites Tumor Model and Therapeutic Experiments. In the present study, stable integrated luciferase gastric undifferentiated NUGC-4-Luc cell lines were established. Then, cells were intraperitoneally injected into nude mice to produce the gastric cancer ascites tumor model in 3–5 days. NUGC-4-luc cells were cultured in RPMI1640 medium + 10% FBS + 1% P/S and cell suspension for ultimate collection was a total of 5×10^6 NUGC-4-luc cells in 50 mL of PBS. The cell suspension was injected into the abdominal cavities of 28 female nude mice [19–21]. These mice underwent in vivo bioluminescence imaging weekly. One week after NUGC-4-Luc cell injection, mice were randomly divided into four groups with seven mice each and were injected intraperitoneally with the following: group 1, cisplatin (purchased from QiLu Pharmaceutical Co., Shandong, China; 1 mg/kg) at days 1–3 + endostar (purchased from Simcere Pharmaceutical Co., Jiangsu, China; 8 mg/kg) at days 4–7; group 2, endostar (8 mg/kg) at days 1–4 + cisplatin (1 mg/kg) at days 5–7; group 3, endostar (8 mg/kg) + cisplatin (1 mg/kg) at days 1, 4 and 7; group 4 (control group), 50 μL of normal saline at days 1–7 [10, 22]. Each group was treated for two consecutive weeks and underwent imaging weekly. One week after the final administration, mice were anesthetized and sacrificed. Peritoneal metastasis of gastric carcinoma was monitored with IVIS.

2.3. Bioluminescence Imaging with IVIS. Mice were anesthetized by isoflurane inhalation and were subsequently injected i.p. with 100 μL of 7.5 mg/mL of D-luciferin (Xenogen). Bioluminescence imaging with a CCD camera (IVIS, Xenogen) was initiated 10 min after injection. Imaging times ranged from 1 to 60 sec, depending on the amount of luciferase activity. Bioluminescence from the region of interest (ROI) was defined manually, and the data were expressed as photon-flux (photons/s/cm^2/steradian). All bioluminescent data were collected and analyzed using IVIS [23].

2.4. Immunohistochemical Staining and Evaluation. Tumor tissue samples were fixed with 10% buffered formalin and embedded in paraffin after routine dehydration. Consecutive 5 μm sections were cut from each block, immunostained, and analyzed for MVD and LVD. Tissue sections were stained with anti-CD34 antibody (rabbit anti-mouse rat anti-mouse monoclonal antibody, 1 : 200; eBioscience, US) and anti-D2-40 antibody (rat anti-mouse monoclonal antibody, 1 : 200; Upstate, US). Biotinylated anti-rat or rabbit antibodies (Beijing Zhongshan Golden Bridge Biological Technology CO., Beijing, China) were used as secondary antibodies. Staining for CD31 was used to evaluate MVD, which were assessed by counting all stained vessels at 6,200x magnification. The mean number of vessels was defined as MVD [19]. Staining for D2-40 was used to evaluate LVD, and the same method was used to evaluate MVD. The stained slides were reviewed and scored independently by two investigators (Drs. Wu and Zhang), who were blinded to the slide identification and clinical data. Disagreements were resolved by discussion to reach a consensus.

2.5. Statistical Analysis. Statistical analysis was performed using the SPSS software package (version 17.0; SPSS Inc., Chicago, IL, USA). Bioluminescence imaging data from IVIS and weights of the nude mice were analyzed by repeated measurements. Analysis of variance in repeated measurement data and comparison of data between various groups were performed by multivariate analysis. One-way analysis of variance (ANOVA) was used to assess the statistical significant differences in MVD among groups. Comparisons of LVD among various groups were performed using a nonparametric Kruskal-Wallis test, followed by the Mann–Whitney test. All P values were two-tailed. P values < 0.05 were considered significant.

3. Results

3.1. Ascites Tumor Model. The background number of cancer cell photons prior to treatment was not significantly different among the four groups ($P > 0.05$). During the treatment, one mouse in the control group died. All of the other mice survived until the experiment was completed. There were no significant differences in nude mice weights between the four treatment groups ($P > 0.05$, Figure 1). After sacrifice, bloody ascites and the small, numerous, and widely distributed peritoneal nodules were observed.

3.2. Drug Efficacy. The group rank of the volume (mL) of ascites in four groups was as follows: group 4 (4.87 ± 0.45) > group 1 (3.1 ± 0.53) > group 2 (2.0 ± 0.08) > group 3 (1.8 ± 0.16) ($P < 0.05$). The group rank for the number of peritoneal nodules was as follows: group 4 (33.75 ± 2.5) > group 2 (21.66 ± 5.77) > group 3 (18.75 ± 2.5) > group 1 (8.75 ± 4.78) ($P < 0.05$).

3.3. The Number of Photons. By using the in vivo imaging processing software, tumor growth curves were plotted according to the number of photons per measurement

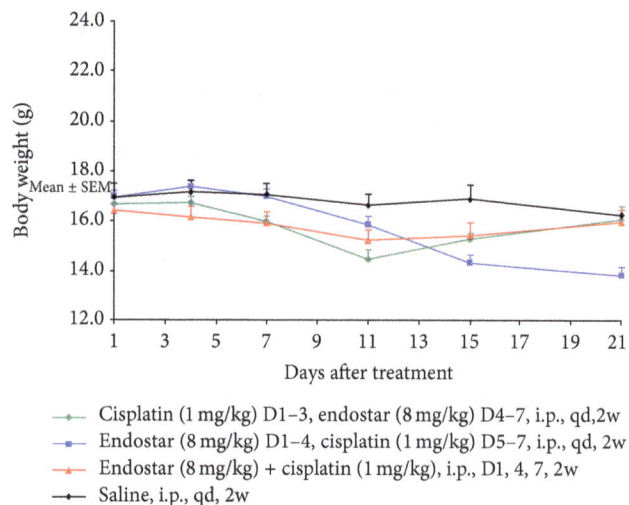

FIGURE 1: The differences in weight changes in nude mice among the four treatment groups as presented by the repeated measures process of the general linear model.

(Figure 2). On days one and eight, there were no significant differences among the four groups ($P > 0.05$).

On days 15 and 21, the number of cancer cell photons in groups 1, 2, and 3 was all less than that in the control group ($P < 0.01$). On day 15 (after two weeks of treatment), the count of cancer cell photons in group 3 (the simultaneous combination of endostar with the cisplatin group) and group 1 (the sequential cisplatin-endostar group) was less than that in group 2 (the endostar sequential cisplatin group) ($P < 0.05$). On day 21, the count in group 3 continued to be less than that in group 2 ($P < 0.05$). However, there was no significant difference between the former two groups ($P > 0.05$). On day 21, the number of cancer cell photons in group 3 (simultaneous combination of endostar with the cisplatin group) continued to be less than that in group 2 (the sequential endostar-cisplatin group) ($P < 0.05$) (Figure 3).

3.4. MVD and LVD. The density of blood vessels and lymphatics was measured by CD34 and D2-40 staining (Figure 4). There were differences in MVD among the four groups ($P < 0.01$). The group rank was as follows: group 4 > group 1 > group 2 ($P < 0.01$); and there was no difference between group 2 and group 3 ($P > 0.05$) (Figure 5). However, there were no statistical differences in LVD among the four groups ($P > 0.05$).

4. Discussion

Due to the reduction in blood supply, cells may not be conducive to chemotherapeutic drug activity. Controlling the timing of administration of the antiangiogenic agent could normalize blood vessels, and chemotherapy during the window period could make it evenly distributed, so as to achieve the maximum effect of chemotherapy. Another rationale for the administration of chemotherapy followed by antivascular treatment is that chemotherapy could minimize tumor burden and reduce VEGF prior to exposure to

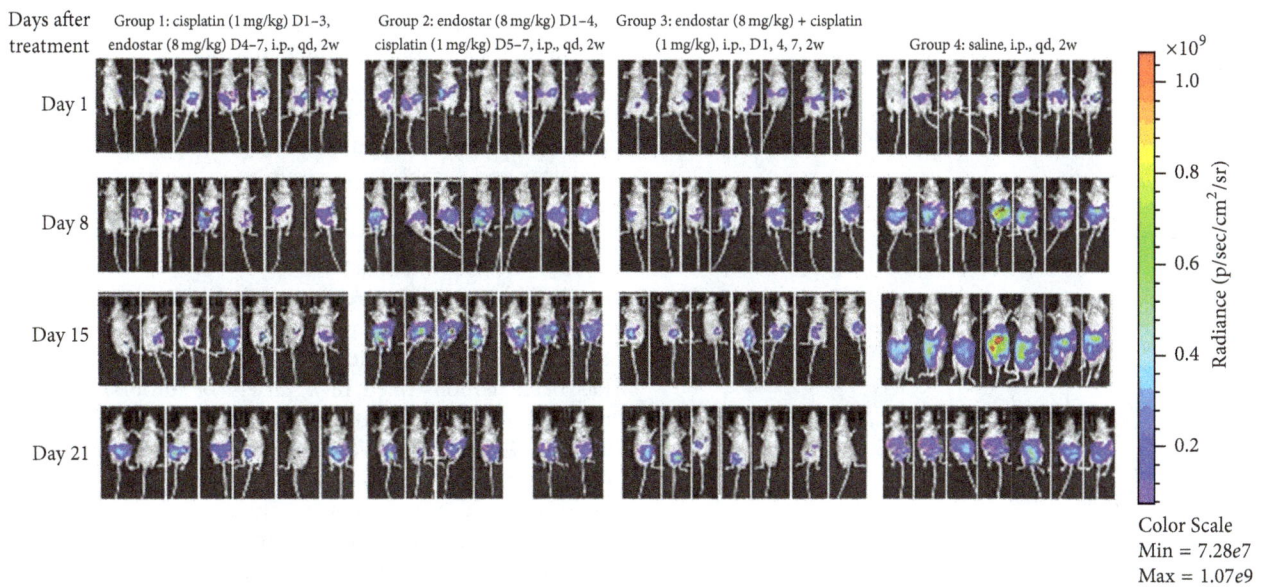

FIGURE 2: Photons analysis of the four experimental groups.

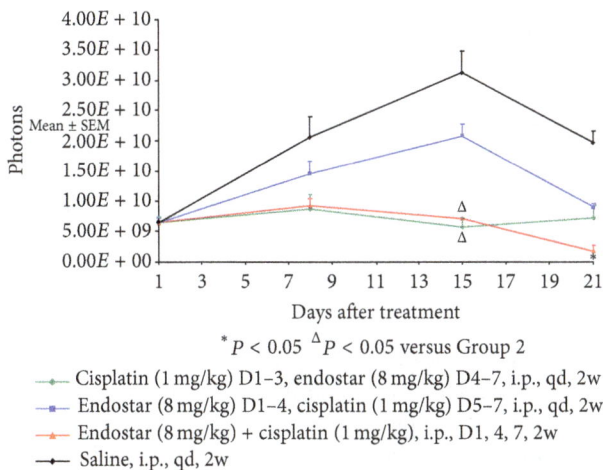

*$P < 0.05$ $^\Delta P < 0.05$ versus Group 2

- Cisplatin (1 mg/kg) D1–3, endostar (8 mg/kg) D4–7, i.p., qd, 2w
- Endostar (8 mg/kg) D1–4, cisplatin (1 mg/kg) D5–7, i.p., qd, 2w
- Endostar (8 mg/kg) + cisplatin (1 mg/kg), i.p., D1, 4, 7, 2w
- Saline, i.p., qd, 2w

FIGURE 3: Photons analysis of the experimental groups by repeated measures process of the general linear model.

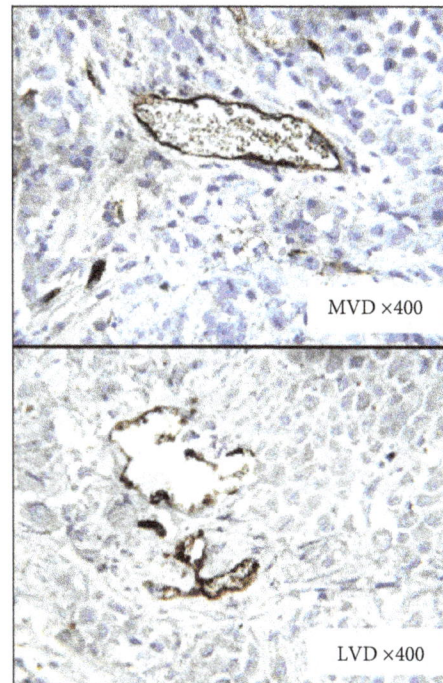

FIGURE 4: Immunohistochemical analysis of MVD and LVD in cancer cells from transplanted peritoneal tumor nodules (CD34-positive blood vessels and D2-40-positive lymphatic vessels in peritoneal nodules).

antiangiogenic therapy, inhibiting blood vessel and tumor growth [24]. Although chemotherapy drugs have different mechanisms of action and doses, the sequence and timing of chemotherapy and antiangiogenic agents need to be tailored to the agents that would be used. The method to determine the lowest effective dose and the window period for the normalization of tumor blood vessels for sequential chemotherapy and antiangiogenic therapy remains unclear. In animal models of solid tumors, the optimal therapeutic window of endostar combined with platinum or paclitaxel has been reported to be approximately 4–6 days by some authors [25] and 3–7 days by other authors [24]. During that time, the tumor normalization of microvascular matures and hypoxia partially improves. Hence, within the time window of antiangiogenic therapy and chemotherapy, the antitumor

effect was found to be the most significant. After that time, antiangiogenic therapy becomes excessive, resulting in the gradual reduction in chemotherapy drug concentration inside the tumor tissue. Patients with solid tumors treated with endostar at 4–6 days prior to chemotherapy have been shown to have had significantly improved antitumor effects.

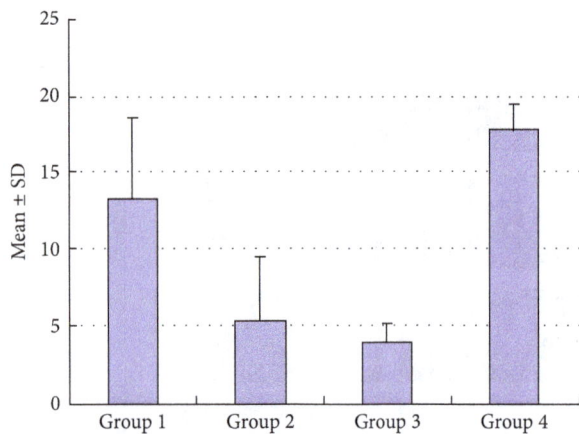

FIGURE 5: Immunohistochemical analysis of MVD in peritoneal tumor nodules (mean ± SD).

These data provides a basis for the proposed sequential use of endostar with cisplatin.

Mouse subcutaneous tumor growth can be easily monitored by caliper measurements. However, in pleural metastasis models, it is difficult to measure tumor growth continuously and evaluate responses to treatment. In vivo optical imaging by bioluminescence or fluorescence can provide real-time observation of gene and cell marker activities in a living animal body. This method has become increasingly used in medical and biological research. Green/red fluorescent protein (GFP/RFP) [26–29] has been widely used because it is suitable for single cell in vitro and in vivo functional testing, and its use could have improved the current study in terms of cellular detail. However, luciferase (Luc) has a longer emission wavelength than GFP and is, therefore, more suitable for examination of small lesions in deep tissue tumors, distant metastases in living body, and monitoring dynamic changes. Compared with orthotopic transplantation models, NUGC-4-Luc peritoneal subcutaneous implants have been reported to better simulate the transfer process in the body and the biological behavior of peritoneal metastasis [30]. The fundamental advantage of Luc-labeled cell in vivo imaging is that the luciferase gene is integrated into the chromosome. When cells divide and differentiate, the luciferase is sustained and stably expressed. The luciferin substrate provided by intraperitoneal or intravenous injection would generate luminescence within minutes. However, this enzyme would only produce luminescence within living cells; and the emitted light intensity is linearly related to the number of labeled cells. By measuring the number of photons, the number of cancer cells can be calculated quantitatively. Currently, Luc-labeled cells have been used previously for solid tumor studies [31] and in the pleural effusion studies of Matsumoto et al. [23], but not in ascites. In the present study, we established the gastric ascites tumor model in nude mice of NUGC-4-Luc cell lines and performed in vivo bioluminescence imaging. Using in vivo imaging techniques to explore the mechanism of growth and metastasis of gastric ascites tumors and the development of anticancer drugs, we provided a stable and reliable, intuitive, convenient, and sensitive animal model.

Compared with orthotopic transplantation models, NUGC-4-Luc peritoneal subcutaneous implants have been reported to better simulate the transfer process in the body and the biological behavior of peritoneal metastasis [30]. The results revealed that 15 days after treatment, cisplatin sequential endostar and combination group were superior to endostar sequential cisplatin in killing cancer cells, while the combined group was still superior to endostar sequential cisplatin group 21 days after treatment.

MVD and LVD are important indicators to evaluate tumor blood vessels and lymphatics. The relationship between MVD, LVD, and poor prognosis of cancer patients has been demonstrated in a variety of tumors. The study counted the number of vessels per unit area by CD34 and D2-40 marker of vascular density MVD and LVD, in order to further explore the relationship between different endostar modes and vessels. These results revealed that endostar sequential cisplatin and the combination group were superior to cisplatin sequential endostar in the inhibitory effect on endothelium. Compared to tumor angiogenesis, little attention has been given to the study of tumor lymphatic angiogenesis. The main reason for this is the fact that no specific markers of lymphatic vessels have been identified. Endostar can reduce vascular permeability, suppress the formation fluid, or inhibit lymph node metastasis in the treatment of serous cavity effusion. Basic research has shown that endostar can inhibit not only MVD, but also LVD [10]. However, the present study found no differences in LVD in peritoneal nodules among the four treatment groups, and there was no difference in the inhibition of lymphatic vessels between endostar with simultaneously and sequentially administered cisplatin. In the future, more studies on vascular morphology in malignant peritoneal effusion would be needed to determine the mechanisms of the effects of endostar and cisplatin.

In conclusion, we established the peritoneal metastasis of a gastric cancer model using NUGC-4-Luc cells and demonstrated that the intrapleural administration of endostar simultaneously and sequentially with cisplatin was a safe and effective treatment for MPE. The results of the simultaneously treated group were superior to that in the sequential groups, in terms of killing cancer cells and inhibiting vascular endothelial growth. Cisplatin-endostar sequential treatment was superior to endostar-cisplatin sequential treatment in killing cancer cells, while the latter was superior to the former in inhibiting peritoneal vascular endothelial growth. It has been suggested that molecular markers can be used to forecast peritoneal vascular endothelial changes, and functional imaging can be used to monitor the number of cancer cells and guide the rational choice of drugs, as well as the timing of administration. In the future, it may be that only molecular markers combined functional imaging techniques would be required for evaluation of treatment efficacy in malignant effusions. There are some limitations to the present study. In the short term, this cell line only formed peritoneal metastasis without involvement of other areas of the body. In addition, there was a lack of controls sacrificed at same time as the test animals and a lack of data on survival. Future research in the screening of different cell lines, peritoneal blood vessels, lymphatic vessels, and the administration of various drug concentrations and survival would be necessary to confirm these current observations. The value of this treatment technique requires confirmation in clinical trials. The future of individualized treatment remains a multidisciplinary, multicenter collaboration, and requires continued translation of basic research into clinical practice.

Competing Interests

The authors declare that there is no conflict of interests regarding the publication of this paper.

References

[1] G. Lombardi, F. Zustovich, M. O. Nicoletto, M. Donach, G. Artioli, and D. Pastorelli, "Diagnosis and treatment of malignant pleural effusion: a systematic literature review and new approaches," *American Journal of Clinical Oncology*, vol. 33, no. 4, pp. 420–423, 2010.

[2] M. Chung and P. Kozuch, "Treatment of malignant ascites," *Current Treatment Options in Oncology*, vol. 9, no. 2-3, pp. 215–233, 2008.

[3] L. Jia, Y. Du, T. Li et al., "Differential expression of vascular endothelial growth factor-A, -C and -D for the diagnosis and prognosis of cancer patients with malignant effusions," *Oncology Letters*, vol. 10, no. 2, pp. 667–674, 2015.

[4] S. Kobold, S. Hegewisch-Becker, K. Oechsle, K. Jordan, C. Bokemeyer, and D. Atanackovic, "Intraperitoneal VEGF inhibition using bevacizumab: a potential approach for the symptomatic treatment of malignant ascites?" *Oncologist*, vol. 14, no. 12, pp. 1242–1251, 2009.

[5] C. S. Grove and Y. C. G. Lee, "Vascular endothelial growth factor: the key mediator in pleural effusion formation," *Current Opinion in Pulmonary Medicine*, vol. 8, no. 4, pp. 294–301, 2002.

[6] O. Pichelmayer, B. Gruenberger, C. Zielinski, and M. Raderer, "Bevacizumab is active in malignant effusion," *Annals of Oncology*, vol. 17, no. 12, p. 1853, 2006.

[7] K. Kitamura, K. Kubota, M. Ando et al., "Bevacizumab plus chemotherapy for advanced non-squamous non-small-cell lung cancer with malignant pleural effusion," *Cancer Chemotherapy and Pharmacology*, vol. 71, no. 2, pp. 457–461, 2013.

[8] N. Du, X. Li, F. Li et al., "Intrapleural combination therapy with bevacizumab and cisplatin for non-small cell lung cancer-mediated malignant pleural effusion," *Oncology Reports*, vol. 29, no. 6, pp. 2332–2340, 2013.

[9] L. Yang, J.-W. Wang, Y. Sun et al., "Randomized phase II trial on escalated doses of Rh-endostatin (YH-16) for advanced non-small cell lung cancer," *Chinese Journal of Oncology*, vol. 28, no. 2, pp. 138–141, 2006.

[10] X. Ma, Y. Yao, D. Yuan et al., "Recombinant human endostatin endostar suppresses angiogenesis and lymphangiogenesis of malignant pleural effusion in mice," *PLoS ONE*, vol. 7, no. 12, Article ID e53449, 2012.

[11] C. H. Contag and M. H. Bachmann, "Advances in in vivo bioluminescence imaging of gene expression," *Annual Review of Biomedical Engineering*, vol. 4, pp. 235–260, 2002.

[12] M. Edinger, Y.-A. Cao, Y. S. Hornig et al., "Advancing animal models of neoplasia through in vivo bioluminescence imaging," *European Journal of Cancer*, vol. 38, no. 16, pp. 2128–2136, 2002.

[13] T. J. Sweeney, V. Mailänder, A. A. Tucker et al., "Visualizing the kinetics of tumor-cell clearance in living animals," *Proceedings of the National Academy of Sciences of the United States of America*, vol. 96, no. 21, pp. 12044–12049, 1999.

[14] M. Vooijs, J. Jonkers, S. Lyons, and A. Berns, "Noninvasive imaging of spontaneous retinoblastoma pathway-dependent tumors in mice," *Cancer Research*, vol. 62, no. 6, pp. 1862–1867, 2002.

[15] J. Y. Adams, M. Johnson, M. Sato et al., "Visualization of advanced human prostate cancer lesions in living mice by a targeted gene transfer vector and optical imaging," *Nature Medicine*, vol. 8, no. 8, pp. 891–896, 2002.

[16] B. Laxman, D. E. Hall, M. S. Bhojani et al., "Noninvasive real-time imaging of apoptosis," *Proceedings of the National Academy of Sciences of the United States of America*, vol. 99, no. 26, pp. 16551–16555, 2002.

[17] P. Ray, H. Pimenta, R. Paulmurugan et al., "Noninvasive quantitative imaging of protein-protein interactions in living subjects," *Proceedings of the National Academy of Sciences of the United States of America*, vol. 99, no. 5, pp. 3105–3110, 2002.

[18] P. Ciana, M. Raviscioni, P. Mussi et al., "In vivo imaging of transcriptionally active estrogen receptors," *Nature Medicine*, vol. 9, no. 1, pp. 82–86, 2003.

[19] K. Yasumoto, K. Koizumi, A. Kawashima et al., "Role of the CXCL12/CXCR4 axis in peritoneal carcinomatosis of gastric cancer," *Cancer Research*, vol. 66, no. 4, pp. 2181–2187, 2006.

[20] M. Kamiyama, Y. Ichikawa, T. Ishikawa et al., "VEGF receptor antisense therapy inhibits angiogenesis and peritoneal dissemination of human gastric cancer in nude mice," *Cancer Gene Therapy*, vol. 9, no. 2, pp. 197–201, 2002.

[21] K. Yasumoto, T. Yamada, A. Kawashima et al., "The EGFR ligands amphiregulin and heparin-binding EGF-like growth factor promote peritoneal carcinomatosis in CXCR4-expressing gastric cancer," *Clinical Cancer Research*, vol. 17, no. 11, pp. 3619–3630, 2011.

[22] F. Fang, P. Chen, X. Wu et al., "Therapeutic effects of recombinant human endostatin adenovirus in a mouse model of malignant pleural effusion," *Journal of Cancer Research and Clinical Oncology*, vol. 135, no. 9, pp. 1149–1157, 2009.

[23] S. Matsumoto, F. Tanaka, K. Sato et al., "Monitoring with a non-invasive bioluminescent in vivo imaging system of pleural metastasis of lung carcinoma," *Lung Cancer*, vol. 66, no. 1, pp. 75–79, 2009.

[24] F. Peng, Z. Xu, J. Wang et al., "Recombinant human endostatin normalizes tumor vasculature and enhances radiation response in xenografted human nasopharyngeal carcinoma models," *PLoS ONE*, vol. 7, no. 4, Article ID e34646, 2012.

[25] G. Xin, J. Du, L. Zhu, Y.-H. Yu, Y. Li, and P.-S. Liu, "Differential anti-tumor effects for various regimens of endostar plus cisplatin in ovarian cancer," *Zhonghua Yi Xue Za Zhi*, vol. 91, no. 47, pp. 3367–3370, 2011.

[26] N. Yamamoto, P. Jiang, M. Yang et al., "Cellular dynamics visualized in live cells in vitro and in vivo by differential dual-color nuclear-cytoplasmic fluorescent-protein expression," *Cancer Research*, vol. 64, no. 12, pp. 4251–4256, 2004.

[27] M. Yang, P. Jiang, and R. M. Hoffman, "Whole-body subcellular multicolor imaging of tumor-host interaction and drug response in real time," *Cancer Research*, vol. 67, no. 11, pp. 5195–5200, 2007.

[28] R. M. Hoffman and M. Yang, "Subcellular imaging in the live mouse," *Nature Protocols*, vol. 1, no. 2, pp. 775–782, 2006.

[29] R. M. Hoffman, "The multiple uses of fluorescent proteins to visualize cancer in vivo," *Nature Reviews Cancer*, vol. 5, no. 10, pp. 796–806, 2005.

[30] T. Furukawa, X. Fu, T. Kubota, M. Watanabe, M. Kitajima, and R. M. Hoffman, "Nude mouse metastatic models of human stomach cancer constructed using orthotopic implantation of histologically intact tissue," *Cancer Research*, vol. 53, pp. 1204–1208, 1993.

[31] Y. Jia, M. Liu, W. Huang et al., "Recombinant human endostatin endostar inhibits tumor growth and metastasis in a mouse xenograft model of colon cancer," *Pathology and Oncology Research*, vol. 18, no. 2, pp. 315–323, 2012.

6

Billroth II with Braun Enteroenterostomy Is a Good Alternative Reconstruction to Roux-en-Y Gastrojejunostomy in Laparoscopic Distal Gastrectomy

Long-Hai Cui, Sang-Yong Son, Ho-Jung Shin, Cheulsu Byun, Hoon Hur, Sang-Uk Han, and Yong Kwan Cho

Department of Surgery, Ajou University School of Medicine, Suwon, Republic of Korea

Correspondence should be addressed to Sang-Yong Son; spy798@gmail.com

Academic Editor: Haruhiko Sugimura

Background. Although Billroth II (BII) reconstruction is simpler and faster than Billroth I or Roux-en-Y (RY) reconstruction in patients undergoing totally laparoscopic distal gastrectomy (TLDG), BII reconstruction is associated with several complications, including more severe bile reflux. BII Braun anastomosis may be a better alternative to RY reconstruction. *Methods.* This retrospective study included 56 consecutive patients who underwent TLDG for gastric cancer, followed by BII Braun or RY reconstruction, between January 2013 and December 2015. Surgical outcomes, including length of operation, quantity of blood lost, and postoperative complications, were compared in the two groups. *Results.* Clinicopathological characteristics did not differ between the BII Braun and RY groups. Mean length of operation was significantly longer in the RY than the BII Braun group (157.3 min versus 134.6 min, $p < 0.010$), but length of hospital stay, blood loss, and complication rate did not differ between the two groups. Ileus occurred in three patients (10.0%) in the RY group. Endoscopic findings 6 months after surgery showed bile reflux in seven (28%) patients in the BII Braun group and five (17.2%) in the RY group ($p = 0.343$), but no significant differences in rate of gastric residue or degree of gastritis in the remnant stomach in the two groups. *Conclusions.* B-II Braun anastomosis is a good alternative to RY reconstruction, reducing length of operation and ileus after TLDG.

1. Introduction

Gastric cancer is one of the most common cancers and the third leading cause of cancer-related deaths worldwide [1]. Surgical resection remains the only definitive treatment of this malignant disease [2]. Early diagnosis of gastric cancer has resulted in a significant improvement in the long-term survival of patients undergoing surgery [3].

Some patients who undergo surgery for gastric cancer experience postgastrectomy complications, including malabsorption, dumping syndrome, reflux esophagitis, alkaline gastritis, and delayed gastric emptying [4–6]. Reflux gastritis, which occurs mainly after Billroth II (BII) reconstruction, causes long-term distress, impairs patient quality of life, and may lead to increased risk of metachronous cancer development [7, 8]. The introduction of Roux-en-Y (RY) reconstruction dramatically reduced the rate of alkaline reflux gastritis [9–13]. Early series reported nearly universal success after Roux diversion, resulting in the suggestion that RY reconstruction be considered a method of primary reconstruction after gastrectomy [14]. However, RY reconstruction has drawbacks, including difficulties performing the procedure and severe complications, such as Roux limb stasis and internal herniation [15–18].

The development of laparoscopic techniques increased the number of patients undergoing totally laparoscopic distal gastrectomy (TLDG) with intracorporeal anastomosis. Use of this surgical method increased the percentage of patients undergoing BII reconstruction, as it is both simple and rapid. BII reconstruction still has limitations, as it can cause more severe bile reflux, increasing the risk of metachronous cancer development [19, 20]. Braun [21] introduced an enteroenterostomy anastomosis in an attempt to divert food from the afferent limb, thus reducing the incidence of the "vicious circle" syndrome. This simple and easy method may be used as a standard method, at least for older patients undergoing TLDG.

It is unclear whether BII Braun anastomosis results in superior perioperative outcomes when compared with RY reconstruction. Few studies to date have compared short-term outcomes and endoscopic findings after 6 months in patients undergoing laparoscopic intracorporeal anastomosis using these two methods. This study therefore compared the short-term surgical outcomes of BII Braun anastomosis and RY reconstruction in patients who underwent laparoscopic distal gastrectomy (LDG) performed by a single surgeon.

2. Material and Methods

2.1. Study Design and Patients. A total of 376 consecutive patients at Ajou University Hospital underwent TLDG by a single surgeon between January 2013 and December 2015. Of these, 167 patients who underwent Billroth I (BI) reconstruction were excluded, as were 153 patients who underwent BII anastomosis alone without the Braun procedure. Of the remaining 56 patients, 26 underwent BII Braun reconstruction and 30 underwent RY reconstruction. Findings in these two groups were evaluated retrospectively.

The evaluated parameters included patient demographics, comorbidities, operative details, time to first flatus, time to sips of water, length of hospital stay, and postoperative complications. Tumor depth, nodal status, and stage were classified according to the 7th American Joint Committee on Cancer Staging System. Lymph node dissection was performed according to the Guidelines of the Japanese Gastric Cancer Association. All patients underwent follow-up upper gastrointestinal endoscopy 6 months postoperatively. Gastric residue, degree of gastritis, and bile reflux (RGB) classification was analyzed, with higher scores indicating worse symptoms or signs in the remnant stomach [22].

The study was reviewed and approved by the Ajou University Hospital Institutional Review Board.

2.2. Surgical Technique. LDG was performed with the patient in the supine position under general anesthesia. The operator and endoscopist stood on the right side of the patient and the first assistant stood on the left side. The method used one 10 mm port for the laparoscope, as well as two 12 mm and two 5 mm ports. The pneumoperitoneum was maintained between 10 and 13 mmHg. Ultrasonically activated shears were used for lymph node dissection.

All patients in our center have undergone reconstruction using intracorporeal anastomosis since April 2010. Following LDG, patients in the BII Braun group underwent gastrojejunostomy about 40 cm from the ligament of Treitz in antecolic and isoperistaltic manners. Braun anastomosis was performed about 25 cm distal to the gastrojejunostomy, using a linear stapler 60 mm in length with white cartilage. Then, entry hole was closed with a 60 mm long linear staple with white cartilage in tangential direction. RY reconstruction was performed with an antecolic route and isoperistaltic Roux limb (length 30 cm) divided 20 cm from the ligament of Treitz. Side-to-side gastrojejunostomy and side-to-side

jejunojejunostomy were performed intracorporeally with a 60 mm long linear stapler with white cartilage. The entry hole was closed by the same technique of Braun anastomosis. In the Roux-en-Y group, mesenteric defect was routinely repaired by a continuous suture with 3-0 Vicryl (Ethicon, Rome, Italy) or V-Loc 90 (Covidien, Mansfield, Massachusetts), whereas Petersen's defect was not repaired in both groups.

2.3. Statistical Analysis. All statistical analyses were performed using SPSS version 20.0 (SPSS Inc., Chicago, IL, USA). Differences between the two groups were assessed using χ^2 tests, Fisher's exact tests, and Student's t-tests, as appropriate. A p value < 0.05 was considered statistically significant.

3. Results

Table 1 shows the demographic and clinical characteristics of the two groups. Age, sex, comorbidities, body mass index (BMI), American Society of Anesthesiologists (ASA) score, extent of surgery, number of retrieved lymph nodes, and pathologic stage were similar in the two groups.

Short-term surgical outcomes and postoperative complications are shown in Table 2. Operation time was significantly longer in the RY than in the BII Braun group (157.3 ± 33.9 min versus 134.6 ± 28.8 min, $p < 0.010$). Time to first sips of water (1.8 ± 0.5 versus 2.0 ± 0.9 days, $p = 0.307$) and length of hospital stay (7.9 ± 8.4 versus 7.0 ± 1.6 days, $p = 0.583$), however, did not differ between the two groups. There were also no significant differences in anesthesia time, blood loss, time to first flatus, and postoperative complications. Ileus occurred in three patients (10.0%) in the RY group.

Functional outcomes were assessed indirectly by weight change and gastrointestinal symptoms (Table 3). The RY group showed a trend of larger weight loss than the BII Braun group, but body mass index of postoperative 3 and 6 months did not differ between the BII Braun and RY groups (22.2 versus 22.0, $p = 0.842$ and 21.9 versus 21.6, $p = 0.680$). Regarding GI symptoms, there was no significant difference in occurrence rate between two groups (11.5% in the BII Braun group versus 30.0% in the RY group, $p = 0.114$). Endoscopic finding was performed at 6 months after surgery in 25 patients (96.1%) in the BII Braun group and 29 (96.6%) in the RY group. The grades of gastric residue, remnant gastritis, and bile reflux did not differ in these two groups (Figure 1).

4. Discussion

Although the number of LDGs has increased worldwide since its introduction in the 1990s [23], there is a lack of consensus among surgeons regarding the choice of reconstructive procedure after LDG. The three methods, BI, BII, and RY, have advantages and disadvantages. The ideal gastrointestinal reconstruction procedure should minimize postoperative morbidity and improve quality of life.

A survey in Korea in 2009 found that BI was the most frequent type of reconstruction after distal gastrectomy (6581 patients, 63.4%), followed by BII reconstruction (3437

TABLE 1: Clinicopathologic characteristics of the patients.

Variable	BII Braun ($n = 26$)	Roux-en-Y ($n = 30$)	p value
Age	60.1 ± 13.3	57.6 ± 12.6	0.466
Sex			0.218
Male	15 (57.7%)	22 (73.3%)	
Female	11 (42.3%)	8 (26.7%)	
BMI (kg/m^2)	23.3 ± 3.3	24.0 ± 3.5	0.491
ASA score			0.453
1	13 (50.0%)	18 (60.0%)	
2	13 (50.0%)	12 (40.0%)	
Comorbidity	12 (46.2%)	12 (40.0%)	0.643
Hypertension	10	6	
Diabetes mellitus	6	7	
Liver diseases	3		
Tuberculosis	2	1	
Myocardial Infarction	1		
Extent of lymph node dissection			0.906
D1+	10 (38.5%)	12 (40.0%)	
D2	16 (61.5%)	18 (60.0%)	
Number of retrieved lymph nodes	36.7 ± 15.4	35.8 ± 10.9	0.793
Pathologic stage			0.043
I	12 (46.2%)	23 (76.6%)	
II	7 (26.9%)	5 (16.7%)	
III	7 (26.9%)	2 (6.7%)	

Values are presented as number (%) or mean ± standard deviation.
BMI = body mass index; ASA = American Society of Anesthesiologists.

TABLE 2: Comparison of surgical outcomes according to the reconstructive procedures.

Variable	BII Braun ($n = 26$)	Roux-en-Y ($n = 30$)	p value
Operating time (min)	134.6 ± 28.8	157.3 ± 33.9	0.010
Blood loss (ml)	89.2 ± 85.5	96.0 ± 89.8	0.773
Sips of water (d)	2.0 ± 0.9	1.8 ± 0.5	0.307
Soft diet (d)	3.2 ± 0.8	3.1 ± 0.8	0.784
Hospital stay (d)	7.0 ± 1.6	7.9 ± 8.4	0.583
Postoperative complications	4 (15.3%)	6 (20.0%)	0.653
Wound	1 (3.8%)		
Intraluminal bleeding	1 (3.8%)	1 (3.3%)	
Ileus		3 (10.0%)	
Leakage		1 (3.3%)	
Pancreatitis	1 (3.8%)	1 (3.3%)	
Other	1 (3.8%)		
Clavien-Dindo classification			1.000
Grades I-II	2 (7.6%)	3 (10.0%)	
Grades III-IV	2 (7.6%)	3 (10.0%)	

Values are presented as number (%) or mean ± standard deviation.

patients, 33.1%), with RY reconstruction rarely performed (332 patients, 3.3%) [24]. Increased experience with TLDG has increased the use of intracorporeal anastomosis, with KLASS 01 data showing that a significantly larger number of patients underwent BII reconstruction than RY following LDG (232 versus 20, $p < 0.001$) [25], because BII was both simpler and faster to perform. In Japan, however, the most common method of reconstruction was BI, followed by RY [26]. BII reconstruction was rarely performed by any Japanese surgeons, because it can cause more severe bile reflux, which may strongly correlate with carcinogenesis in the gastric remnant [26]. The results of our study suggest that

TABLE 3: Comparison of postoperative weight change and gastrointestinal symptoms.

Variable	BII Braun ($n = 26$)	Roux-en-Y ($n = 30$)	p value
Length of resected stomach (cm)			
Lesser curvature	12.4 ± 2.6	13.7 ± 2.6	0.086
Greater curvature	19.0 ± 3.9	22.0 ± 4.9	0.016
Body weight (kg)			
Preoperative	61.9 ± 10.7	67.3 ± 13.1	0.102
Postoperative 3 months	58.9 ± 10.3	61.8 ± 12.0	0.334
Postoperative 6 months	58.3 ± 10.3	60.7 ± 12.2	0.424
BMI (kg/m^2)			
Preoperative	23.3 ± 3.3	24.0 ± 3.5	0.491
Postoperative 3 months	22.2 ± 3.1	22.0 ± 3.2	0.842
Postoperative 6 months	21.9 ± 3.0	21.6 ± 3.2	0.680
Postoperative GI symptoms	3 (11.5%)	9 (30.0%)	0.114
Diarrhea	3	3	
Constipation		2	
Dyspepsia		1	
Gas bloating		1	
Reflux/soreness		2	

Values are presented as number (%) or mean ± standard deviation.
BMI = body mass index; GI = gastrointestinal.

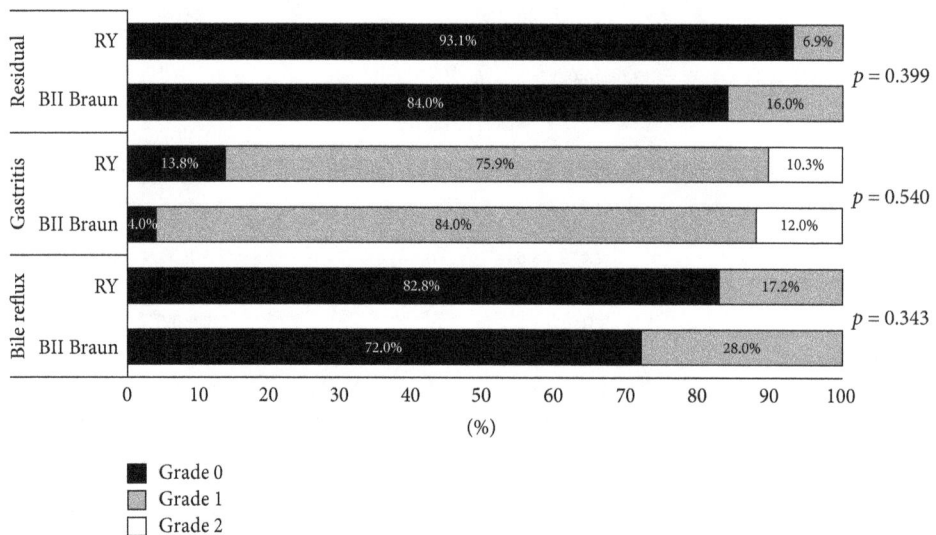

FIGURE 1: RGB score of gastroscopy at postoperative 6 months.

BII Braun reconstruction after LDG for gastric cancer has perioperative outcomes similar to those of RY reconstruction, as shown by rates of postoperative complications and 6-month postoperative bile reflux (RGB) scores. These findings indicate that BII Braun anastomosis successfully diverts a substantial amount of bile from the remnant stomach and therefore may be an alternative to RY reconstruction in treating bile reflux.

Postoperative complications leading to malnutrition, such as delayed gastric emptying, anastomotic leak, and dumping syndrome, may require enteral nutritional support, prolong hospital stay, and increase health care costs. A comparison of patients who underwent BII or RY reconstruction found no differences in the rates of postgastrectomy diarrhea (9.1% versus 9.7%), dumping syndrome (6% versus 3.2%), and weight gain (78.8% vs. 90.3%) [27]. Although our retrospective registry did not include specific information on dumping syndrome and relevant quality-of-life parameters, we evaluated length of hospital stay, discharge destination, and hospital readmission as indirect measures of potential postoperative gastrointestinal dysfunction. We found all of these parameters were similar in the BII Braun and RY groups.

A retrospective study from Memorial Sloan Kettering Cancer Center compared outcomes in 122 patients who underwent RY reconstruction and 588 who underwent classic BII reconstruction after pancreaticoduodenectomy [28]. There were no differences in the rates of delayed gastric emptying (10.1% versus 10.3%), reoperation (9.1% *vs.* 6.9%), interventional radiology procedures (9.8% versus 6.8%), length of hospital stay (11 days versus 10 days), and mortality (0.9% versus 2.6%), findings similar to the results of our study.

Theoretically, LDG with BII Braun anastomosis may also minimize specific complications such as afferent loop syndrome and roux stasis syndrome. Braun anastomosis can divert a substantial amount of bile from the remnant stomach to the efferent loop; thereby it may reduce the afferent loop syndrome compared with BII without Braun anastomosis [29]. In our study, three patients in the RY group experienced ileus, indicating the roux stasis syndrome. Roux stasis syndrome is characterized by symptoms such as nausea, vomiting, epigastric pain, fullness, and difficulties in eating after Roux-en-Y gastrojejunostomy. However, the clinical definition of the roux stasis syndrome is ambiguous, sometimes confusing with postoperative ileus. Thus, more study is required to clarify the reality of roux stasis syndrome.

This study had several limitations, including its retrospective design. It was difficult to identify intraoperative factors that may have influenced the choice of BII Braun or RY reconstruction, but a certain selection bias might influence the present study. For instance, in the size of resected specimen, the mean length of greater curvature is significantly longer in the RY than in the BII Braun group (22.0 cm *vs.* 19.0 cm, $p = 0.016$). However, this was not a direct evidence that RY group has larger remnant stomach than BII Braun group and its clinical influence might be limited because the BMI were not different during postoperative 6 months. Moreover, the patient population was relatively small. Furthermore, it is difficult to discern retrospectively whether specific complications were directly related to the type of reconstruction. However, BII Braun anastomosis successfully diverted a substantial amount of bile from the remnant stomach, making this outcome comparable in the two groups.

5. Conclusions

The type of reconstruction after LDG had no effect on the rate or distribution of postoperative complications, length of hospital stay, or postoperative bile reflux scores. As BII Braun anastomosis successfully diverted a substantial amount of bile from the remnant stomach, this method may be a good alternative to RY reconstruction in preventing bile reflux. Short-term perioperative outcomes showed that BII Braun anastomosis and RY reconstruction can be considered equally acceptable restorative options following LDG for gastric cancer.

Ethical Approval

All procedures performed in studies involving human participants were in accordance with the ethical standards of the institutional and/or national research committee and with the 1964 Helsinki declaration and its later amendments or comparable ethical standards. For this type of study formal consent is not required.

Consent

Informed consent was obtained from all individual participants included in the study.

Disclosure

The funding source hand no role in the design of this article and will not have any role during its execution or publication.

Competing Interests

The authors declared no potential conflict of interests relevant to this article.

Authors' Contributions

Study conception and design were done by Sang-Uk Han, Sang-Yong Son, and Yong Kwan Cho. Acquisition of data was done by Long-Hai Cui. Analysis and interpretation of data were done by Sang-Yong Son and Sang-Uk Han. Drafting of manuscript was done by Long-Hai Cui. Critical revision of manuscript was done by Ho-Jung Shin, Cheulsu Byun, and Hoon Hur.

Acknowledgments

This study was supported by a grant from the National R & D Program for Cancer Control, Ministry of Health & Welfare, Republic of Korea (1320270).

References

[1] L. A. Torre, F. Bray, R. L. Siegel, J. Ferlay, J. Lortet-Tieulent, and A. Jemal, "Global cancer statistics, 2012," *CA Cancer Journal for Clinicians*, vol. 65, no. 2, pp. 87–108, 2015.

[2] J.-P. Kim, "Current status of surgical treatment of gastric cancer," *Journal of Surgical Oncology*, vol. 79, no. 2, pp. 79–80, 2002.

[3] D. H. Roukos, "Current advances and changes in treatment strategy may improve survival and quality of life in patients with potentially curable gastric cancer," *Annals of Surgical Oncology*, vol. 6, no. 1, pp. 46–56, 1999.

[4] C.-W. Wu, M.-C. Hsieh, S.-S. Lo, W.-Y. Lui, and F.-K. P'Eng, "Quality of life of patients with gastric adenocarcinoma after curative gastrectomy," *World Journal of Surgery*, vol. 21, no. 7, pp. 777–782, 1997.

[5] R. Tomita, K. Tanjoh, S. Fujisaki, and M. Fukuzawa, "Relation between gastroduodenal interdigestive migrating motor complex and postoperative gastrointestinal symptoms before and after cisapride therapy following distal gastrectomy for early

gastric cancer," *World Journal of Surgery*, vol. 24, no. 10, pp. 1250–1257, 2000.

[6] E. R. Woodward and M. P. Hocking, "Postgastrectomy syndromes," *The Surgical Clinics of North America*, vol. 67, no. 3, pp. 509–520, 1987.

[7] A. C. Fiore, M. A. Malangoni, T. A. Broadie, J. A. Madura, and J. E. Jesseph, "Surgical management of alkaline reflux gastritis," *Archives of Surgery*, vol. 117, no. 5, pp. 689–694, 1982.

[8] T. C. Northfield and C. N. Hall, "Carcinoma of the gastric stump: risks and pathogenesis," *Gut*, vol. 31, no. 11, pp. 1217–1219, 1990.

[9] M. K. Bartlett and J. D. Burrington, "Bilious vomiting after gastric surgery. Experience with a modified Roux-Y loop for relief," *Archives of Surgery*, vol. 97, no. 1, pp. 34–39, 1968.

[10] J. A. van Heerden, J. T. Priestley, G. M. Farrow, and S. F. Phillips, "Postoperative alkaline reflux gastritis. Surgical implications," *The American Journal of Surgery*, vol. 118, no. 3, pp. 427–433, 1969.

[11] J. A. van Heerden, S. F. Phillips, M. A. Adson, and D. C. McIlrath, "Postoperative reflux gastritis," *The American Journal of Surgery*, vol. 129, no. 1, pp. 82–88, 1975.

[12] F. L. Bushkin and E. R. Woodward, "Alkaline reflux gastritis," *Major Problems in Clinical Surgery*, vol. 20, pp. 48–63, 1976.

[13] T. Kennedy and R. Green, "Roux diversion for bile reflux following gastric surgery," *The British Journal of Surgery*, vol. 65, no. 5, pp. 323–325, 1978.

[14] J. L. Herrington Jr., "Roux-en-Y diversion as an alternate method of reconstruction of the alimentary tract after primary resection of the stomach," *Surgery Gynecology & Obstetrics*, vol. 143, no. 1, pp. 92–93, 1976.

[15] L. H. Karlstrom, N. J. Soper, K. A. Kelly, and S. F. Phillips, "Ectopic jejunal pacemakers and enterogastric reflux after Roux gastrectomy: effect of intestinal pacing," *Surgery*, vol. 106, no. 3, pp. 486–495, 1989.

[16] L. E. Perino, K. A. Adcock, and J. S. Goff, "Gastrointestinal symptoms, motility, and transit after the Roux-en-Y operation," *The American Journal of Gastroenterology*, vol. 83, no. 4, pp. 380–385, 1988.

[17] W. D. Harrison, M. P. Hocking, and S. B. Vogel, "Gastric emptying and myoelectric activity following Roux-en-Y gastrojejunostomy," *The Journal of Surgical Research*, vol. 49, no. 5, pp. 385–389, 1990.

[18] M. P. Hocking, R. G. Carlson, and S. B. Vogel, "Does selective vagotomy prevent delayed gastric emptying and altered myoelectric activity following Roux-en-Y gastrojejunostomy?" *The American Journal of Surgery*, vol. 163, no. 1, pp. 32–36, 1992.

[19] K. Fukuhara, H. Osugi, N. Takada, M. Takemura, M. Higashino, and H. Kinoshita, "Reconstructive procedure after distal gastrectomy for gastric cancer that best prevents duodenogastroesophageal reflux," *World Journal of Surgery*, vol. 26, no. 12, pp. 1452–1457, 2002.

[20] Y. Sugiyama, H. Sohma, M. Ozawa et al., "Regurgitant bile acids and mucosal injury of the gastric remnant after partial gastrectomy," *The American Journal of Surgery*, vol. 153, no. 4, pp. 399–403, 1987.

[21] H. Braun, "Ueber die Gastro-enterostomie und Gleichzeutig Ausgefuhrte," *Langenbecks Archiv für Chirurgie*, vol. 45, no. 2, p. 361, 1893.

[22] M. Kubo, M. Sasako, T. Gotoda et al., "Endoscopic evaluation of the remnant stomach after gastrectomy: proposal for a new classification," *Gastric Cancer*, vol. 5, no. 2, pp. 83–89, 2002.

[23] S. Kitano, Y. Iso, and K. Sugimachi, "Laparoscopy-assisted billroth I gastrectomy," *Surgical Laparoscopy & Endoscopy*, vol. 4, no. 2, pp. 146–148, 1994.

[24] O. Jeong and Y.-K. Park, "Clinicopathological features and surgical treatment of gastric cancer in South Korea: the results of 2009 nationwide survey on surgically treated gastric cancer patients," *Journal of Gastric Cancer*, vol. 11, no. 2, pp. 69–77, 2011.

[25] W. Kim, H.-H. Kim, S.-U. Han et al., "Decreased morbidity of laparoscopic distal gastrectomy compared with open distal gastrectomy for stage I gastric cancer: short-term outcomes from a multicenter randomized controlled trial (KLASS-01)," *Annals of Surgery*, vol. 263, no. 1, pp. 28–35, 2016.

[26] K. Kumagai, K. Shimizu, N. Yokoyama, S. Aida, S. Arima, and T. Aikou, "Questionnaire survey regarding the current status and controversial issues concerning reconstruction after gastrectomy in Japan," *Surgery Today*, vol. 42, no. 5, pp. 411–418, 2012.

[27] A. Csendes, A. M. Burgos, G. Smok, P. Burdiles, I. Braghetto, and J. C. Díaz, "Latest results (12–21 years) of a prospective randomized study comparing billroth ii and roux-en-y anastomosis after a partial gastrectomy plus vagotomy in patients with duodenal ulcers," *Annals of Surgery*, vol. 249, no. 2, pp. 189–194, 2009.

[28] S. R. Grobmyer, S. T. Hollenbeck, D. P. Jaques et al., "Roux-en-Y reconstruction after pancreaticoduodenectomy," *Archives of Surgery*, vol. 143, no. 12, pp. 1184–1188, 2008.

[29] S. B. Vogel, W. E. Drane, and E. R. Woodward, "Clinical and radionuclide evaluation of bile diversion by braun enteroenterostomy: prevention and treatment of alkaline reflux gastritis. An alternative to Roux-en-Y diversion," *Annals of Surgery*, vol. 219, no. 5, pp. 458–465, 1994.

7

Veronicastrum axillare Alleviates Ethanol-Induced Injury on Gastric Epithelial Cells via Downregulation of the NF-kB Signaling Pathway

Wei-chun Zhao,[1] Yan-shan Xu,[1] Gang Chen,[2] Yan Guo,[1] Dan-yi Wang,[1] and Gui-bin Meng[1]

[1]*College of Life Sciences, Zhejiang Chinese Medical University, Hangzhou 310053, China*
[2]*Department of Chemistry, Simon Fraser University, Burnaby, BC, Canada V5A 1S6*

Correspondence should be addressed to Wei-chun Zhao; weichunzhao@hotmail.com

Academic Editor: Kazuhiko Uchiyama

We used human gastric epithelial cells (GES-1) line in an ethanol-induced cell damage model to study the protective effect of *Veronicastrum axillare* and its modulation to NF-κB signal pathway. The goal was to probe the molecular mechanism of *V. axillare* decoction in the prevention of gastric ulcer and therefore provide guidance in the clinical application of *V. axillare* on treating injuries from chronic nephritis, pleural effusion, gastric ulcer, and other ailments. The effects of *V. axillare*-loaded serums on cell viability were detected by MTT assays. Enzyme-linked immunosorbent assay (ELISA) and Real-Time PCR methods were used to analyze the protein and mRNA expression of TNF-α, NF-κB, IκBα, and IKKβ. The results showed that *V. axillare*-loaded serum partially reversed the damaging effects of ethanol and NF-κB activator (phorbol-12-myristate-13-acetate: PMA) and increased cell viability. The protein and mRNA expressions of TNF-α, NF-κB, IκBα, and IKKβ were significantly upregulated by ethanol and PMA while they were downregulated by *V. axillare*-loaded serum. In summary, *V. axillare*-loaded serum has significantly protective effect on GES-1 against ethanol-induced injury. The protective effect was likely linked to downregulation of TNF-α based NF-κB signal pathway.

1. Introduction

Gastric ulcer is one of the most common clinical conditions of the digestive system. Globally, more than 14 million people are diagnosed with gastric ulcer annually, and about 4 million people would die from related complications [1]. Human gastric epithelial tissue is in constant turn-over, maintaining a balance between cell death and new cell formation. It has some capacity to repair food-oriented chemical and physical damage [2–4]. However when the damage exceeds the self-repair capacity, the structure and function of the gastric epithelial tissue can be compromised, leading to an imbalance between cell generation and cell death, which in turn can cause gastric inflammation and ulcer.

Alcohol is an indispensable part in many people's life. It is even dubbed as catalyst to build relationships and make deals amongst businessmen. Although alcohol in moderation has health benefits, elevated alcohol consumption has been linked to GI track disorders, and acute GI epithelial tissue alcohol damage is on the rise [5]. Excessive consumption of hard liquor can directly cause gastric epithelial cell damage, resulting in inflammation, congestion, edema, bleeding, erosion, and ulcer in the GI track. Chronic alcoholism has strong ties to GI disorders, atrophic gastritis, and cancer [5, 6]. Therefore, alcohol has been recognized as a key pathogen in gastric epithelial tissue damage. Methods for the prevention and treatment of such damage and deduction of protective mechanisms have been the focus of many research projects [7].

Veronicastrum axillare (Sieb. et Zucc) Yamazaki (Scrophulariaceae) has been widely used both alone and in conjugation with other herbs in Chinese folk medicines to treat injuries from chronic nephritis, pleural effusion, gastric ulcer, furunculosis, burns, snake bites, and other ailments [8–13]. Our preliminary studies showed that the water extract of *V. axillare* significantly reduced ethanol-induced gastric damage in a rat model and downregulation of the expression of the key factors of NF-κB signaling pathway [14–19]. In this study we used human GES-1 cell line in an ethanol-induced cell damage model to study the protective effect of *V. axillare* and its modulation to NF-κB signal pathway. The goal was to probe the molecular mechanism of *V. axillare* decoction in the prevention of gastric ulcer and therefore provide guidance in the clinical application of *V. axillare* on treating injuries from chronic nephritis, pleural effusion, gastric ulcer, furunculosis, and other ailments.

2. Materials and Methods

2.1. Materials and Reagents. *V. axillare* was picked from Lishui in Zhejiang province of China, which was identified as Scrophulariaceae, *V. axillare* plant by Professor Zhensheng Yao (Zhejiang Chinese Medical University). The preparation of high-dose decoction (0.14 g dried plant per mL) followed the protocol of Du [6]. The high-dose decoction was diluted 1:1 and 1:3 with water to prepare medium-dose and low-dose solutions, respectively. Ranitidine capsule (Shanghai Modern HaSen (Shangqiu) Pharmaceutical Co., Ltd., lot 14071604) was made into 0.18% suspension based on the labeled API content just before use. Other reagents and supplies were obtained from their respective commercial suppliers: absolute ethanol, Hangzhou Shuanglin Chemicals (lot 20140820); GES-1 cell line: immortalized human gastric epithelial cell line, Cancer Hospital Chinese Academy of Medical Sciences; DMEM high glucose culture medium, HyClone; PMA (phorbol-12-myristate-13-acetate), Sigma-Aldrich; NF-κB/TNF-α ELISA kit (lot 20150701A) and IκBα/IKKβ ELISA kit (lot 20150801A), Shanghai Yuanye Biotech Ltd.; PrimeScript™ RT Master Mix (RR036A) and SYBR Premix Ex Taq™ II (lot RR820A), Takara.

2.2. Equipment. Thermo 3111 CO_2 incubator (Thermo, USA), TE2000-S inverted phase differential microscope (Nikon, Japan), Milli-Q water purification station (Millipore), 3K15 refrigerated centrifuge (Sigma, Germany), Tanon 2500 gel imaging station (Tianneng Scientific Co. Ltd.), Q5000 micro UV-Vis spectrophotometer (Quawell, USA), StepOnePlus™ Real-Time PCR system (ABI Co.), and Multiskan Flash microplate reader (Thermo, USA) were used.

2.3. Drug-Loaded Serum Preparation. 20 male SD rats (SPF grade, 200 ± 20 g, Shanghai Sciple Biky Company, certificate SCXK (Hu) 2013-0003) were randomly divided into normal group, Ranitidine group, *V. axillare* high-dose, medium-dose, and low-dose groups, four in each group. The rats were hosted at 23 ± 2°C, 50–70% RH. The rats were daily intragastrically given at 20 mL/kg the following solutions, respectively: 0.9% saline, 0.027 g/kg Ranitidine (equivalent to 3 times the human clinical dose), and *V. axillare* decoction (0.140 g/mL, 0.070 g/mL, and 0.035 g/mL for high-/medium-/low-dose group, resp.). The animals had access to water and food *ad libitum* during the first 13 days and were denied food for the 14th day while they still have free access to water. Two hours after the final dosing, the animals were euthanized by giving 3.0 mL/kg of 10% chloral hydrate subcutaneously,

and blood was taken from the abdominal aorta. The blood samples were left at room temperature for 1 h and then centrifuged at 3500 rpm for 10 min. The resulting supernatants were passed through 0.22 μm sterile filters to yield the drug-loaded serums (4-5 mL/rat), which were divided into small aliquots and stored at −20°C.

2.4. Cell Subculture. GES-1 cell lines were cultured in 10% FBS supplemented DMEM medium in 25T culturing flasks at 37°C/5% CO_2, and the medium was changed every other day. When the cells have fully covered the flask bottom, 1 mL of 0.25% Trypsin was added to digest the monolayer and cells were subcultured at 1 : 3 ratio.

2.5. In Vitro Model. Cultured GES-1 were aliquoted to 10 groups, that is, normal group, model group, Ranitidine group (positive control), *V. axillare* high-/medium-/low-dose groups, PMA group, and *V. axillare* high-/medium-/low-dose + PMA groups. GES-1 culture in its logarithmic growth phase was used to inoculate normal growth medium in a cell cultural plate (six-well plate: 2 mL/well, 1.2×10^6 cells; 96-well plate: 100 μL/well, 4×10^4 cells). After the cells have adhered to the bottom of the wells for 24 h, the mediums were removed, washed twice with PBS, and then replaced with DMEM medium supplemented with 10% drug-loaded rat serum prepared above (drug-loaded DMEM medium). The cells were further cultured for 24 h, and then the mediums in all but the normal group wells were replaced with drug-loaded DMEM medium containing 5% ethanol [3]. After 4 h, cells in wells were used for the subsequent experiments [3].

2.6. Cell Viability Assay. MTT stock solution (5 mg/mL, 20 μL/well) was added to GES-1 cell cultures in a 96-well plate prepared in 2.5, and the cells were further cultured for 4 h. The supernatants were removed, and 150 μL of DMSO was added to each well. The optical absorption was measured at 490 nm on a microplate reader.

2.7. Measurement of NF-κB, TNF-α, IκBα, and IKKβ Protein Expression by ELISA. The supernatants from different groups of GES-1 cell cultures in a 6-well plate described in 2.5 were placed in sterile microcentrifuge tubes and centrifuged at 3000 rpm for 10 min. The supernatants were transferred to new tubes and the amounts of NF-kB, TNF-α, IκBα, and IKKβ were measured according to manufacturers' protocols.

2.8. Measurement of NF-κB, TNF-α, IκBα, and IKKβ mRNA Expression by RT-PCR. After removing the supernatant, the cells remaining in the 6-well plate (described in 2.7) were treated with Trizol reagent to extract the total RNA [20, 21]. A 0.5 μg aliquot of each RNA sample was reverse transcribed with PrimeScript RT Master Mix kit (Takara Co.). A 2 μL aliquot of each reverse transcription product was amplified with SYBR Prime Ex Tag™ II kit following the manufacturer's protocol to obtain target cDNA (primer sequences see Table 1): predenature at 95°C for 30 sec, followed by 40 cycles of 95°C, 5 sec, then 60°C, 30 sec. The relative amounts of

TABLE 1: Forward and reverse primers for β-actin, NF-κB, TNF-α, IκBα, and IKKβ.

	Forward primer 5′–3′	Reverse primer 5′–3′	Fragment (bp)
β-actin	CCTGGCACCCAGCACAAT	GGGCCGGACTCGTCATAC	144
NF-κB	ACTGTGAGGATGGGATCTGC	TCTGTCATTCGTGCTTCCAG	127
TNF-α	GGCGTGGAGCTGAGAGATAA	GTGTGGGTGAGGAGCACAT	119
IκBα	CCACTCCATCCTGAAGGCTA	CATTGACATCAGCACCCAAG	116
IKKβ	CCTGGTAGAACGGATGATGG	GTACAGCTCCCTTGCTTGCT	118

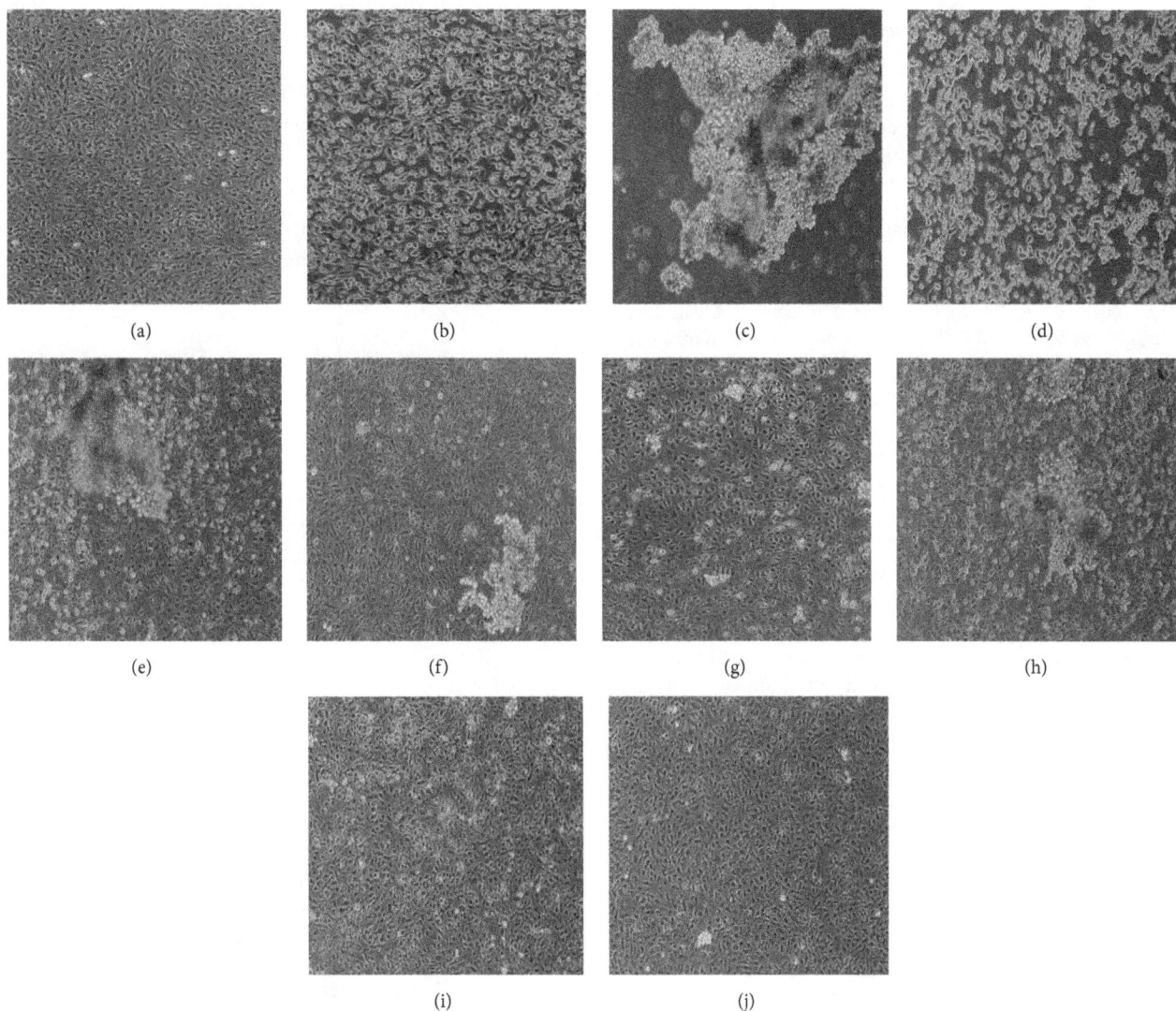

FIGURE 1: Effect of *Veronicastrum axillare*-loaded serum on cellular morphology of GES-1 injured by ethanol. Note: (a) normal; (b) model; (c) PMA; (d) low dosage of *V. axillare* + PMA; (e) medium dosage of *V. axillare* + PMA; (f) high dosage of *V. axillare* + PMA; (g) Ranitidine; (h) low dosage of *V. axillare*; (i) medium dosage of *V. axillare*; (j) high dosage of *V. axillare*.

NF-κB, TNF-α, IκBα, and IKKβ mRNA were calculated with $2^{-\Delta\Delta Ct}$ method, using β-actin as the internal standard.

2.9. Statistical Analysis. All results were analyzed using SPSS v. 18.0 (IBM) and expressed as average ± standard error ($\overline{x}\pm S$). Intergroup differences were analyzed by one-way ANOVA, and group-wise comparisons were made using Tukey HSD protocol, with $P < 0.05$ as being statistically significant.

3. Results

3.1. Effect of V. axillare-Loaded Serum on Cell Viability after Ethanol Damage. As seen in Figure 1, normal cells appeared as a dense monolayer that adhered to the bottom and maintained their healthy, cuboidal shapes. In the ethanol model group, most cells had swollen to round shape, and significant numbers dissociated from the wall. Intercellular space increased, connections decreased, and cells separated

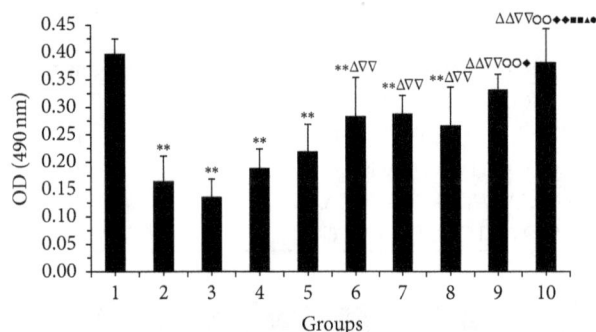

Figure 2: Effect of *Veronicastrum axillare*-loaded serum on cell viability in GES-1 injured by ethanol test by MTT method. Note: 1. normal; 2. model; 3. PMA; 4. low dosage of *V. axillare* + PMA; 5. medium dosage of *V. axillare* + PMA; 6. high dosage of *V. axillare* + PMA; 7. Ranitidine; 8. low dosage of *V. axillare*; 9. medium dosage of *V. axillare*; 10. high dosage of *V. axillare*. Compared with normal, $^{*}P < 0.05$, $^{**}P < 0.01$; compared with model, $^{\triangle}P < 0.05$, $^{\triangle\triangle}P < 0.01$; compared with PMA, $^{\triangledown\triangledown}P < 0.01$; compared with low dosage of *V. axillare* + PMA, $^{\circ\circ}P < 0.01$; compared with medium dosage of *V. axillare* + PMA, $^{\blacklozenge}P < 0.05$, $^{\blacklozenge\blacklozenge}P < 0.01$; compared with high dosage of *V. axillare* + PMA, $^{\blacksquare\blacksquare}P < 0.01$; compared with Ranitidine, $^{\blacktriangle}P < 0.05$; compared with low dosage of *V. axillare*, $^{\bullet}P < 0.05$.

from each other. In the PMA group, cells formed globular aggregates and almost completely floated to the surface. Cell morphology was even worse than the ethanol model group, suggesting PMA could further stimulate dissociation of cells from each other. In *V. axillare* groups, as the dosing increased, cell morphology improved and eventually got close to normal cells. In low-dose *V. axillare* group, although cells were still swollen, the severity was reduced, and they remained adhered to the culturing dish. In the medium-dose group, cell swelling was greatly reduced, and half of the view field showed normal cell morphology. In the high-dose group, almost no cell swelling was observed. The high-dose group appeared better than the Ranitidine group (positive control). In *V. axillare* + PMA groups, there were also improvements to cell morphology and cell adhesion as the dose increased, but overall cells appeared weaker than the *V. axillare* groups without PMA. Compared with the normal group, cell in the model group, PMA group, and *V. axillare* + PMA groups all showed significant lower viability (Figure 2, $P < 0.05$, $P < 0.01$). Cell viabilities for *V. axillare* high- and medium-dose groups, Ranitidine group, and *V. axillare* high-dose + PMA group were significantly higher than those for the PMA group, *V. axillare* low-dose + PMA group, and *V. axillare* medium-dose + PMA group ($P < 0.05$, $P < 0.01$). Cell viability enhancement in the *V. axillare* high-dose group was much better than those in the *V. axillare* + PMA groups, Ranitidine group, and *V. axillare* low-dose group. This indicated *V. axillare*-loaded serum reduced GES-1 cell damage from PMA treatment.

3.2. Effect of *V. axillare*-Loaded Serum on NF-κB, TNF-α, IκBα, and IKKβ Level.
As shown in Figure 3, when compared with the normal group, the NF-κB, TNF-α, IκBα, and IKKβ levels in the model group and the PMA group all increased

($P < 0.05$, $P < 0.01$). Compared with the model group, *V. axillare* groups and Ranitidine group had significant downregulation of NF-κB, TNF-α, IκBα, and IKKβ ($P < 0.05$, $P < 0.01$); the effects in the *V. axillare* groups tend to be dose-dependent, with the high-dose group being the most significant. *V. axillare* high-dose + PMA group, *V. axillare* groups, and Ranitidine group all had significant inhibition on the expression of NF-κB, TNF-α, IκBα, and IKKβ when compared with the PMA group ($P < 0.05$, $P < 0.01$). The inhibition of TNF-α was stronger in the *V. axillare* high- and medium-dose groups compared with that of *V. axillare* low-dose + PMA group ($P < 0.05$, Figure 3(b)). The downregulation of IkBα in the *V. axillare* high- and medium-dose groups and *V. axillare* high-dose + PMA group was more significant than that of *V. axillare* medium-dose + PMA group ($P < 0.05$, $P < 0.01$; Figure 3(c)). The downregulation of IKKβ in the *V. axillare* high- and medium-dose groups, *V. axillare* medium-dose + PMA group, and Ranitidine group was stronger than that of the *V. axillare* low-dose + PMA group ($P < 0.01$, $P < 0.05$; Figure 3(d)).

3.3. Extraction of Total RNA and Analysis of the DNA Amplification Product.
The extracted RNA was subjected to nondenaturing agarose gel electrophoresis (2%), and the 5S, 18S, and 28S RNA bands were well defined, proving the integrity of the extracted RNA (Figure 4). Electrophoresis of the PCR products and subsequent fluorescent quantification showed the PCR products were uniform and in agreement with the expected product size, indicating NF-κB, TNF-α, IkBα, and IKKβ gene and β-actin primers participated in the reactions and the PCR amplifications were successful (Figure 5).

3.4. Effect of *V. axillare*-Loaded Serum on the Expression of NF-κB, TNF-α, IκBα, and IKKβ mRNA.
Figure 6 showed that the model group and PMA group had upregulation of NF-κB, TNF-α, IκBα, and IKKβ mRNA compared with the normal group ($P < 0.01$). Moreover, the upregulation of NF-κB in the PMA group was significantly higher than that of the model group ($P < 0.01$, Figure 6(a)), indicating the activation of NF-κB by PMA. The expression of NF-κB, TNF-α, IκBα, and IKKβ mRNA were significantly downregulated by high/medium/low dose of *V. axillare* and Ranitidine ($P < 0.05$, $P < 0.01$; Figures 6(a) and 6(c)). Compared with the PMA group, the expression of NF-κB, TNF-α, IκBα, and IKKβ mRNA was significantly reduced in *V. axillare* groups, *V. axillare* + PMA groups, and Ranitidine group ($P < 0.01$; Figures 6(a)–6(c)). Compared with the *V. axillare* high-dose + PMA group, *V. axillare* high-dose group further reduced the expression of TNF-α, IκBα, and IKKβ mRNA ($P < 0.05$, $P < 0.01$; Figures 6(b)–6(d)), and the downregulation of NF-κB and IKKβ was more than that of the *V. axillare* low-dose group ($P < 0.05$; Figures 6(a) and 6(d)).

4. Discussion

Alcoholic gastric epithelial injury refers to conditions caused by excessive alcohol consumption that induced damage to

(a)

(b)

(c)

(d)

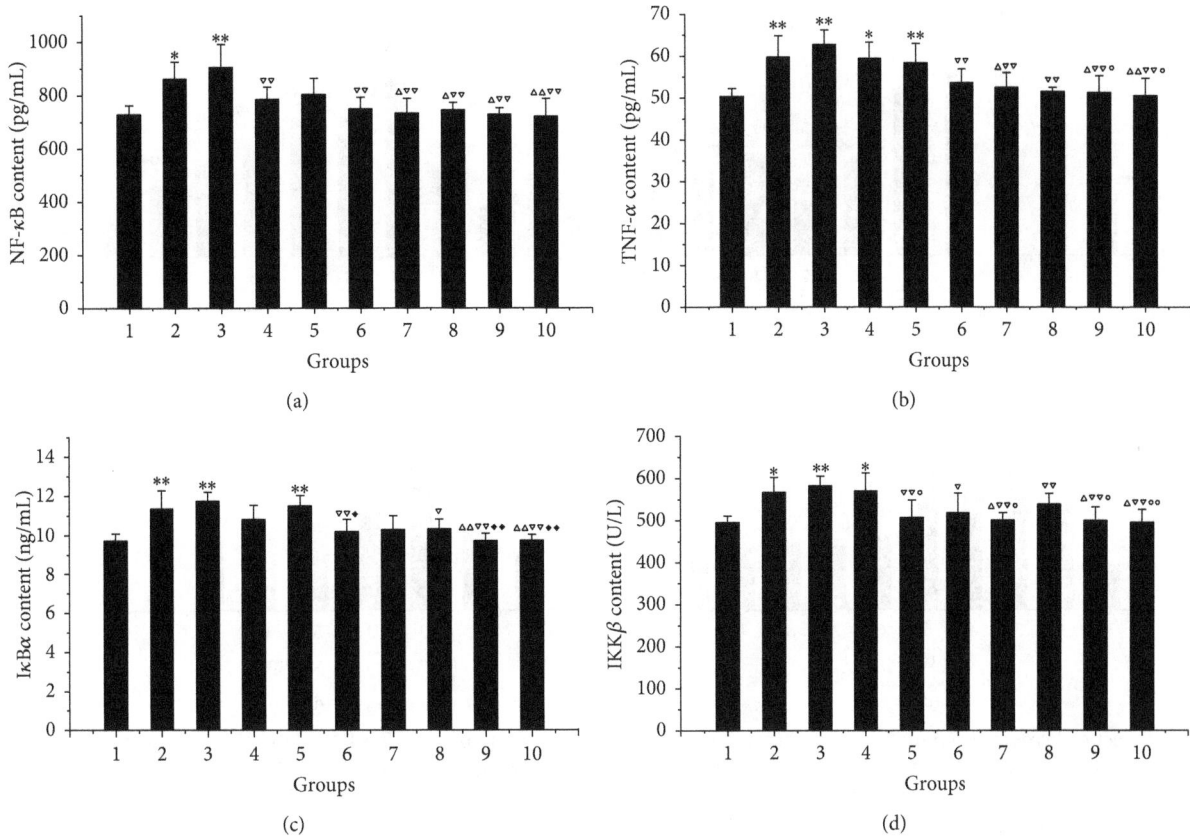

FIGURE 3: Effect of *Veronicastrum axillare*-loaded serum on NF-κB, TNF-α, IκBα, and IKKβ content in GES-1 injured by ethanol. Note: 1. normal; 2. model; 3. PMA; 4. low dosage of *V. axillare* + PMA; 5. medium dosage of *V. axillare* + PMA; 6. high dosage of *V. axillare* + PMA; 7. Ranitidine; 8. low dosage of *V. axillare*; 9. medium dosage of *V. axillare*; 10. high dosage of *V. axillare*. Compared with normal, $^*P < 0.05$, $^{**}P < 0.01$; compared with model, $^{\triangle}P < 0.05$, $^{\triangle\triangle}P < 0.01$; compared with PMA, $^{\triangledown}P < 0.05$, $^{\triangledown\triangledown}P < 0.01$; compared with low dosage of *V. axillare* + PMA, $^{\circ}P < 0.05$, $^{\circ\circ}P < 0.01$; compared with medium dosage of *V. axillare* + PMA, $^{\blacklozenge}P < 0.05$, $^{\blacklozenge\blacklozenge}P < 0.01$.

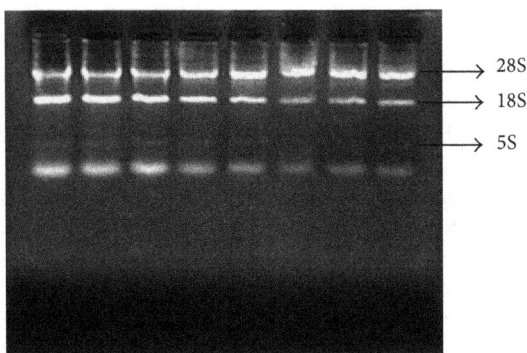

FIGURE 4: RNA integrity check: nondenaturing agarose gel electrophoresis.

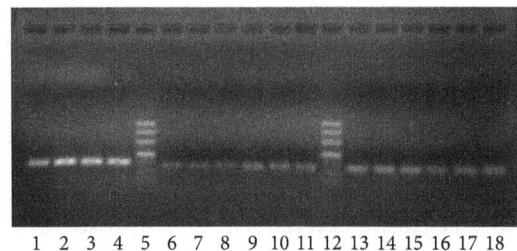

FIGURE 5: Agarose gel electrophoresis of qRT-PCR products. Note: Lanes 5 and 12: DL500 DNA Ladder Marker (500, 400, 300, 200, 150, 100, and 50 bp in turn from the top down). Lanes 1–4: β-actin (144 bp). Lanes 6–8: NF-κB (127 bp). Lanes 9–11: TNF-α (119 bp). Lanes 13–15: IκBα (116 bp). Lanes 16–18: IKKβ (118 bp).

the gastric epithelial tissues (such as gastric ulcer and gastrorrhagia). The clinical symptoms include abdominal pain, fullness, vomiting, and heartburn [3]. The injury caused by alcohol is typically exerted by inducing epithelial cell damage and apoptosis. Our preliminary *in vivo* results showed that the water extract of *V. axillare* significantly inhibited ethanol-induced gastric epithelial cell damage [14, 15, 19]. The ulcer

inhibition rates of low, middle, and high dosage (0.7 g/kg, 1.4 g/kg, and 2.8 g/kg) group were 47.9%, 71.4%, and 89.4%, respectively [15]. The current study used MTT assay to examine the effect on cell viability under ethanol assault by pretreatment of GES-1 with *V. axillare*-loaded serum. The results showed that *V. axillare*-loaded serum had protective effects and reduced the damage caused by ethanol. This is the first evidence at the cellular level that *V. axillare*-loaded serum

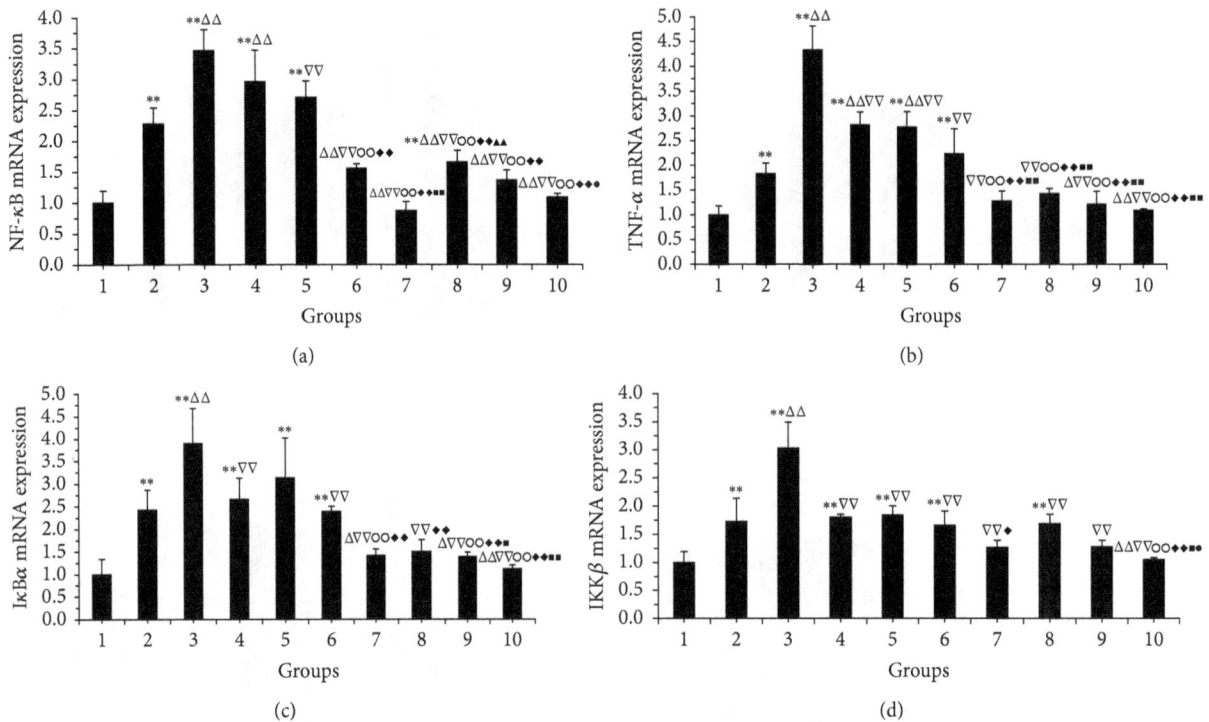

FIGURE 6: Effect of *Veronicastrum axillare*-loaded serum on NF-κB, TNF-α, IκBα, and IKKβ mRNA in GES-1 injured by ethanol. Note: 1. normal; 2. model; 3. PMA; 4. low dosage of *V. axillare* + PMA; 5. medium dosage of *V. axillare* + PMA; 6. high dosage of *V. axillare* + PMA; 7. Ranitidine; 8. low dosage of *V. axillare*; 9. medium dosage of *V. axillare*; 10. high dosage of *V. axillare*. Compared with normal, $^{**}P < 0.01$; compared with model, $^{\triangle}P < 0.05$, $^{\triangle\triangle}P < 0.01$; compared with PMA, $^{\triangledown\triangledown}P < 0.01$; compared with low dosage of *V. axillare* + PMA, $^{\circ\circ}P < 0.01$; compared with medium dosage of *V. axillare* + PMA, $^{\blacklozenge}P < 0.05$, $^{\blacklozenge\blacklozenge}P < 0.01$; compared with high dosage of *V. axillare* + PMA, $^{\blacksquare}P < 0.05$, $^{\blacksquare\blacksquare}P < 0.01$; compared with Ranitidine, $^{\blacktriangle\blacktriangle}P < 0.01$; compared with low dosage of *V. axillare*, $^{\blacklozenge}P < 0.05$.

is effective against damage induced by ethanol as a model of alcoholic gastric ulcer [14–19].

Alcohol can cause gastric epithelial injury by inducing apoptosis through the TNF-α pathway and through the formation of ROS, which causes cellular damage through oxidative stress [3]. At the same time, the expression of TNF-α is under the control of NF-κB signal pathway. NF-κB signaling pathway is involved in controlling the gene expression of multiple factors and plays an important role in immune response, inflammation, stress response, cell apoptosis, cancer, and ontogenetic development [22–24]. Excessive activation of the NF-κB pathway will trigger body's specific and nonspecific immune response and cause tissue damage and organ dysfunction. The three key factors in the NF-κB pathway are IκBα, IKKβ, and NF-κB [25]. When IKKβ is activated by inter- or intracellular stimulations, it causes IκBα phosphorylation and ubiquitination. Ubiquitinated IκBα can be degraded by a 28S small proteasome, which causes the nucleic acid binding domain in NF-κB to be exposed, and the translocation of NF-κB into the nucleus. This in turn will change the chemical structure of IκB, causing a series of biological responses, thus controlling the gene expression of TNF-α [17, 26]. Studies have shown that Tong Xin Luo Capsule can protect the retina in a mouse diabetic model by downregulating IκBα, IKKβ, and NF-κB expressions [27]. Severe liver damage was observed in IKKβ-knockout mice, and IL-1β and TNF-α induced NF-κB activity was

significantly reduced [28]. An earlier *in vivo* study has shown that the protective effect of *V. axillare* on ethanol-induced gastric ulcer of SD rats is intimately linked to TNF-α mediated NF-κB signaling pathway [15, 17]. Compared with the ethanol injury model group, the expressions of TNF-α, NF-κB, TNFR-1, RIP1, IκBα, and IL-1β in rats gastric tissue are downregulated by *V. axillare*. The current study has shown that, in the model group, the mRNA expression of NF-κB, TNF-α, IκBα, and IKKβ of GES-1 cell lines increased significantly, and the protein concentrations of them in GES-1 supernatant also increased remarkably, while different doses of *V. axillare* downregulated these factors in GES-1 and supernatant to various degrees. Those indicated that *V. axillare* likely exerted the protective effect on GES-1 against ethanol damage through the NF-κB pathway by downregulating the expressions of NF-κB, TNF-α, IκBα, and IKKβ. The concentrations of NF-κB, IκBα, and IKKβ in supernatant increased after the GES-1 were damaged by 5% ethanol. This increase was likely due to increased cell membrane permeability from the swelling and cell damage, although there is possibility that these factors are actively secreted. Further studies will be needed to discern the exact mechanism.

PMA can activate protein kinase C (PKC), thus activating NF-κB [29]. Under resting conditions, NF-κB and IκB exist as an inactive complex in the cytoplasm. When cells are stimulated by a PKC agonist, PKC is activated, with the concomitant activation of IKKβ. IKKβ can act as the kinase of IκB to cause its phosphorylation and dissociation from NF-κB. IκBα contains a gene promoter domain that binds NF-κB, the binding of which causes IκBα gene expression to increase rapidly. At the same time, the dissociated NF-κB is activated to display the transcription modulating activity [30–34]. The gene of the proinflammatory cellular factor TNF-α has a κB-binding domain. When NF-κB is activated, it will bind to the κB domain and promote its transcription, thus aggravating the inflammation [35, 36]. Study has shown that, with increasing concentration of PMA, the concentration of NF-κB protein in astrocytes also increased [37]. In another study, the damage to myocytes from Doxorubicin was linked to the overactivation of NF-κB and TNF-α [38]. This study showed that the expressions of NF-κB, TNF-α, IκBα, and IKKβ in the PMA group were significantly higher than those of the normal group and the model group. This may indicate that when PMA activated PKC, it also activated IKKβ. This would cause the phosphorylation of IκBα and its dissociation from NF-κB. The dissociated NF-κB displayed TNF-α modulating activity, which affected the NF-κB signaling pathway. Compared with the PMA group, V. axillare high-dose + PMA group had significantly lower NF-κB, TNF-α, IκBα, and IKKβ levels, which indicated V. axillare inhibited the activation of NF-κB pathway by PMA, and in turn supported that V. axillare protected GES-1 from alcohol damage by blocking the NF-κB pathway.

Chinese herbal medicines and their active compounds have become an active research field because of their advantages of multitarget, multichannel activities and less recurrence and play an irreplaceable role in the treatment of gastric ulcer. Our preliminary studies showed that the decoction of V. axillare can significantly reduce the acute gastric mucosal injury in SD rats induced by ethanol, improving the pathological state of the gastric mucosa, and regulating the secretion of gastric juice and gastric acid [14]. Compared with the ethanol injury model group, the concentrations or activities of multiple protective factors such as NO [12], iNOS [12], superoxide dismutase (SOD) [10], cyclooxygenase 2 (COX2) (unpublished data), prostaglandin E2 (PGE2) (unpublished data), and aquaporins (AQP1) [14] in rat gastric epithelial tissues are upregulated by pretreatment of V. axillare, while the activities of pepsin [14] and the expression of endothelin 1 (ET-1) [11], AQP3 [14], and AQP4 [14] are downregulated. The concentrations of EGF [10] and VEGF [12] between the ethanol-injured model group and V. axillare group are not significantly different. In this experiment, Ranitidine was used as the positive control. This is because Ranitidine is a commonly used drug in the treatment of gastric ulcer. Ranitidine is a histamine H2 receptor antagonist (H2RA). It can effectively inhibit the secretion of gastric acid caused by histamine, pentapeptide gastrin, and the stimulation of food and reduce the activity of pepsin. Our prior results showed that Ranitidine can significantly reduce ethanol-induced gastric ulcer, increase the level of PGE2, and upregulate the expression of COX-2 protein and mRNA. But the antiulcer effect of Ranitidine was weaker than V. axillare. This may be related to their different antiulcer mechanisms. As the antiulcer mechanism of V. axillare is not clear, other antiulcer

drugs, such as Omeprazole (a proton pump inhibitors, PPIs), Colloidal Bismuth Subcitrate (gastric mucosal protective agent), Dexamethasone (anti-inflammatory drugs), Weikangling Capsule (Chinese medicine), could be included as positive controls in further studies.

In summary, V. axillare-loaded serum significantly protected GES-1 against ethanol-induced damage. This effect is likely linked to the downregulation of the expression of NF-κB, TNF-α, IκBα, and IKKβ. The exact mechanism remains to be elucidated.

Competing Interests

The authors declare that they have no conflict of interests.

Acknowledgments

This study was undertaken with support from "Natural Science Foundation of Zhejiang Province (no. LY14H280006)" and "Founds of Zhejiang Provincial Educational Department (no. Y201121241)". The authors wish to express their special thanks to Professor Robert N. Young, Kun-yan Zhu, Qin Yu, and Min-li Chen for their helpful comments on experimental designs and an earlier draft of the manuscript. They also thank Yue-qin Cai for providing technical assistance.

References

[1] B. M. Srikanta, M. N. Siddaraju, and S. M. Dharmesh, "A novel phenol-bound pectic polysaccharide from Decalepis hamiltonii with multi-step ulcer preventive activity," World Journal of Gastroenterology, vol. 13, no. 39, pp. 5196–5207, 2007.

[2] I. Sobhani, A. Bado, C. Vissuzaine et al., "Leptin secretion and leptin receptor in the human stomach," Gut, vol. 47, no. 2, pp. 178–183, 2000.

[3] C. L. Liu, The Mechanism Research of Astragalus Glysosides's Protecting Effect on Ethanol-induced GES-1 Cells Injury, Guangzhou University of Chinese Medicine, GuangDong, China, 2014.

[4] S. Y. She, D. Y. Liu, M. Chen et al., "Effect of fungus infection on gastric epitheial cell apoptosis and proliferation in gastric ulcer patients," Guangxi Medical Journal, vol. 24, no. 10, pp. 1525–1526, 2002.

[5] Y. X. Lou and Y. Peng, "Progress of mechanism researching of gastric mucosa," Journal of Military Surgeon in Southwest China, vol. 13, no. 1, pp. 122–123, 2011.

[6] M. Li, "Diagnosis and treatment of 76 cases of acute gastric mucosal lesion caused by acute alcoholism," Contemporary Medicine, vol. 18, no. 33, pp. 52–53, 2012.

[7] Y. B. Zhang, Y. S. Ruan, X. H. Zhao et al., "Alcohol—induced gastric mucosal injury and its protective effect," Journal of Food Safety and Food Quality, vol. 4, no. 4, pp. 1239–1244, 2013.

[8] X. Dang, B. Zhao, A. Gao et al., "Pharmaceutical research of Veronicastrum," Journal of Anhui Agricultural Sciences, vol. 32, pp. 19801–19802, 2011.

[9] X. Q. Zeng, "Folk remedies for treatment of acute and chronic nephritis," New Rural Technology, vol. 21, article 44, 2010.

[10] J. H. Wu, "Veronicastrum axillare treatment of acute and chronic nephritis," Zhejiang Journal of Traditional Chinese Medicine, no. 11, p. 516, 1997.

[11] J. H. Wu, "*Veronicastrum axillare* treatment of pleural effusion," *Zhejiang Journal of Traditional Chinese Medicine*, vol. 1, article 33, 2003.

[12] J. Shu, "Treatment of 110 cases of liver cirrhosis with *Lysimachia christinae* Hance and *Veronicastrum axillare* (Sieb.et Zucc) Yamazaki," *Journal of Practical Traditional Chinese Internal Medicine*, vol. 19, no. 2, p. 148, 2005.

[13] C. J. Zheng, X. H. Deng, Y. Wu et al., "Antiinflammatory effects and chemical constituents of *Veronicastrum axillare*," *Phytotherapy Research*, vol. 28, no. 10, pp. 1561–1566, 2014.

[14] G. F. Shen, W. Guo, W. C. Zhao et al., "Antiulcer effects and action pathways of *Veronicastrum axillare* on gastric ulcer in rat induced by ethanol," *Chinese Journal of Integrated Traditional and Western Medicine*, vol. 32, no. 10, pp. 1370–1373, 2012.

[15] Y. Du, W. C. Zhao, L. L. Lu et al., "Study on the antiulcer effects of *Veronicastrum axillare* on gastric ulcer in rats induced by ethanol based on tumor necrosis factor-α (TNF-α) and endothelin-1 (ET-1)," *Asian Pacific Journal of Tropical Biomedicine*, vol. 3, no. 12, pp. 925–930, 2013.

[16] Y. Du, W. C. Zhao, W. W. Shen et al., "Antiulcer effects of *Veronicastrum axillare* on gastric ulcer in rats induced by ethanol and the effect on the expression of NO, iNOS and VEGF," *Journal of Chinese Medical University*, vol. 37, no. 10, pp. 1151–1155, 2013.

[17] Y. Du, *Study on Molecular Mechanism of Veronicastrum axillare (Sieb.et Zucc) Yamazaki against Gastric Ulcer by Intervening Inflammatory Response*, Zhejiang Chinese Medical University, Zhejiang, China, 2014.

[18] Q. J. Lou, Y. S. Xu, W. C. Zhao et al., "Study on the regulation roles of water metabolism in gastric mucosa injury induced by ethanol and the effect of *Veronicastrum axillare*," *Journal of Zhejiang Chinese Medical University*, vol. 40, no. 1, pp. 13–18, 2016.

[19] Y. S. Xu, W. C. Zhao, D. Y. Wang et al., "Protective effect of *Veronicastrum axillare* on human gastric epithelial cells (GES-1) and its modulation on the PKA, CREB and AQP1," *Journal of Zhejiang Chinese Medical University*, vol. 40, no. 3, pp. 173–178, 2016.

[20] A. B. Hummon, S. R. Lim, M. J. Difilippantonio, and T. Ried, "Isolation and solubilization of proteins after TRIzol® extraction of RNA and DNA from patient material following prolonged storage," *BioTechniques*, vol. 42, no. 4, pp. 467–472, 2007.

[21] P. Chomczynski, "A reagent for the single-step simultaneous isolation of RNA, DNA and proteins from cell and tissue samples," *BioTechniques*, vol. 15, no. 3, pp. 532–536, 1993.

[22] F. Chen, V. Castranova, and X. Shi, "New insights into the role of nuclear factor-κB in cell growth regulation," *The American Journal of Pathology*, vol. 159, no. 2, pp. 387–397, 2001.

[23] S. Ghosh, M. J. May, and E. B. Kopp, "NF-κB and rel proteins: evolutionarily conserved mediators of immune responses," *Annual Review of Immunology*, vol. 16, pp. 225–260, 1998.

[24] A. S. Baldwin Jr., "The NF-κB and IκB proteins: new discoveries and insights," *Annual Review of Immunology*, vol. 14, pp. 649–681, 1996.

[25] C. Chen, R. Moreno, B. Samikannu et al., "Improved intraportal islet transplantation outcome by systemic IKK-beta inhibition: NF-κB activity in pancreatic islets depends on oxygen availability," *American Journal of Transplantation*, vol. 11, no. 2, pp. 215–224, 2011.

[26] T. Zhao, *Expression and Significance of IKK, IκB, and NF-κB in NSCLC*, Qingdao University, Shandong, China, 2012.

[27] X. Wang, C. Wang, H. Y. Xing et al., "Effects of Tongxinluo capsule on retina through IKKβ /IκBα /NF-κB pathway in diabetic mouse," *Recent Advances in Ophthalmology*, vol. 34, no. 11, pp. 1005–1008, 2014.

[28] M. Tanaka, M. E. Fuentes, K. Yamaguchi et al., "Embryonic lethality, liver degeneration, and impaired NF-kappaB activation in IKK-beta-deficient mice," *Immunity*, vol. 10, no. 4, pp. 421–429, 1999.

[29] X. Y. Yang, *The Effect of Triptolide on the COX-2 Expression in A431 Cell Line and PMA-Treated HaCaT Cell Line*, Central South University, Hunan, China, 2007.

[30] M. A. Huber, A. Denk, R. U. Peter et al., "The IKK-2/Ikappa Balpha/NF-kappa B pathway plays a key role in the regulation of CCR3 and eotaxin-1 in fibroblasts. A critical link to dermatitis in IκBα-deficient mice," *The Journal of Biological Chemistry*, vol. 277, no. 2, pp. 1268–1275, 2002.

[31] J. S. Zhang, X. Y. Wang, Y. A. Shan et al., "Research progress of transcription factor NF-κB," *Chinese Science Bulletin*, vol. 47, no. 5, pp. 323–329, 2002.

[32] N. Sizemore, N. Lerner, N. Dombrowski et al., "Distinct roles of the IkappaB kinase alpha and beta subunits in liberating nuclear factor kappaB (NF-kappaB) from IkappaB and in phosphorylating the p65 subunit of NF-kappaB," *Journal of Biological Chemistry*, vol. 277, no. 6, pp. 3863–3869, 2002.

[33] B. H. B. Kwok, B. Koh, M. I. Ndubuisi et al., "The anti-inflammatory natural product parthenolide from the medicinal herb Feverfew directly binds to and inhibits IκB kinase," *Chemistry and Biology*, vol. 8, no. 8, pp. 759–766, 2001.

[34] P. J. Chiao, S. Miyamoto, and I. M. Verma, "Autoregulation of I kappa B alpha activity," *Proceedings of the National Academy of Sciences*, vol. 91, no. 1, pp. 28–32, 1994.

[35] W. G. van Eyndhoven, C. J. Gamper, E. Cho et al., "TRAF-3 mRNA splice-deletion variants encode isoforms that induce NF-kappaB activation," *Molecular Immunology*, vol. 36, no. 10, pp. 647–658, 1999.

[36] J. S. Kim and C. Jobin, "Role of NF-kappaB in inflammatory disorders: just when you thought you knew everything," *Journal of Pediatric Gastroenterology and Nutrition*, vol. 38, no. 1, pp. 109–110, 2004.

[37] W. Mo, B. Chen, X. H. Zhou et al., "Effect of different concentration of PMA and PDTC on the expression of NF-κB in astrocytes," *Hainan Medical Journal*, vol. 23, no. 7, pp. 15–17, 2012.

[38] J. Shu, W. H. Yan, H. B. Wang et al., "Research on TLR4/NF-κB expression of cardiac cells and signal-transduction pathway of DOX in newborn rats the intervention of dexam ethasone," *Journal of Jiangsu University (Medicine Edition)*, vol. 19, no. 6, pp. 480–484, 2009.

8

Clinical Outcomes and Safety of Partial Full-Thickness Myotomy versus Circular Muscle Myotomy in Peroral Endoscopic Myotomy for Achalasia Patients

Chenyu Li,[1] **Aixia Gong,**[1] **Jingwen Zhang,**[1] **Zhijun Duan,**[2] **Linmei Ge,**[1] **Nan Xia,**[1] **Jing Leng,**[1] **Mei Li,**[1] **and Yanjie Liu**[1]

[1]*Department of Digestive Endoscopy, The First Affiliated Hospital of Dalian Medical University, Dalian, Liaoning 116000, China*
[2]*Department of Gastroenterology, The First Affiliated Hospital of Dalian Medical University, Dalian, Liaoning 116000, China*

Correspondence should be addressed to Aixia Gong; gongaixiadmu@163.com

Academic Editor: Mihir S. Wagh

Background. Here we aimed to evaluate and compare the efficacy and safety between partial full-thickness myotomy and circular muscle myotomy during POEM procedure in achalasia patients. *Methods.* Clinical data of achalasia of cardia (AC) patients who underwent POEM in our center during January 2014 to January 2015 was collected (34 cases). 19 patients who received partial full-thickness myotomy were assigned to group A and 14 patients who received circular muscle myotomy were assigned to group B. The procedure-related parameters between the two groups were compared. Symptom relief rate and postprocedure manometry outcomes were compared to evaluate the efficacy. Procedure-related adverse events and complications were compared to evaluate the safety. *Results.* (1) Mean operation times were significantly shorter in group A than group B (62.42 ± 23.17 *vs* 87.86 ± 26.44 min, $p < 0.01$). (2) Symptom relief rate and postprocedure manometry outcomes had no statistical differences when compared between the two groups (all $p > 0.05$). (3) Comparison of procedure-related adverse events and complications had no statistical differences (all $p > 0.05$). *Conclusion.* Partial full-thickness myotomy had no significant differences in efficacy or safety with circular myotomy, but partial full-thickness myotomy significantly reduced the procedure time.

1. Introduction

Achalasia (AC) is a primary motility disease of the esophagus which presents with symptoms such as dysphagia, chest pain, regurgitation, and weight loss [1]. Without effective medical intervention, the symptoms tend to aggravate and are often associated with esophageal morphological changes which may lead to negative prognosis [2].

In the year 2010, Inoue carried out peroral endoscopic myotomy (POEM), a novel endoscopic procedure, which incorporated methods of endoscopic submucosal dissection (ESD) and natural orifice transluminal endoscopic surgery (NOTES) [3]. By comparing different surgical methods, to explore more effective and safer therapy, with an acceptable safety profile and excellent symptoms relief rate, POEM has been established as one of the best therapies for AC patients [4]. With the advantages of being less invasive, less costly, and

shorter hospital stay, its preliminary efficacy such as short-term remission rate showed no difference with laparoscopic Heller myotomy (LHM) [5, 6]. However, there still exist some challenges which need further attention, such as the method of myotomy during the procedure. Theoretically, completeness of lower esophageal sphincter (LES) myotomy is the key for better outcomes. But gastroesophageal reflux disease (GERD) has always been a potential complication of the POEM procedure. It is reported that postprocedure gastroesophageal reflux rate of POEM can fluctuate between 16.5% and 60%, mostly higher than 30% [7]. Another concern has been the risk of perforation which may refer to full-thickness myotomy.

The POEM procedure has been operational in the First Affiliated Hospital of the Dalian Medical University since the year 2013, and the circular method was solely used. However, from January 2014 to January 2015, partial full-thickness

TABLE 1: Preoperative patients characteristics.

Patients characteristics	Group A (n = 19)	Group B (n = 14)	p value
Age, y	45.37 ± 12.28	46.07 ± 15.43	0.89
Symptom duration, y	6.36 ± 7.44	5.04 ± 4.19	0.56
LESP (mmH$_2$O)	27.71 ± 15.60	37.37 ± 17.41	0.19
IRP (mmH$_2$O)	19.36 ± 14.10	12.60 ± 5.94	0.20
LES length (cm)	3.17 ± 1.47	3.39 ± 0.70	0.70
Prior history of treatment			
Heller	0 (0.0%)	0 (0.0%)	1.00
Pneumatic balloon dilation	2 (10.5%)	3 (21.4)	0.63
Botox	2 (10.5%)	1 (7.1%)	0.55
POEM	0 (0.0%)	0 (0.0%)	1.00

LESP: lower esophageal sphincter pressure, IRP: integrated relaxation pressure, LES: lower esophageal sphincter, and POEM: peroral endoscopic myotomy.

myotomy was introduced as well. The focus of this retrospective study was to compare the efficiency and safety of the two methods.

2. Patients and Methods

2.1. Enrolling Criteria. Eckardt symptom score was used to select the study participant [8]. Patients with other organic diseases such as esophageal or upper gastric tumors (by esophagogastroduodenoscopy) were excluded. Diagnosis of AC was also based on at least one of other accessory examinations (esophageal manometry, barium esophagogram).

2.2. Exclusion Criteria. The exclusion criteria encompassed patients who had recently taken anticoagulant or hormonal drugs. Also, patients with severe cardiopulmonary dysfunction and impaired blood clotting function were exempted from the study. Likewise, patients with serious erosion or fibrosis in lower segment of esophagus or severe sigmoid-shaped esophagus were excluded [4, 9].

2.3. Grouping Situation. By the different methods of myotomy, 19 patients who received partial full-thickness myotomy were assigned to group A and 14 patients who received circular myotomy were assigned to group B.

2.4. Patients Characteristics. Patients characteristics are as summarized in Table 1. As showed, there were no significant differences (all *p* value > 0.05) in mean age, symptom duration, LESP (lower esophageal sphincter pressure), IRP (integrated relaxation pressure), length of LES (lower esophageal sphincter), and prior history of treatment between the two groups.

2.5. Instruments. The instruments used for POEM procedure include Olympus -260 main engine, esophagogastroduodenoscopy (GIF-Q260J, Olympus), ERBE VIO300 system,

OFP water insufflation, UCR CO2 insufflator, transparent cap (D-201-11804), injection needle (NM-4L-1, Olympus), IT2 knife (KD-611), dual knife (KD-650L), hook knife (KD-620LR), biopsy forceps (FD-410LR), clips (HX-610-135, Olympus), and other accessories.

2.6. Procedures. All patients were admitted three day prior to the scheduled surgery. During those three days, the patients underwent electrocardiogram (ECG), routine blood analysis, blood electrolytes analysis, routing urine analysis, blood typing, chest X-ray examination, and general physical examination to ensure their suitability to go through the procedure. Patients were restricted to a clear liquid diet for 48 hours and kept 12 hours fasting water before the procedure. Prophylactic intravenous antibiotics were administered 30 minutes before the commencement of the procedure. To reduce the risk of aspiration and enhance clarity during surgery, suction by endoscopy was performed before trachea cannula.

After general anesthesia, the esophagogastric junction (EGJ) was reached with the transparent cap attached to the distal of endoscopy, and the distance from EGJ to incisors was measured by the scale along the scope. The transparent cap was used to help maintain a clear field of view [10]. Submucosal injection was then performed (at the position of 6 o'clock) approximately 10 cm proximal to EGJ (Figure 1(a)). The electrocautery knife was then used to create a 1-2 cm incision. The endoscopy was maneuvered through the incision into the submucosa (Figure 1(b)). The injection was repeated until a submucosal tunnel was created (Figure 1(c)), passing over the EGJ, for a distal tunnel of 2-3 cm into the stomach. Spindle vessels narrowing followed by widening of the submucosal tunnel at the EGJ were used as markers of entry into the gastric side [11]. The myotomy began at about 2 cm distal to the mucosal entry, approximately 8 cm above the EGJ, and the distal was extended to the fundus of the stomach in all patients.

In group B, selective dissection of the circular muscular layer was done with careful protection of the longitudinal muscular layer (Figures 1(d) and 2(b-1)). In group A, a partial full-thickness myotomy was adopted. In this method, only circular muscle layer was cut from approximately 8 cm to 2 cm above the EGJ. Then both inner circular muscular layer and outer longitudinal muscular layer were cut from 2 cm above the EGJ to the fundus of the stomach (Figures 1(e) and 2(a-1)). After the myotomy was completed, the endoscopy was withdrawn and passed through the stomach to ensure that adequate increase in EGJ compliance has been achieved. The submucosal tunnel was then irrigated with antibiotic solution and the incision was closed with endoscopic metallic clips (Figures 1(f), 2(a-2), and 2(b-2)).

2.7. Measurements. Procedure-related parameters are operation success rate (percentage of patients who successfully received tunnel creation and myotomy), procedure time, and length of myotomy. Efficacy was compared by short-term remission rate (Eckardt score ≤ 3), recurrence rate [12], and postoperative manometry outcomes. Safety parameters

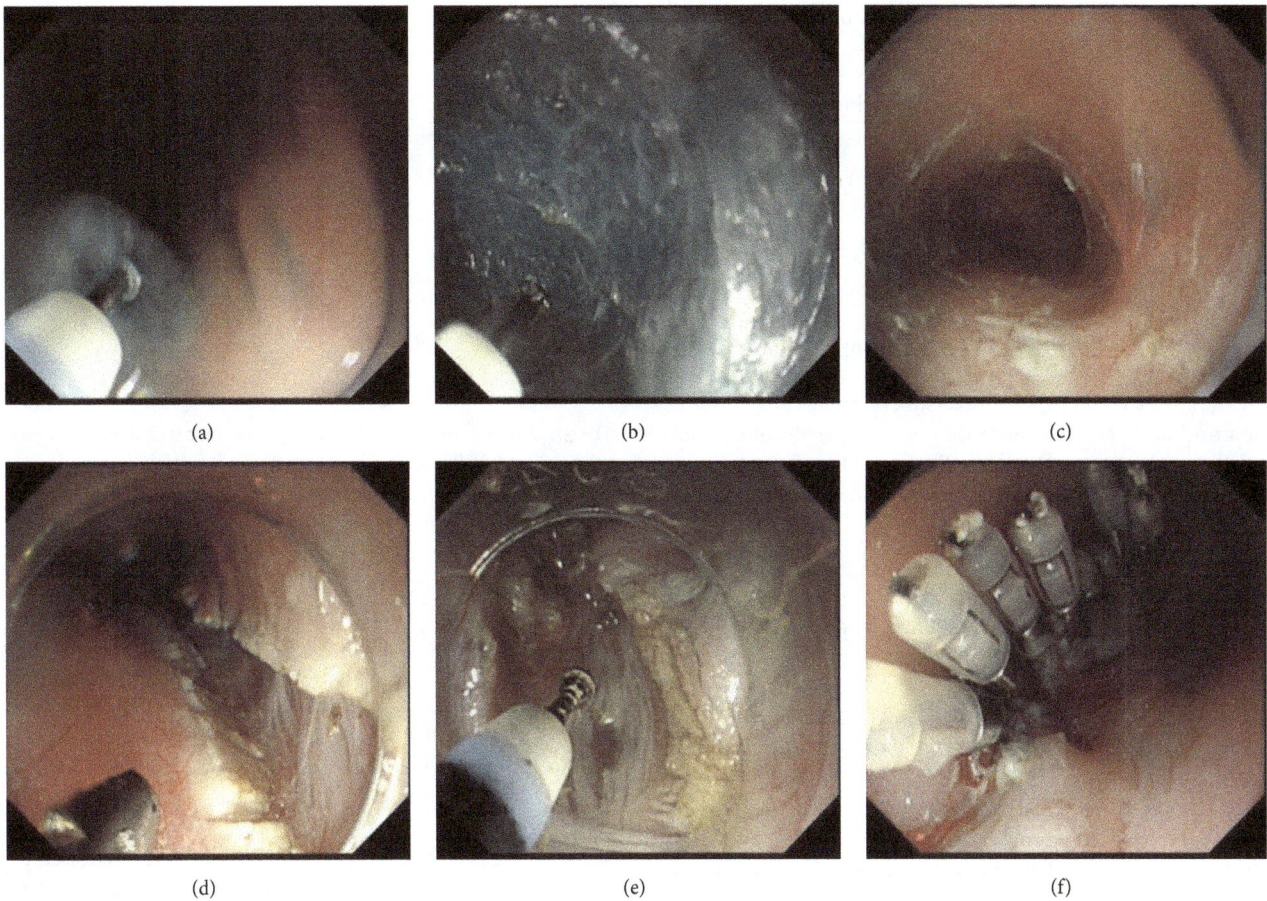

FIGURE 1: (a) Submucosal injection. (b) Creating submucosal tunnel. (c) Submucosal tunnel was dissected. (d) Circular muscle myotomy. (e) full-thickness muscle myotomy. (f) Closure of the mucosal entry site (with metallic clips).

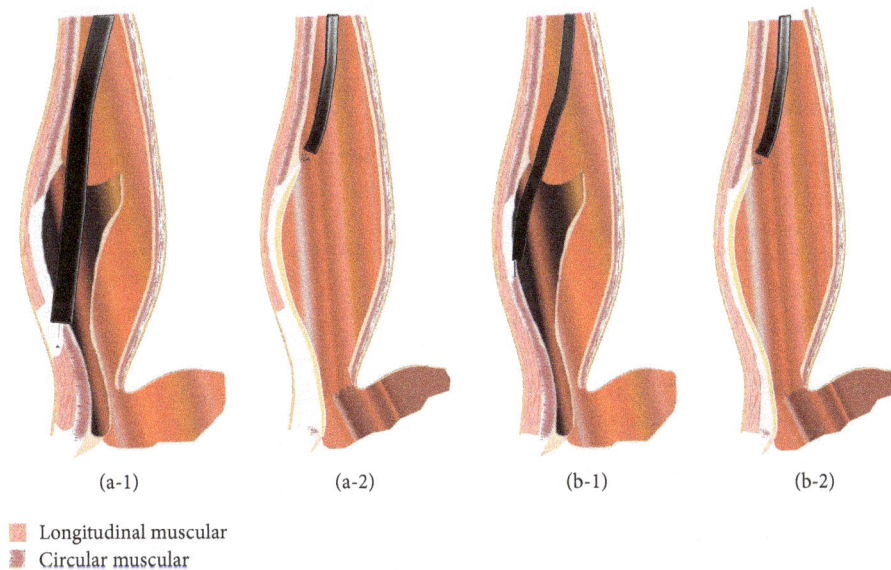

Longitudinal muscular
Circular muscular

FIGURE 2: (a-1) The myotomy was begun at about 2 cm distal to the mucosal entry. In partial full-thickness myotomy, not only the circular muscle layer but also the longitudinal muscle layer was cut at 2 cm above the EGJ. (a-2) Distal of full-thickness myotomy was extended to the fundus of the stomach. Incision was closed by endoscopic metallic clips. (b-1) The myotomy was begun at about 2 cm distal to the mucosal entry in partial full-thickness myotomy. In circular muscle myotomy, only circular muscle layer was resected and the longitudinal muscle layer was carefully protected. (b-2) Distal of circular muscle myotomy was extended to the fundus of the stomach. Incision was closed by endoscopic metallic clips.

TABLE 2: Eckardt symptom score.

Score	Symptoms			
	Weight loss (Kg)	Dysphagia	Chest pain	Regurgitation
0	None	None	None	None
1	<5	Occasional	Occasional	Occasional
2	5~10	Daily	Daily	Daily
3	>10	Every meal	Every meal	Every meal

TABLE 3: Procedure-related parameters.

Parameters	Group A (n = 19)	Group B (n = 14)	p value
Operation success rate	100%	100%	1.00
Operation time (min)	56.73 ± 20.51	88.21 ± 27.08	**<0.01**
Tunnel creation time (min)	15.24 ± 2.81	16.93 ± 3.43	0.16
Myotomy time (min)	41.49 ± 19.71	71.29 ± 24.68	**<0.01**
Myotomy length (cm)	10.33 ± 0.90	9.86 ± 1.70	0.36

are procedure-related adverse events: delayed bleeding (24 h after surgery) [13], mucosal injury, fever (temperature > 37.6°C), air related complications (subcutaneous emphysema, pneumothorax, and pneumoperitoneum), pneumonia, pleural effusion, and mediastinal effusion [14]. Clinical reflux complications are based on symptoms and endoscopic evidence (erosion).

2.8. Postprocedure Management. Patients were kept in supine position for 4 h. For most patients, a postoperative CT scan was performed on the first day after POEM to evaluate procedure-related adverse events such as subcutaneous emphysema, pneumothorax, and pneumoperitoneum. Patients were kept 48~72 h fasting water and on a liquid diet for an additional 1 to 2 weeks, after which soft food were introduced. All patients, postoperatively, were given prophylactic proton pump inhibitor (PPI). Oral administration was continued for at least one month after hospital discharged. Routine follow-up was undertaken for 12 months. All patients' Eckardt scores were collected (Table 2). Patients who underwent partial full-thickness myotomy were examined by manometry, upper endoscopy, and barium esophagram at 6–12 months after procedure.

2.9. Statistical Analysis. IBM SPSS 23.0 software was used for the statistical analysis. Measured values were expressed as means with standard deviations. Statistical significance of normally distributed data was evaluated using Student's *t*-test for independent parameters or paired *t*-test for paired samples. All reported p values were 2-tailed, and statistical significance was considered when p values were <0.05.

3. Results

3.1. Procedure-Related Parameters. The POEM procedure was accomplished successfully (tunnel creation and muscle layer myotomy) in all cases (100%). While mean tunnel creation times were similar (15.24 ± 2.81 versus 16.93 ± 3.43, p = 0.16), mean myotomy time and mean procedure time were significantly shorter in group A compared to group B (p < 0.01), as indicated in Table 3.

3.2. Comparison of Efficiency. The overall efficiency was notable; Eckardt score for postoperative symptom verses preoperative was 0.45 ± 0.83 versus 6.52 ± 1.82, p < 0.01. Postoperative Eckardt score showed no difference between the two groups (0.47 ± 0.77 versus 0.50 ± 0.94, p = 0.93).

Treatment success rate (postoperative Eckardt score < 3 at 1st month) was 100% in both groups.

Comparisons of efficiency follow-up of short-term remission rates (Eckardt score ≤ 3) in a total 33 patients at the 1st, 3rd, 6th, and 12th month were 97.0% (32 of 33), 97.0% (32 of 33), 91.1% (30 of 33), and 87.9% (29 of 33), respectively. Accomplished with manometry and gastroscopes as accessory examinations, recurrence rate was 0% in patients who underwent partial full-thickness myotomy. Remission rates in group A at 1st, 3rd, 6th, and 12th months were 100% (19 of 19), 94.7% (18 of 19), and 89.4% (17 of 19) respectively, while that in group B were 92.9% (13 of 14), 85.7% (12 of 14), and 85.7% (12 of 14), respectively. There was no significant difference between the two groups (p > 0.05 for all time points between the groups). Nine patients underwent postoperative manometry, 5 patients from group A and 4 patients from group B (Table 4(b)). Postoperative IRP (integrated relaxation pressure) and LESP (lower esophageal sphincter pressure) were significantly reduced compared to preoperative data (p < 0.01). Figure 3 Showed the preoperative manometry and postoperative manometry micrographs of representative cases. Outcomes of postoperative IRP were similar between the two groups (3.18 ± 1.97 versus 3.05 ± 1.32, p = 0.91).

3.3. Comparison of Adverse Events. Three patients in group A and 1 patient in group B had mucosal injury (p = 0.62); 1 or 2 metallic clips were used for closing each of the perforations. Seven patients from group A (36.8%) and 4 patients from group B (28.6%) experienced fever on the second day after operation, while 2 patients in group A and 1 in group B developed pneumonia. No significant differences in these events were observed between the two groups. Comparisons of gas related adverse events were subcutaneous emphysema: 2 [10.5%] versus 3 [21.4%], p = 0.63; pneumomediastinum: 3 [15.7%] versus 2 [14.3%], p = 0.97; pneumoperitoneum: 3 [15.7%] versus 2 [14.3%], p = 0.97; and comparison of effusion were 8 [42.1%] versus 6 [42.8%], p = 0.96. No delayed bleeding or pneumothorax was observed (Table 5).

Detection of reflux was based on symptoms such as heartburns, regurgitation, and chest pains. During follow-up, the reflux complication rate was 10.5% (2 of 19) at 6th month and 31.5% (6 of 19) at 12th month for group A and for group B, respectively, and the corresponding incidences were 14.2% (2 of 14) and 35.7% (5 of 14), Table 6. Thus, no statistical significance existed between the groups. Ten

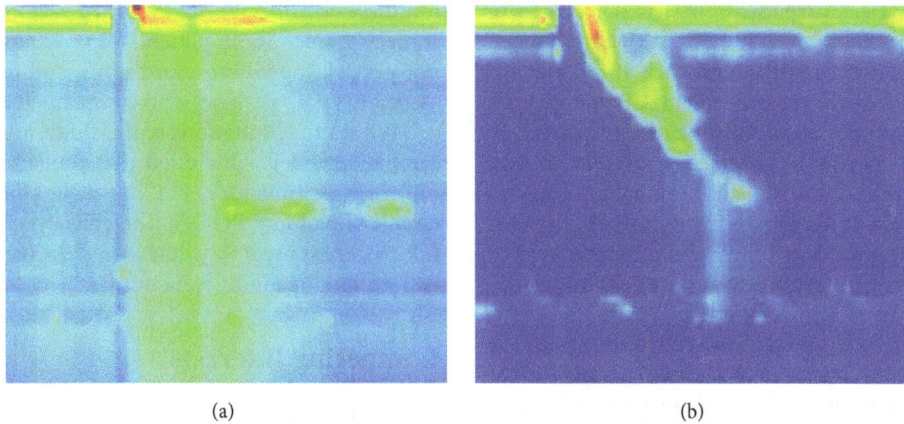

(a)   (b)

FIGURE 3: (a) A case of preoperative manometry showed Type II (absence of normal peristalsis and panoesophageal pressurization with ≥20% of swallows). (b) Postoperative manometry showed significant amelioration of panoesophageal pressurization.

TABLE 4: (a) Comparison of symptom relief (by Eckardt). (b) Preoperative and postoperative IRP and LESP Comparison (mmH$_2$O).

(a)

Parameters	Group A (n = 19)	Group B (n = 14)	p value
Preoperative symptom score	6.74 ± 1.79	6.64 ± 1.86	0.89
Postoperative symptom score	0.47 ± 0.77	0.50 ± 0.94	0.93
1-month remission rate	100% (19/19)	92.9% (13/14)	0.42
6-month remission rate	94.7% (18/19)	85.7% (12/14)	0.56
12-month remission rate	89.4% (17/19)	85.7% (12/14)	0.61

(b)

Parameters	Totally (n = 9)	Group A (n = 5)	Group B (n = 4)
IRP			
Preoperative	16.47 ± 4.89	16.30 ± 5.05	19.17 ± 1.65
Postoperative	3.12 ± 1.61	3.18 ± 1.97	3.05 ± 1.32
p value	**<0.01**	**0.04**	**<0.01**
LESP			
Preoperative	34.72 ± 18.58	37.60 ± 20.50	32.80 ± 10.91
Postoperative	10.49 ± 11.92	12.56 ± 15.21	9.10 ± 10.54
p value	**<0.01**	**0.021**	**<0.01**

IRP: integrated relaxation pressure and LESP: lower esophageal sphincter pressure.

TABLE 5: Comparison of procedure related adverse events.

Variable	Group A (n = 19)	Group B (n = 14)	p value
Mucosal injury	3 (15.7%)	1 (7.1%)	0.62
Fever	7 (36.8%)	4 (28.6%)	0.45
Pneumonia	2 (10.5%)	1 (7.1%)	0.55
Air-related complications	4 (21.1%)	5 (35.7%)	0.44
Subcutaneous emphysema	2 (10.5%)	3 (21.4%)	0.63
Pneumomediastinum	3 (15.7%)	2 (14.3%)	0.97
Pneumoperitoneum	3 (15.7%)	2 (14.3%)	0.97
Pneumothorax	0 (0.0%)	0 (0.0%)	1.00
Delayed bleeding	0 (0.0%)	0 (0.0%)	1.00
Effusion	8 (42.1%)	6 (42.8%)	0.96

TABLE 6: Comparison of reflux complication.

Variable	Group A	Group B	p value
Reflux rate by symptom at 6th	10.5% (2 of 19)	14.2% (2 of 14)	0.63
Reflux rate by symptom at 12th	31.5% (6 of 19)	35.7% (5 of 14)	0.71
Reflux rate base on endoscopy at 12th	26.7% (4 of 15)	25% (3 of 12)	0.96

4. Discussion

Achalasia (AC) is an idiopathic disease of the esophagus characterized by inability of the LES to relax while swallowing. This condition weakens the quality of life of sufferers. Treatments for AC patients mostly aim at decreasing the residual pressure of the LES so that ingested material can pass into the stomach unimpeded. Previous study has showed that both endoscopic pneumatic dilation and LHM were effective in correcting the disorder [11]. Since 2010 when POEM was first applied in humans, study has confirmed its excellent outcome and advantages as compared to laparoscopic myotomy and

out of the 27 (37.0%) patients who underwent postoperative esophagogastroscopy complained about reflux symptoms. Comparing group A with group B (through endoscopic findings of reflux esophagitis), the reflux rate was 26.6% (4 of 15) versus 25% (3 of 12), $p = 0.96$.

pneumatic dilation [15]. Currently, POEM is performed in multiple centers worldwide as the first-line therapy of AC. However, some aspects or modifications such as the method of myotomy still need further improvement. Compared with circular muscle myotomy, partial full-thickness myotomy in POEM surgery also begins with selective circular muscle bundle myotomy from 2 cm distal to the mucosal entry to approximately 2 cm above the EGJ. A myotomy of both inner circular muscle layer and outer longitudinal muscle layer is then performed during partial full-thickness myotomy.

This study discussed two methods of POEM by comparing the operation success rate, procedure time, surgery efficacy, and safety. Success rates of the two groups (of the different methods) were 100% each. Mean procedure time was significantly shorter in partial full thickness myotomy group than circular muscle myotomy group. During circular muscle myotomy, much time is consumed by carefully distinguishing and protecting the longitudinal bundles. In full-thickness myotomy, however, both circular and longitudinal layers are craved in corresponding sections, and this could be the source of time saving.

As shown in Tables 4(a) and 4(b), the overall efficiency was notable. The postoperative Eckardt score significantly reduced from 6.52 ± 1.82 to 0.45 ± 0.83, $p < 0.01$, but the efficacy was equivalent between the two groups. Five patients in group A and four in group B underwent postoperative manometry, as compared with preoperative data. IRP reduced from 16.30 ± 5.05 mmH$_2$O to 3.18 ± 1.97 mmH$_2$O in group A ($p = 0.04$), and from 19.17 ± 1.65 mmH$_2$O to 3.05 ± 1.32 mmH$_2$O in group B ($p = 0.01$). It is worth noting that there was no statistical difference between the two groups with regard to postoperative esophageal pressure ($p = 0.91$), which meant that partial full thickness myotomy might not increase the incidence of postoperative reflux rate. As compared with circular muscle myotomy, partial full-thickness myotomy did not significantly reduce IRP and did not increase reflux rate.

As shown in Tables 5 and 6, there were no statistical differences in procedure-related adverse events or complications between the two groups. In total, 11 cases developed fever on the first day after the procedure. The temperature of these cases fluctuated between 37.6°C and 38.1°C. Diagnosis from routine blood test and CT revealed that two patients had aspiration pneumonia. Nine of the patients exhibited postoperative absorption heat. However, body temperatures returned to normal after the administration of intravenous antibiotic infusion combined with physical hypothermia method. Other patients with fever were asymptomatic, and no drug intervention but physical hypothermia method was used. There were three patients in group A of mucosal injury during the surgery. Two of the cases had preoperative esophagitis in lower segment. Adhesion and fibrosis due to previous esophagitis may refer to the mucosal injury during tunnel creation period. Mucosal integrity was repaired with metallic clips during the surgery.

The overall reflux complication rate by symptoms was 34.4%; the rate was 25.9% by endoscopic findings of reflux esophagitis, with no statistical difference between the two groups (all $p > 0.05$). Factors that might have accounted

for these include the ingestion of acid-inhibitory drug by some patients. Some patients were exposed in acid reflux, not yet developed into esophagitis, and neurosis which was associated with patients who complained about chest pain.

Within the limitations of the study, especially the limited sample size, it is concluded that procedure time of partial full-thickness myotomy POEM was significantly shorter than circular myotomy POEM. The efficacy and safety of partial full-thickness myotomy POEM and circular myotomy POEM had no significant differences.

Competing Interests

The authors declare that there is no conflict of interests regarding the publication of this paper.

References

[1] S. P. Shin, G. W. Song, and W. J. Ko, "Clinical outcomes of Peroral endoscopic myotomy for achalasia depend on manometric subtype," *Gastrointestinal Endoscopy*, vol. 5, no. 84, p. 494, 2015.

[2] M. E. Allaix and M. G. Patti, "New trends and concepts in diagnosis and treatment of achalasia," *Cirugía Española*, vol. 91, no. 6, pp. 352–357, 2013.

[3] H. Inoue, H. Minami, Y. Kobayashi et al., "Peroral endoscopic myotomy (POEM) for esophageal achalasia," *Endoscopy*, vol. 42, no. 4, pp. 265–271, 2010.

[4] S. N. Stavropoulos, D. J. Desilets, K.-H. Fuchs et al., "Per-oral endoscopic myotomy white paper summary," *Gastrointestinal Endoscopy*, vol. 80, no. 1, pp. 1–15, 2014.

[5] M. Min, L. H. Peng, Y. S. Yang et al., "Characteristics of achalasia subtypes in untreated chinese patients: a high-resolution manometry study," *Journal of Digestive Diseases*, vol. 13, no. 10, pp. 504–509, 2012.

[6] A. J. Bredenoord, M. Fox, P. J. Kahrilas, J. E. Pandolfino, W. Schwizer, and A. J. P. M. Smout, "Chicago classification criteria of esophageal motility disorders defined in high resolution esophageal pressure topography," *Neurogastroenterology and Motility*, vol. 24, no. 1, pp. 57–65, 2012.

[7] S. Roman, F. Zerbib, L. Queneherve, H. Clermidy, S. B. D. Varannes, and F. Mion, "The Chicago classification for achalasia in a French multicentric cohort," *Digestive and Liver Disease*, vol. 44, no. 12, pp. 976–980, 2012.

[8] Y. Zhong, Q. Shi, P.-H. Zhou, and L. I.-Q. Yao, "Su1542 the application value of endoscopic ultrasonography (EUS) before peroral endoscopic myotomy (POEM) for esophageal achalasia (EA)," *Gastrointestinal Endoscopy*, vol. 77, no. 5, p. 362, 2013.

[9] M. A. Barnes, A. S. Ho, P. S. Malhotra, P. J. Koltai, and A. Messner, "The use of botulinum toxin for pediatric cricopharyngeal achalasia," *International Journal of Pediatric Otorhinolaryngology*, vol. 75, no. 9, pp. 1210–1214, 2011.

[10] A. S. Yague, T. Kaltenbach, and H. Yamamoto, "The endoscopic cap that can," *Gastrointestinal Endoscopy*, vol. 1, no. 76, pp. 169–178, 2012.

[11] H. Inoue, H. Sato, H. Ikeda et al., "Per-oral endoscopic myotomy: a series of 500 patients," *Journal of the American College of Surgeons*, vol. 221, no. 2, pp. 256–264, 2015.

[12] A. Fovos, O. Jarral, V. Patel, T. Podas, D. Spalding, and E. Zacharakis, "Does Heller's myotomy provide superior clinical

outcome in comparison to botulinum toxin injection for treatment of achalasia? Best evidence topic (BET)," *International Journal of Surgery*, vol. 10, no. 3, pp. 120–123, 2012.

[13] G. E. Boeckxstaens, V. Annese, S. B. Des Varannes et al., "Pneumatic dilation versus laparoscopic Heller's myotomy for idiopathic achalasia," *New England Journal of Medicine*, vol. 364, no. 19, pp. 1807–1816, 2011.

[14] A. Khafagy and I. Abdelnaby, "Efficacy of pneumatic dilatation as a definitive therapeutic modality for classic achalasia," *Egyptian Journal of Ear, Nose, Throat and Allied Sciences*, vol. 14, no. 3, pp. 161–168, 2013.

[15] D. Von Renteln, H. Inoue, H. Minami et al., "Peroral endoscopic myotomy for the treatment of achalasia: a prospective single center study," *American Journal of Gastroenterology*, vol. 107, no. 3, pp. 411–417, 2012.

9

Platelet Count to Spleen Diameter Ratio for the Diagnosis of Gastroesophageal Varices in Liver Cirrhosis

Runhua Chen,[1] Han Deng,[2] Xia Ding,[3] Chune Xie,[4] Wei Wang,[5] and Qian Shen[6]

[1] Department of Gastroenterology, Dongfang Hospital, Beijing University of Chinese Medicine, Beijing, China
[2] Postgraduate College, Dalian Medical University, Dalian, China
[3] Department of Hospital Administration, Beijing University of Chinese Medicine, Beijing, China
[4] Department of Personnel, Dongfang Hospital, Beijing University of Chinese Medicine, Beijing, China
[5] Department of Cardiology, Wangjing Hospital, China Academy of Chinese Medical Sciences, Beijing, China
[6] Department of Massage and Physiotherapy, Dongfang Hospital, Beijing University of Chinese Medicine, Beijing, China

Correspondence should be addressed to Qian Shen; rbd144@163.com

Academic Editor: Nianping Feng

Platelet count to spleen diameter ratio (PSR) was studied extensively as a noninvasive method of diagnosis for varices. The present study aimed to systematically assess the performance of PSR in the diagnosis of varices. PubMed, EMBASE, and article references were searched. The summary receiver operating characteristic curves (AUSROCs), sensitivities, specificities, positive and negative likelihood ratio, and diagnostic odds ratio were calculated. The heterogeneity, quality, and publication bias of studies were evaluated. Subgroup and sensitivity analyses were performed. A total of 49 papers were included. The AUSROCs of PSR for any varices and high-risk varices were 0.8719 and 0.8132, respectively. The summary sensitivities of PSR for any varices and high-risk varices were 0.84 and 0.78, respectively. The summary specificities of PSR for any varices and high-risk varices were 0.78 and 0.67, respectively. The AUSROC of PSR for any varices at the threshold of 909 was 0.8867. The AUSROC of PSR for any varices in viral liver cirrhosis was 0.8675. The overall quality of studies was moderate. Significant heterogeneity and publication bias existed in the study. In conclusion, PSR can be used to identify varices in liver cirrhosis. PSR had a high sensitivity in viral liver cirrhosis.

1. Introduction

Gastroesophageal varices are one of the major complications of liver cirrhosis. Early detection of varices in cirrhotic patients is crucial to ensure timely initiation of prophylactic therapies. Platelet count to spleen diameter ratio (PSR) was first proposed by Giannini et al. to predict the presence of varices in 2003 [1]. An increasing number of studies have since evaluated the accuracy of PSR in the detection of varices, albeit drawing inconsistent conclusions. In two previous meta-analyses regarding the diagnostic accuracy of PSR in predicting the presence of varices, Ying et al. [2] recommended using PSR to identify varices to decrease the use of upper gastrointestinal endoscopy, while Chawla et al. [3] found that PSR has low grade evidence to replace upper gastrointestinal endoscopy as a noninvasive method

for varices. The performance of PSR for varices is still not unified at present, which has limited the use of PSR in clinical practice. Thus, we conducted this systematic review and meta-analysis to evaluate the performance of PSR for varices.

2. Methods

Selection, data extraction, and quality assessment of studies were conducted by two investigators (RC and QS) independently. Disagreement between the two investigators was resolved by a consensus.

2.1. Search Strategy and Selection Criteria. PubMed and EMBASE were searched on May 27, 2016. The search terms were as follows: (((((((platelet count to spleen diameter ratio)

OR PSR) OR PC/SD)) OR ((((platelet) OR platelet count)) AND ((spleen) OR spleen diameter)))) AND liver cirrhosis) AND varices. Relevant references were also screened. Duplicates, commentaries, reviews, case reports, letters, meta-analyses, book sections, and meeting abstracts were excluded. The inclusion criteria were as follows: (1) participants should be diagnosed with liver cirrhosis; (2) upper gastrointestinal endoscopy should be performed as the reference tests for the diagnosis of varices; (3) PSR should be performed as alternative tests for the diagnosis of varices; (4) diagnostic accuracy data of PSR on the diagnosis of varices were available. The language and publication year were not limited.

2.2. Data Extraction. The following data from each study was extracted: the first author, publication year, region, study design, total number of patients, age, sex, etiology of liver cirrhosis, hepatocellular carcinoma (HCC), Child-Pugh class, location of varices (i.e., esophageal varices [EV] and/or gastric varices [GV]), prevalence of any varices and/or high-risk (or large) varices, cut-off value, true positive (TP) value, false positive (FP) value, false negative (FN) value, and true negative (TN) value. Missing values were calculated using the following formulae: sensitivity = TP/(TP + FN), and specificity = TN/(TN + FP). The raw TP, FN, FP, and TN numbers of included studies were shown in Supplementary Table 1 (see Supplementary Material available online at https://doi.org/10.1155/2017/7407506).

2.3. Quality Assessment. The quality of each study was assessed by QUADAS-2 (Quality Assessment of Diagnostic Accuracy Studies-2) tool [4]. This tool comprises four domains: patient selection, index test, reference standard, and flow and timing. The risk of bias in each domain was rated as "low risk," "high risk," and "unclear risk" with signaling questions. The applicability concerns in the first three domains were assessed as "low concern," "high concern," and "unclear concern." If the total number of "low risk" and "high concern" was equal or greater than 6 in a study, the study was considered as high quality.

2.4. Statistical Analysis. The area under the summary receiver operating characteristic curves (AUSROCs) with standard errors (SEs) and Q indexes with SEs, summary sensitivities and specificities with 95% confidence intervals (CIs), summary positive and negative likelihood ratios (PLRs and NLRs) with 95% CIs, and summary diagnostic odds ratios (DORs) with 95% CIs were calculated using statistical software (Meta-Disc software version 1.4). We analyzed these data using the random-effects model. The diagnostic threshold was analyzed by Spearman correlation coefficient and p value. $p < 0.05$ showed a statistically significant diagnostic threshold effect. Therefore, only AUSROCs with SEs and Q indexes with SEs were calculated. The heterogeneity among studies was evaluated by Chi-square test and inconsistency index. A statistically significant heterogeneity was defined as $p < 0.1$ and/or $I^2 > 50\%$.

To explore the publication bias, we performed Deeks' funnel plot asymmetry test in Stata 12.0 (College Station, TX,

USA). Sensitivity analyses were performed via removing each study to evaluate the impact on the pooled results of the removed study.

We calculated the diagnostic accuracy of PSR for various cut-off values in predicting the presence of any and high-risk varices. If there were multiple different cut-off values in the same paper, we selected the optimal cut-off values. PSR for any varices at threshold of 909 was the most generally accepted cut-off value at present. Thus, we performed subgroup analyses using the cut-off value of 909. In addition, we performed subgroup analyses based on the etiology of cirrhosis, region, study design, prevalence of varices, sample size, and study quality for any varices.

3. Results

3.1. Selection of Studies. A total of 345 papers were selected from PubMed ($n = 120$), EMBASE ($n = 218$), and manual search ($n = 7$). The flow diagram of study selection was shown in Figure 1. 112 duplicates and 145 irrelevant papers were excluded. Then, we screened 88 full-text articles for eligibility. 39 papers which lacked relevant diagnostic data were excluded. Among them, 28 papers were applied only with abstracts. Finally, 49 papers [1, 5–52] were included in our study. 42 and 16 papers were about any varices and high-risk varices, respectively.

3.2. Characteristics of Studies. The characteristics of studies were shown in Table 1. Our meta-analysis included a total of 6274 patients. 22 papers were prospective studies. 2 papers [10, 20] were published in abstracts and 47 papers were full-texts. The etiologies of cirrhosis were alcohol, schistosomiasis, and viral hepatitis in 1 [12], 2 [5, 32], and 13 [9, 19, 22, 26, 27, 30, 33, 36, 39, 40, 42–44] papers, respectively. Two papers were about EV and GV [8, 12], and the rest of the papers were about EV alone. In two papers, all patients had Child-Pugh A [22, 40]. The diagnostic accuracy of PSR for any varices at threshold of 909 was reported in 19 papers.

3.3. Quality Assessment of Studies. The overall quality of the included studies was not very high (Supplementary Table 2). In the patient selection domain, only 17 papers were rated as "low risk." In the index test and reference standard domains, 10 and 14 papers were rated as "low risk." Most papers had not reported whether investigators were blinded when interpreting the results of index test and reference standard. 2 papers were rated as "high risk" in flow and timing domain as the interval time between index test and reference standard was greater than 3 months. 44 papers have "high concern" in patient selection domain. In addition, all papers were rated as "high concern" in index test and reference standard domains. 11 papers were considered with high quality.

3.4. Overall Results. Significant threshold effect was not found in overall meta-analyses.

Diagnostic accuracy of PSR for the presence of any varices was pooled from 42 papers [1, 5–10, 13, 14, 16–19, 21–34, 36–40, 42–50, 52]. The AUSROC was 0.8719 (Figure 2(a)). The summary sensitivity and specificity were 0.84 (95%

Records identified through database searching
(i) PubMed ($n = 120$)
(ii) EMBASE ($n = 218$)

Additional records identified through manual search ($n = 7$)

233 records screened after duplicates removed

145 excluded
(i) Reviews ($n = 6$)
(ii) Case reports ($n = 20$)
(iii) Commentary ($n = 3$)
(iv) Letter ($n = 9$)
(v) Meta-analyses ($n = 2$)
(vi) Book section ($n = 1$)
(vii) Meeting abstracts ($n = 2$)
(viii) Unrelated to varices, PSR, and/or cirrhosis ($n = 102$)

88 full-text articles assessed for eligibility

Excluded
Lack of relevant data ($n = 39$)

49 studies included in meta-analysis

Predict the presence of varices ($n = 42$)

Predict the presence of high-risk varices ($n = 16$)

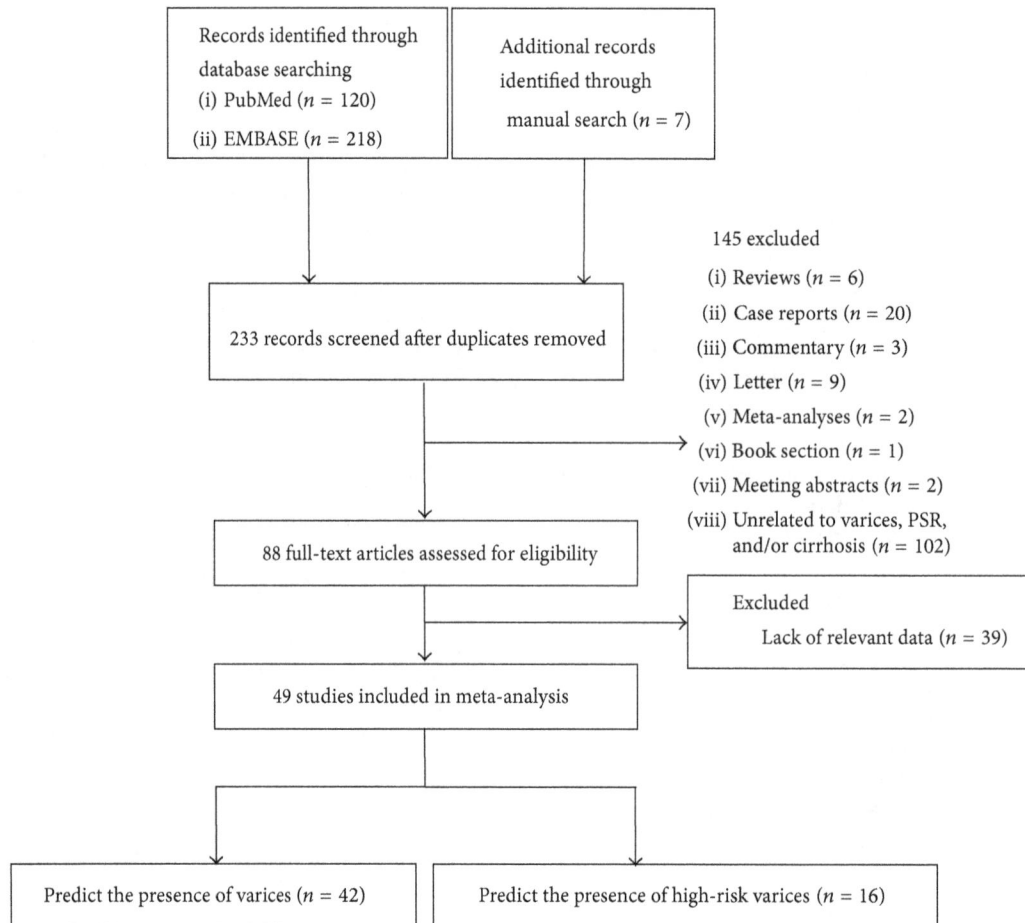

FIGURE 1: Flowchart of study selection.

CI: 0.83–0.85) and 0.78 (95% CI: 0.76–0.79), respectively (Figure 3). The summary PLR, NLR, and DOR were 3.54 (95% CI: 2.75–4.56), 0.17 (95% CI: 0.12–0.23), and 25.32 (95% CI: 15.72–40.77), respectively.

Diagnostic accuracy of PSR for the presence of high-risk varices was pooled from 16 papers [6, 7, 11–13, 15, 17, 19, 20, 22, 25, 29, 30, 35, 41, 51]. The AUSROC was 0.8132 (Figure 2(b)). The summary sensitivity and specificity were 0.78 (95% CI: 0.75–0.81) and 0.67 (95% CI: 0.64–0.71), respectively (Figure 4). The summary PLR, NLR, and DOR were 2.54 (95% CI: 1.99–3.24), 0.32 (95% CI: 0.24–0.44), and 9.08 (95% CI: 5.33–15.47), respectively. The diagnostic accuracy of PSR for high-risk varices was lower than PSR for any varices.

3.5. Subgroup Results. The subgroup results were summarized in Table 2. Significant threshold effect was found in the subgroup of South America. Thus, their diagnostic accuracy was not combined.

3.6. Heterogeneity. Significant heterogeneity between papers was found in most analyses except for the subgroup of North America and sample size less than 100.

3.7. Sensitivity Analyses. Sensitivity analysis results were similar to the overall meta-analysis results. The heterogeneity remained significant (data not shown).

3.8. Publication Bias. The publication bias existed in the study ($p = 0.007$).

4. Discussions

In our study, the AUSROC of PSR for any varices was 0.8719. The summary sensitivity and specificity were 0.84 and 0.78, respectively. The diagnostic accuracy of PSR for high-risk varices was lower than PSR for any varices. The diagnostic accuracy of PSR for varices at threshold of 909 was similar to PSR at various thresholds. While the summary sensitivity (0.92) in viral liver cirrhosis was improved over that of mixed etiologies, they had the same summary specificities (0.78). The subgroup analysis of Asia had the highest AUSROC (0.9195).

The high diagnostic accuracy of PSR for varices can be explained as follows. Varices and hypersplenism are the results of portal hypertension. The platelet count can be influenced by many factors in cirrhotic patients other than hypersplenism. The decreased thrombopoietin production is the reason. Thrombopoietin is mainly produced by hepatocytes and the quantity can be largely reduced when the hepatocytes was damaged. In addition, the shortened platelet mean lifetime and myelotoxic effects of alcohol or hepatitis viruses also reduced the platelet count. Splenomegaly is the clinical manifestation of hypersplenism. Thus, a combined

TABLE 1: Characteristics of studies.

First author (year)	Regions	Study design	Number of total Pts	Age (year)	Male (%)	Etiology of cirrhosis	HCC (%)	Child-Pugh class (%)	Location of varices	Prevalence of varices (%)	Prevalence of high-risk/large varices (%)	Cut-off of varices
Karatzas (2016)	Greece	Prospective	38	63	78.9%	Alcohol 47.4% Viral hepatitis 34.2% Others 18.4%	NA	A, 55.3% B, 28.9% C, 15.8%	EV + GV	63.2%	10.5%	1310.597 (optimal) 909
Kim (2016)	South Korea	Retrospective	103	53.5 ± 11.8	65.0%	Alcohol 28.2% HBV 50.5% HCV 8.7% HBV and alcohol 7.8% Others 4.9%	NA	NA	EV	38.8%	12.6%	860
Takuma (2016)	Japan	Prospective	60	70.8 ± 9.9	56.7%	Alcohol 10% HBV 13.3% HCV 58.3% Others 18.3%	NA	A, 68.3% B, 30% C, 1.7%	EV	40.0%	26.7%	3.36
Xu (2016)	China	Prospective	236	61.4 ± 10.2	43.2%	Schistosomiasis 100%	NA	NA	EV	40.3%	NA	1004 (optimal) 909
Albreedy (2015)	Egypt	Prospective	100	44.24 ± 7.05	58.0%	NA	0%	A, 41% B, 33% C, 26%	EV	66.0%	47.0%	979.9
Cho (2015)	South Korea	Retrospective	219	52/50*	91.8%	Alcohol 100%	0%	A, 59.4% B, 36.1% C, 4.6%	EV + GV	NA	33.3%	NA
Stefanescu (2015)	Romania	Cross-sectional	90	56.47 ± 9.38/54.98 ± 8.42*	55.6%	Alcohol 33.3% HBV 13.3% HCV 33.3% Others 20%	0%	A, 62.2% B, 35.6% C, 2.2%	EV	81.1%	52.2%	NA
Valero (2015) (abstract)	Philippines	Retrospective	101	64.8/61.6	NA	NA	0%	NA	EV	85.1%	NA	1.86
Zhao (2015)	China	Retrospective	124	51.34 ± 11.089	57.3%	HCV 100%	NA	NA	EV	51.6%	NA	909

TABLE 1: Continued.

First author (year)	Regions	Study design	Number of total Pts	Age (year)	Male (%)	Etiology of cirrhosis	HCC (%)	Child-Pugh class (%)	Location of varices	Prevalence of varices (%)	Prevalence of high-risk/large varices (%)	Cut-off of varices
Chiodi (2014)	Uruguay	Retrospective	125	54	56.8%	Alcohol 40% HBV 3.2% HCV 16.8% Autoimmune 12% Others 19.2% Unknown 8.8	0%	NA	EV	63.2%	42.4%	1010%
González-Ojeda (2014)	Mexico	Cross-sectional	91	53.75 ± 12	54.9%	Alcohol 52.7% HCV 26.4% Others 11% Unknown 10%	0%	A, 18.7% B, 40.7% C, 40.7%	EV	80.2%	57.1%	884
Wang (2014)	China	Retrospective	104	59	56.7%	Alcohol 17.3% HBV 66.3% Alcohol and HBV 12.5% Unknown 3.8%	NA	A, 24% B, 35.6% C, 40.4%	EV	99.0%	51.9%	NA
Zafar (2014)	Pakistan	Prospective	215	46.93 ± 13.22	42.3%	NA	NA	NA	EV	60.9%	NA	909
Calvaruso (2013)	Italy	Prospective	96	63.2 ± 9.5	69.8%	HCV 100%	0%	A, 100%	EV	56.3%	27.1%	800
Masjedizadeh (2013)	Iran	Prospective	140	57/53	70.0%	Alcohol 3.6% HBV 36.4% HCV 17.1% Autoimmune 8.6% Others 5.7% Unknown 28.6%	NA	A, 43.6% B, 42.1% C, 14.3%	EV	85.0%	33.6%	663
Rajendran (2013) (abstract)	India	Cross-sectional	101	NA	93.1%	Alcohol 85% HBV 9% HCV 5%	NA	NA	EV	95.0%	65.0%	NA
Saad (2013)	Egypt	NA	32	55 ± 6.6/49.5 ± 4.7/ 48.9 ± 4.7*	62.5%	HCV 100%	0%	A, 71.9% B, 28.1%	EV	62.5%	31.3%	545
Sharma (2013)	India	NA	174	49.3 ± 11.7	88.5%	Alcohol 44.3% HBV 13.2% HCV 16.7% Unknown 25.9%	0%	A, 31.6% B, 56.9% C, 11.5%	EV	71.3%	44.8%	1023.2 (optimal) 909
Al-Dahshan (2012)	Egypt	NA	60	52.62 ± 8.22	78.3%	HBV 81.7% HCV 18.3%	0%	NA	EV	66.7%	NA	1023

Table 1: Continued.

First author (year)	Regions	Study design	Number of total Pts	Age (year)	Male (%)	Etiology of cirrhosis	HCC (%)	Child-Pugh class (%)	Location of varices	Prevalence of varices (%)	Prevalence of high-risk/large varices (%)	Cut-off of varices
Colecchia (2012)	Italy	Prospective	100	54	71.0%	HCV 100%	0%	A, 68% B, 32%	EV	53.0%	49.0%	1883 (optimal) 513
Mahassadi (2012)	Cote d'Ivoire	NA (training sample)	111	49	70.3%	Alcohol 20.7% HBV 61.3% HCV 12.6% Others 5.4%	0%	A, 22.5% B, 35.1% C, 42.3%	EV	76.6%	70.3%	868
		NA (validation sample)	91	50	64.2%	Alcohol 26.4% HBV 58.2% HCV 15.4%	0%	A, 19.8% B, 52.7% C, 22% Unknown, 5.5%	EV	79.1%	65.9%	868
Mangone (2012)	Italy	Prospective	87	62.8	58.6%	Alcohol 8% HBV 10.5% HCV 63.2% Others 18.3%	NA	A, 90.8% B, 6.9% Unknown, 2.3%	EV	35.6%	NA	936.364 (optimal) 909
Nisar (2012)	Pakistan	Cross-sectional	150	50.99 ± 12.99	54.0%	NA	NA	NA	EV	68.0%	NA	909
Abu El Makarem (2011)	Egypt	Prospective	175	48	65.7%	HCV 100%	NA	A, 26.3% B, 33.7% C, 40%	EV	74.9%	NA	939.7
Agha (2011)	Italy	Prospective	43	61	70.0%	Schistosomiasis 100%	NA	NA	EV	72.1%	44.2%	885
Cherian (2011)	India	Prospective	229	42	61.6%	Alcohol 42.4% HBV 15.3% HCV 10% Others 12.7% Unknown 19.7%	0%	A, 18.3% B, 55.5% C, 26.2%	EV	77.7%	35.4%	666
Esmat (2011)	Egypt	Prospective	100	49.2 ± 8	48.0%	HCV 100%	NA	A, 20% B, 31% C, 49%	EV	82.0%	60.0%	1326.6 (optimal) 909
Mosqueira (2011)	Peru	Retrospective	47	60.74	50.0%	Alcohol 25.5% HBV 2.1% HCV 14.9% Autoimmune 8.5% Unknown 48.9%	NA	NA	EV	74.5%	46.8%	909
Stefanescu (2011)	Romania	Prospective	137	56	56.2%	Alcohol/HCV 100%	NA	A, 64.9% B, 28.4% C, 6.8%	EV	84.9%	44.0%	1068
Barikbin (2010)	Iran	Prospective	50	52.1 ± 16.2	82.0%	Alcohol 4% HBV 38% HCV 14% Others 6% Unknown 38%	0%	A, 10% B, 28% C, 62%	EV	74.0%	62.0%	921

TABLE 1: Continued.

First author (year)	Regions	Study design	Number of total Pts	Age (year)	Male (%)	Etiology of cirrhosis	HCC (%)	Child-Pugh class (%)	Location of varices	Prevalence of varices (%)	Prevalence of high-risk/large varices (%)	Cut-off of varices
De Mattos (2010)	Brazil	NA	164	56.6 ± 11.6	56.7%	Alcohol 29.3% Viral hepatitis 43.9% Viral hepatitis and alcohol 10.4% Others 16.5%	NA	A, 57.6% B, 37.7% C, 4.6%	EV	73.2%	40.8%	909
Nashaat (2010)	Egypt	NA	50	49.6 ± 8.8	74.0%	HBV 20% HCV 70% HBV and HCV 10%	NA	A, 38% B, 42% C, 20%	EV	88.0%	NA	820
Sarangapani (2010)	India	Prospective	106	45	67.9%	Alcohol 58.5% HBV 21.7% Others 19.8%	0%	NA	EV	72.6%	48.1%	NA%
Schwarzenberger (2010)	US	Retrospective	137	56	64.0%	Alcohol 18% HBV 23% HCV 34% Others 17% Unknown 9	NA	NA	EV	55.5%	18.2%	909
Agha (2009)	Pakistan	Prospective	311	49	55.6%	HCV 100%	0%	A, 25.8% B, 58.6% C, 15.6%	EV	49.5%	12.9%	909
Barrera (2009)	Chile	Prospective	67	66 ± 12.2	43.3%	Alcohol 26.9% Viral hepatitis 7.5% PBC 14.9% Others 26.8% Unknown 26.9%	NA	A, 46.2% B, 38.8% C, 15%	EV	85.1%	49.3%	NA
Cammà (2009)	Italy	Prospective	104	61.4 ± 9.5	57.7%	HCV 100%	0%	A, 100%	EV	60.6%	NA	792
Sharif (2009)	Pakistan	Cross-sectional	100	NA	56.0%	HBV 29% HCV 71%	NA	NA	EV	50.0%	NA	2200
Baig (2008)	India	Prospective	150	51	84.0%	Alcohol 48.7% HBV 26% HCV 9.3% Others 7.3% Unknown 8.7%	NA	A, 64.7% B, 21.3% C, 14%	EV	70.7%	46.7%	1014 (optimal) 909

TABLE 1: Continued.

First author (year)	Regions	Study design	Number of total Pts	Age (year)	Male (%)	Etiology of cirrhosis	HCC (%)	Child-Pugh class (%)	Location of varices	Prevalence of varices (%)	Prevalence of high-risk/large varices (%)	Cut-off of varices
Parrino (2008)	Italy	NA	158	66.6 ± 9.6	63.3%	NA	0%	A, 64% B, 31% C, 5%	EV	74.1%	19.6%	1300
Tao (2008)	China	NA	69	53	63.8%	HBV 100%	NA	A, 20.3% B, 63.8% C, 15.9%	EV	78.3%	NA	909
Yu (2008)	China	Retrospective	89	53	82.0%	HBV 100%	NA	A, 29.2% B, 42.7% C, 28.1%	EV	75.3%	29.2%	909
Lei (2007)	China	Retrospective	326	55	77.3%	Alcohol 4.3% HBV 90.8% HBV and HBV 1.5% Others 3.4%	NA	A, 14.7% B, 67.5% C, 17.8%	EV	41.7%	15.6%	0.55 (optimal) 0.42
Giannini (2006)	Italy	Prospective	218	58/54*	58.7%	Alcohol 18.8% Viral hepatitis 48.2% PBC 16.1% Viral hepatitis and alcohol 12.4% Others 4.6%	8.7%	A, 50.9% B, 34.4% C, 14.7%	EV	54.1%	21.6%	909
Legasto (2006)	Philippines	Cross-sectional	150	51/57*	70.7%	Alcohol 90% HBV 10%	0%	NA	EV	46.0%	NA	160 (optimal) 909
Sethar (2006)	Pakistan	Cross-sectional	113	37.1 ± 14.85	69.0%	HBV 33.6% HCV 52.2% HBV + HCV 7.1% Others 7.1%	NA	A, 13.3% B, 60.2% C, 26.6%	EV	58.4%	NA	1445
Giannini (2005)	Italy	Prospective	68	65 ± 10	63.2%	Viral, 77.9% Nonviral, 22.1%	NA	A, 35.3% B, 41.2% C, 23.5%	EV	40.0%	5.9%	909

TABLE 1: Continued.

First author (year)	Regions	Study design	Number of total Pts	Age (year)	Male (%)	Etiology of cirrhosis	HCC (%)	Child-Pugh class (%)	Location of varices	Prevalence of varices (%)	Prevalence of high-risk/large varices (%)	Cut-off of varices
Pleština (2005)	Croatia	NA	99	53.6 ± 9.76	78.8%	HCV/HBV 13.1% Alcohol 83.9% PBC 3%	0%	A, 20.2% B, 53.5% C, 25.3% Unknown, 1%	EV	100.0%	53.5%	NA
			145	61	71.0%	Alcohol 16.6% HBV 11% HCV 53.8% Others 18.6%	NA	A, 37% B, 36% C, 27%	EV	61.0%	20.0%	909
Giannini (2003)	Italy	Retrospective	121	64	65.3%	Alcohol 24% HBV 5% HCV 63.6% Others 7.4%	NA	A, 41.3% B, 42.1% C, 16.5%	EV	58.7%	15.7%	909

EV, esophageal varices; GV, gastric varices; HBV, hepatitis B virus; HCC, hepatocellular carcinoma; HCV, hepatitis C virus; NA, not available; PBC, primary biliary cirrhosis; Pts, patients. *Notes*. ∗, age of patients was applied according to grade of varices or severity of cirrhosis.

TABLE 2: Results of meta-analyses in subgroups for any varices.

Groups	AUSROC	Sensitivity (95% CI)	Specificity (95% CI)	PLR (95% CI)	NLR (95% CI)	DOR (95% CI)
Threshold of 909	0.8867	0.84 (0.82–0.86)	0.80 (0.78–0.82)	3.95 (2.66–5.86)	0.21 (0.13–0.32)	25.06 (11.84–53.03)
Patients with viral hepatitis	0.8675	0.92 (0.90–0.94)	0.78 (0.74–0.81)	3.80 (2.04–7.08)	0.11 (0.06–0.23)	37.76 (14.43–98.84)
High quality studies	0.876	0.84 (0.81–0.87)	0.77 (0.74–0.8)	3.64 (2.11–6.3)	0.15 (0.07–0.33)	23.79 (10.35–54.7)
Prospective studies	0.8748	0.86 (0.84–0.88)	0.76 (0.73–0.79)	3.59 (2.39–5.39)	0.12 (0.07–0.22)	33.85 (15.67–73.15)
Region						
Europe	0.8289	0.83 (0.8–0.86)	0.65 (0.61–0.7)	2.58 (1.81–3.69)	0.2 (0.11–0.38)	15.46 (7.07–33.79)
Asia	0.9195	0.86 (0.84–0.87)	0.86 (0.84–0.88)	5.18 (3.5–7.65)	0.11 (0.06–0.2)	55.48 (24.27–126.81)
Africa	0.8537	0.87 (0.84–0.9)	0.71 (0.64–0.77)	3.28 (1.74–6.16)	0.16 (0.08–0.34)	23.31 (9.2–59.09)
North America	NA	0.82 (0.75–0.88)	0.67 (0.56–0.77)	2.45 (1.76–3.4)	0.27 (0.18–0.39)	9.06 (4.73–17.36)
Sample size						
<100	0.7895	0.81 (0.77–0.84)	0.7 (0.65–0.75)	2.57 (2.01–3.3)	0.25 (0.15–0.4)	12.58 (6.34–24.97)
≥100	0.9012	0.85 (0.83–0.86)	0.79 (0.77–0.81)	4.1 (2.92–5.77)	0.14 (0.09–0.22)	34.51 (18.84–63.2)
Prevalence of varices						
<50%	0.8804	0.91 (0.88–0.93)	0.86 (0.83–0.88)	5.29 (3.03–9.23)	0.11 (0.04–0.3)	54.16 (14.29–205.25)
≥50%	0.8633	0.83 (0.81–0.84)	0.73 (0.7–0.75)	3.15 (2.45–4.05)	0.19 (0.13–0.26)	21.12 (12.85–34.71)

AUSROC, area under the summary receiver operating characteristic curves; CI, confidence interval; DOR, diagnostic odds ratios; NLR, negative likelihood ratio; PLR, positive likelihood ratio.

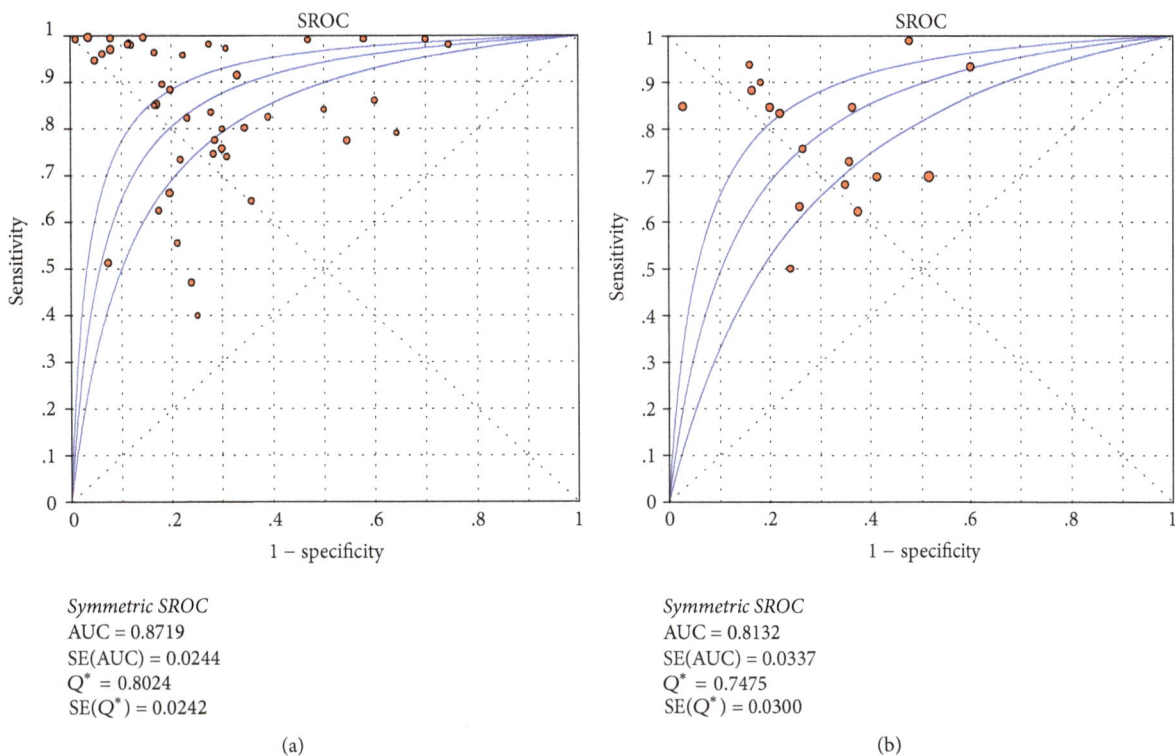

Symmetric SROC
AUC = 0.8719
SE(AUC) = 0.0244
$Q^* = 0.8024$
SE(Q^*) = 0.0242

(a)

Symmetric SROC
AUC = 0.8132
SE(AUC) = 0.0337
$Q^* = 0.7475$
SE(Q^*) = 0.0300

(b)

FIGURE 2: AUSROCs of PSR for varices in liver cirrhosis. (a) Any size varices; (b) high-risk varices.

index of platelet count and spleen diameter has much more relevance with portal hypertension and varices than the sole decreased platelet count [1].

In clinic practice, the measure of spleen diameter and platelet count is easily obtainable during the routine ultrasonography and serum examination. PSR is convenient, cheap, and noninvasive. Based on our study, we recommend that those patients whose PSR is less than 909 should undergo

upper gastrointestinal endoscopy to evaluate the grade of varices. 80% of patients whose value of PSR is greater than 909 can avoid unnecessary upper gastrointestinal endoscopic examination.

Compared with the two previous studies, our metaanalysis included a greater number of studies without limiting the publication language and cut-off values. Compared with other noninvasive methods, PSR has an upper-middle

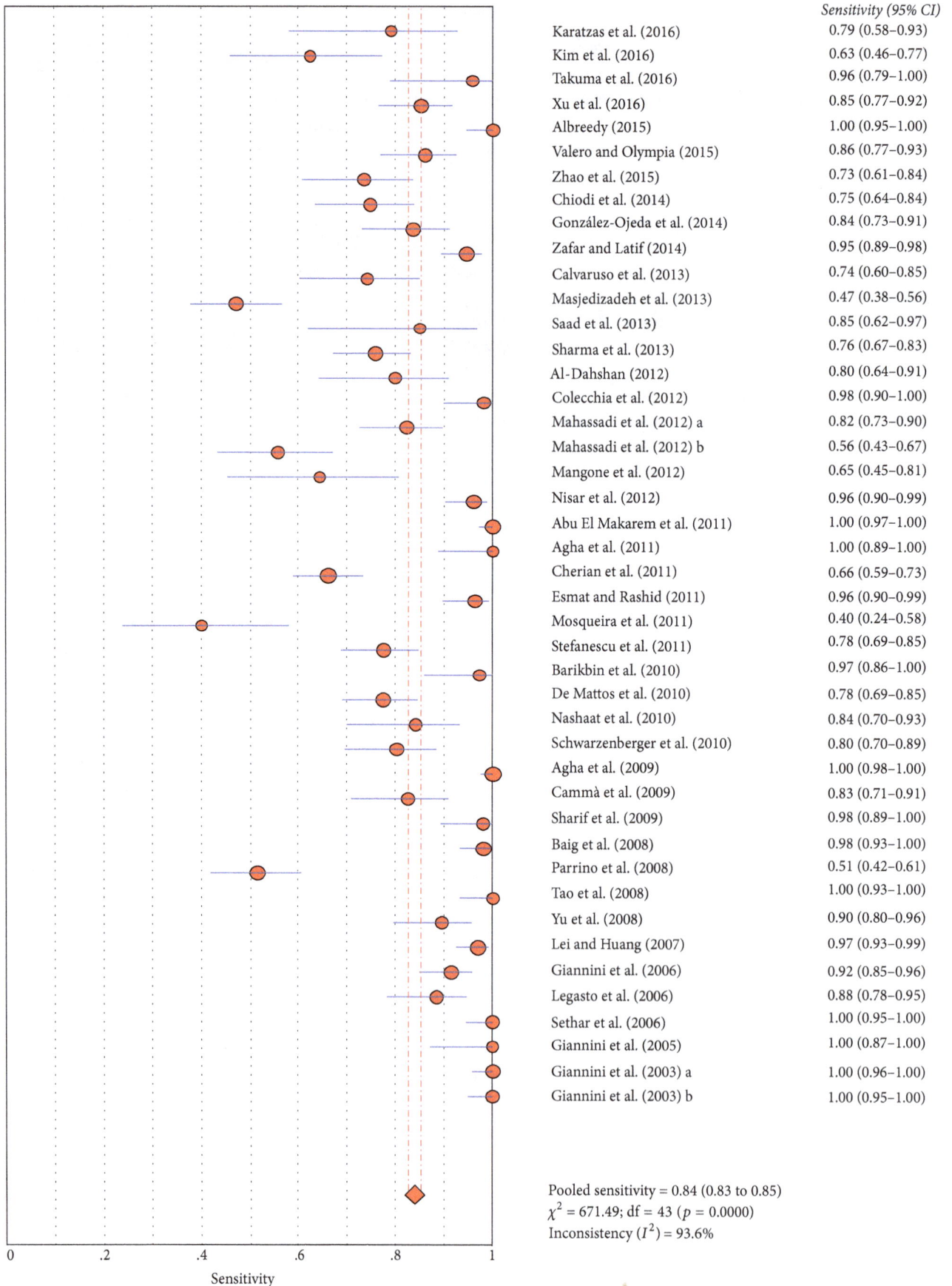

	Sensitivity (95% CI)
Karatzas et al. (2016)	0.79 (0.58–0.93)
Kim et al. (2016)	0.63 (0.46–0.77)
Takuma et al. (2016)	0.96 (0.79–1.00)
Xu et al. (2016)	0.85 (0.77–0.92)
Albreedy (2015)	1.00 (0.95–1.00)
Valero and Olympia (2015)	0.86 (0.77–0.93)
Zhao et al. (2015)	0.73 (0.61–0.84)
Chiodi et al. (2014)	0.75 (0.64–0.84)
González-Ojeda et al. (2014)	0.84 (0.73–0.91)
Zafar and Latif (2014)	0.95 (0.89–0.98)
Calvaruso et al. (2013)	0.74 (0.60–0.85)
Masjedizadeh et al. (2013)	0.47 (0.38–0.56)
Saad et al. (2013)	0.85 (0.62–0.97)
Sharma et al. (2013)	0.76 (0.67–0.83)
Al-Dahshan (2012)	0.80 (0.64–0.91)
Colecchia et al. (2012)	0.98 (0.90–1.00)
Mahassadi et al. (2012) a	0.82 (0.73–0.90)
Mahassadi et al. (2012) b	0.56 (0.43–0.67)
Mangone et al. (2012)	0.65 (0.45–0.81)
Nisar et al. (2012)	0.96 (0.90–0.99)
Abu El Makarem et al. (2011)	1.00 (0.97–1.00)
Agha et al. (2011)	1.00 (0.89–1.00)
Cherian et al. (2011)	0.66 (0.59–0.73)
Esmat and Rashid (2011)	0.96 (0.90–0.99)
Mosqueira et al. (2011)	0.40 (0.24–0.58)
Stefanescu et al. (2011)	0.78 (0.69–0.85)
Barikbin et al. (2010)	0.97 (0.86–1.00)
De Mattos et al. (2010)	0.78 (0.69–0.85)
Nashaat et al. (2010)	0.84 (0.70–0.93)
Schwarzenberger et al. (2010)	0.80 (0.70–0.89)
Agha et al. (2009)	1.00 (0.98–1.00)
Cammà et al. (2009)	0.83 (0.71–0.91)
Sharif et al. (2009)	0.98 (0.89–1.00)
Baig et al. (2008)	0.98 (0.93–1.00)
Parrino et al. (2008)	0.51 (0.42–0.61)
Tao et al. (2008)	1.00 (0.93–1.00)
Yu et al. (2008)	0.90 (0.80–0.96)
Lei and Huang (2007)	0.97 (0.93–0.99)
Giannini et al. (2006)	0.92 (0.85–0.96)
Legasto et al. (2006)	0.88 (0.78–0.95)
Sethar et al. (2006)	1.00 (0.95–1.00)
Giannini et al. (2005)	1.00 (0.87–1.00)
Giannini et al. (2003) a	1.00 (0.96–1.00)
Giannini et al. (2003) b	1.00 (0.95–1.00)

Pooled sensitivity = 0.84 (0.83 to 0.85)
$\chi^2 = 671.49$; df = 43 ($p = 0.0000$)
Inconsistency (I^2) = 93.6%

(a)

FIGURE 3: Continued.

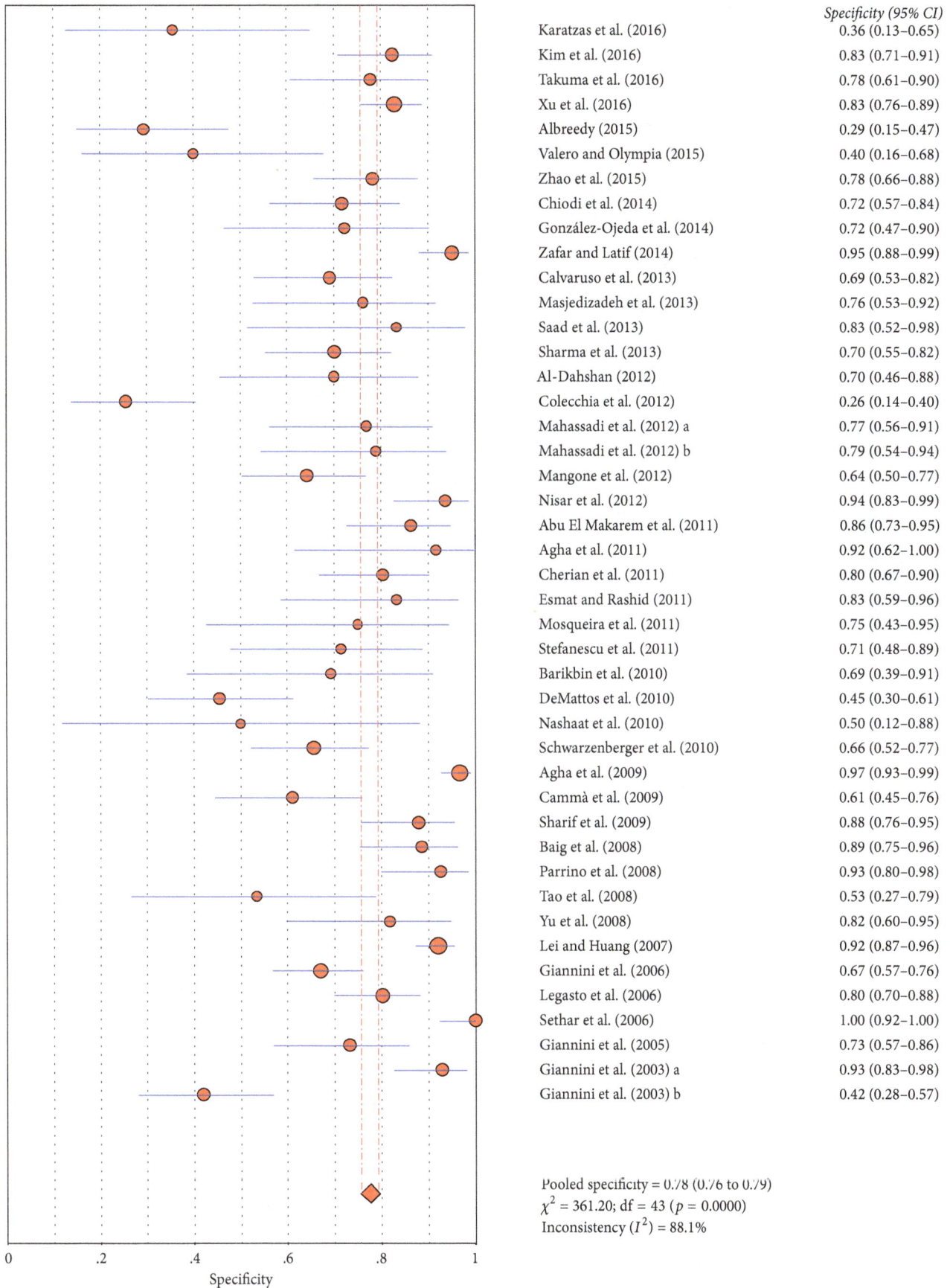

	Specificity (95% CI)
Karatzas et al. (2016)	0.36 (0.13–0.65)
Kim et al. (2016)	0.83 (0.71–0.91)
Takuma et al. (2016)	0.78 (0.61–0.90)
Xu et al. (2016)	0.83 (0.76–0.89)
Albreedy (2015)	0.29 (0.15–0.47)
Valero and Olympia (2015)	0.40 (0.16–0.68)
Zhao et al. (2015)	0.78 (0.66–0.88)
Chiodi et al. (2014)	0.72 (0.57–0.84)
González-Ojeda et al. (2014)	0.72 (0.47–0.90)
Zafar and Latif (2014)	0.95 (0.88–0.99)
Calvaruso et al. (2013)	0.69 (0.53–0.82)
Masjedizadeh et al. (2013)	0.76 (0.53–0.92)
Saad et al. (2013)	0.83 (0.52–0.98)
Sharma et al. (2013)	0.70 (0.55–0.82)
Al-Dahshan (2012)	0.70 (0.46–0.88)
Colecchia et al. (2012)	0.26 (0.14–0.40)
Mahassadi et al. (2012) a	0.77 (0.56–0.91)
Mahassadi et al. (2012) b	0.79 (0.54–0.94)
Mangone et al. (2012)	0.64 (0.50–0.77)
Nisar et al. (2012)	0.94 (0.83–0.99)
Abu El Makarem et al. (2011)	0.86 (0.73–0.95)
Agha et al. (2011)	0.92 (0.62–1.00)
Cherian et al. (2011)	0.80 (0.67–0.90)
Esmat and Rashid (2011)	0.83 (0.59–0.96)
Mosqueira et al. (2011)	0.75 (0.43–0.95)
Stefanescu et al. (2011)	0.71 (0.48–0.89)
Barikbin et al. (2010)	0.69 (0.39–0.91)
DeMattos et al. (2010)	0.45 (0.30–0.61)
Nashaat et al. (2010)	0.50 (0.12–0.88)
Schwarzenberger et al. (2010)	0.66 (0.52–0.77)
Agha et al. (2009)	0.97 (0.93–0.99)
Cammà et al. (2009)	0.61 (0.45–0.76)
Sharif et al. (2009)	0.88 (0.76–0.95)
Baig et al. (2008)	0.89 (0.75–0.96)
Parrino et al. (2008)	0.93 (0.80–0.98)
Tao et al. (2008)	0.53 (0.27–0.79)
Yu et al. (2008)	0.82 (0.60–0.95)
Lei and Huang (2007)	0.92 (0.87–0.96)
Giannini et al. (2006)	0.67 (0.57–0.76)
Legasto et al. (2006)	0.80 (0.70–0.88)
Sethar et al. (2006)	1.00 (0.92–1.00)
Giannini et al. (2005)	0.73 (0.57–0.86)
Giannini et al. (2003) a	0.93 (0.83–0.98)
Giannini et al. (2003) b	0.42 (0.28–0.57)

Pooled specificity = 0.78 (0.76 to 0.79)
$\chi^2 = 361.20$; df = 43 ($p = 0.0000$)
Inconsistency (I^2) = 88.1%

(b)

FIGURE 3: Summary sensitivity and specificity of PSR for any size varices in liver cirrhosis. (a) Summary sensitivity; (b) summary specificity.

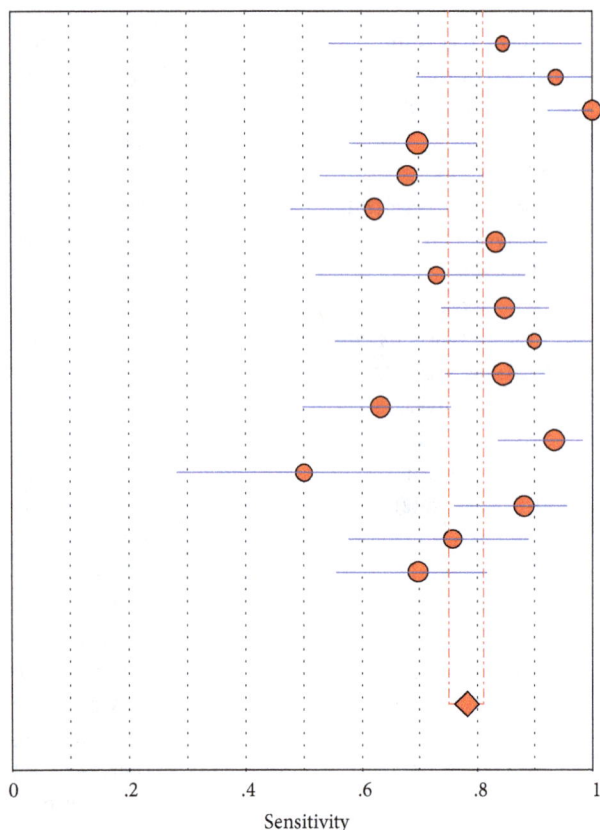

	Sensitivity (95% CI)
Kim et al. (2016)	0.85 (0.55–0.98)
Takuma et al. (2016)	0.94 (0.70–1.00)
Albreedy (2015)	1.00 (0.92–1.00)
Cho et al. (2015)	0.70 (0.58–0.80)
Stefanescu et al. (2015)	0.68 (0.53–0.81)
Chiodi et al. (2014)	0.62 (0.48–0.75)
Wang et al. (2014)	0.83 (0.71–0.92)
Calvaruso et al. (2013)	0.73 (0.52–0.88)
Rajendran et al. (2013)	0.85 (0.74–0.92)
Saad et al. (2013)	0.90 (0.55–1.00)
Mahassadi et al. (2012) a	0.85 (0.75–0.92)
Mahassadi et al. (2012) b	0.63 (0.50–0.75)
Esmat and Rashid (2011)	0.93 (0.84–0.98)
Mosqueira et al. (2011)	0.50 (0.28–0.72)
Sarangapani et al. (2010)	0.88 (0.76–0.96)
Barrera et al. (2009)	0.76 (0.58–0.89)
Pleština et al. (2005)	0.70 (0.56–0.82)

Pooled sensitivity = 0.78 (0.75 to 0.81)

$\chi^2 = 75.98$; df = 16 ($p = 0.0000$)

Inconsistency (I^2) = 78.9%

(a)

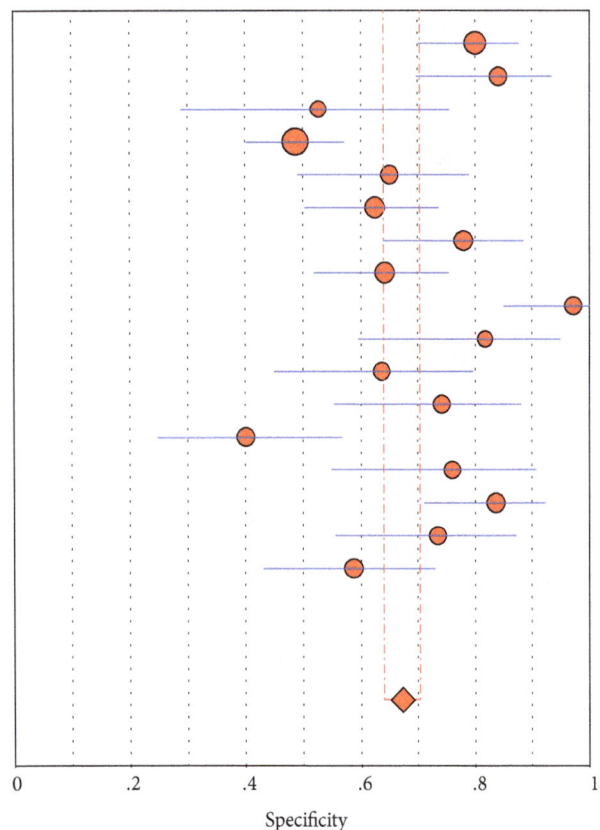

	Specificity (95% CI)
Kim et al. (2016)	0.80 (0.70–0.88)
Takuma et al. (2016)	0.84 (0.70–0.93)
Albreedy (2015)	0.53 (0.29–0.76)
Cho et al. (2015)	0.49 (0.40–0.57)
Stefanescu et al. (2015)	0.65 (0.49–0.79)
Chiodi et al. (2014)	0.63 (0.50–0.74)
Wang et al. (2014)	0.78 (0.64–0.88)
Calvaruso et al. (2013)	0.64 (0.52–0.75)
Rajendran et al. (2013)	0.97 (0.85–1.00)
Saad et al. (2013)	0.82 (0.60–0.95)
Mahassadi et al. (2012) a	0.64 (0.45–0.80)
Mahassadi et al. (2012) b	0.74 (0.55–0.88)
Esmat and Rashid (2011)	0.40 (0.25–0.57)
Mosqueira et al. (2011)	0.76 (0.55–0.91)
Sarangapani et al. (2010)	0.84 (0.71–0.92)
Barrera et al. (2009)	0.74 (0.56–0.87)
Pleština et al. (2005)	0.59 (0.43–0.73)

Pooled specificity = 0.67 (0.64 to 0.71)

$\chi^2 = 87.21$; df = 16 ($p = 0.0000$)

Inconsistency (I^2) = 81.7%

(b)

FIGURE 4: Summary sensitivity and specificity of PSR for high-risk varices in liver cirrhosis. (a) Summary sensitivity; (b) summary specificity.

performance for varies. As previous studies have shown [53–55], serum markers cannot be used to identify varices for the low-moderate diagnostic accuracy. Computer tomography has similar summary sensitivity (0.896) and specificity (0.723) compared to PSR [56]. In addition, the diagnostic accuracy of PSR for varices was slightly higher than spleen stiffness measurement [57] and liver stiffness measurement [58]. Their summary sensitivities were 0.78 and 0.87, respectively. The summary specificities were 0.76 and 0.53, respectively. While the diagnostic accuracy of PSR for varices was slightly lower than capsule endoscopy [59], its summary sensitivity and specificity were 0.85 and 0.84, respectively. Some studies reported that splenoportal index and congestion index have high diagnostic accuracy. Their sensitivities and specificities were both greater than 80% [60, 61]. However, there are no systematic studies to evaluate their performance of varices.

Our study has some limitations. (1) 39 papers lacking relevant data were excluded, out of which some reported that PSR had no statistically significant difference in predicting the presence of varices. (2) Most analyses had significant heterogeneity. It may be attributed to the different selection criteria of patients, such as the prevalence of decompensated cirrhosis, etiologies of cirrhosis, and history of variceal bleeding. We have no evidence to support this assumption. The same situation was also found in the previous meta-analyses [2, 3]. (3) The publication bias exists in the study. (4) Most TP, FP, FN, and TN were recalculated using sensitivities and specificities, which may introduce some errors. (5) PSR is not applicable to patients with a history of splenectomy.

In conclusion, PSR can be used to identify varices in liver cirrhosis. PSR had a high sensitivity in viral liver cirrhosis.

Abbreviations

PSR: Platelet count to spleen diameter ratio
HCC: Hepatocellular carcinoma
TP: True positive
FP: False positive
FN: False negative
TN: True negative
AUSROC: Area under the summary receiver operating characteristic curve
SE: Standard error
CI: Confidence interval
PLR: Positive likelihood ratio
NLR: Negative likelihood ratio
DOR: Diagnostic odds ratio.

Competing Interests

The authors declare that they have no competing interests.

References

[1] E. Giannini, F. Botta, P. Borro et al., "Platelet count/spleen diameter ratio: proposal and validation of a non-invasive parameter to predict the presence of oesophageal varices in patients with liver cirrhosis," *Gut*, vol. 52, no. 8, pp. 1200–1205, 2003.

[2] L. Ying, X. Lin, Z.-L. Xie, Y.-P. Hu, and K.-Q. Shi, "Performance of platelet count/spleen diameter ratio for diagnosis of esophageal varices in cirrhosis: a meta-analysis," *Digestive Diseases and Sciences*, vol. 57, no. 6, pp. 1672–1681, 2012.

[3] S. Chawla, A. Katz, B. M. Attar, A. Gupta, D. S. Sandhu, and R. Agarwal, "Platelet count/spleen diameter ratio to predict the presence of esophageal varices in patients with cirrhosis: a systematic review," *European Journal of Gastroenterology and Hepatology*, vol. 24, no. 4, pp. 431–436, 2012.

[4] P. F. Whiting, A. W. S. Rutjes, M. E. Westwood et al., "Quadas-2: a revised tool for the quality assessment of diagnostic accuracy studies," *Annals of Internal Medicine*, vol. 155, no. 8, pp. 529–536, 2011.

[5] X.-D. Xu, C.-F. Xu, J.-J. Dai, J.-Q. Qian, and X. Pin, "Ratio of platelet count/spleen diameter predicted the presence of esophageal varices in patients with schistosomiasis liver cirrhosis," *European Journal of Gastroenterology & Hepatology*, vol. 28, no. 5, pp. 588–591, 2016.

[6] Y. Takuma, K. Nouso, Y. Morimoto et al., "Portal hypertension in patients with liver cirrhosis: diagnostic accuracy of spleen stiffness," *Radiology*, vol. 279, no. 2, pp. 609–619, 2016.

[7] T. Y. Kim, T. Y. Kim, Y. Kim, S. Lim, W. K. Jeong, and J. H. Sohn, "Diagnostic performance of shear wave elastography for predicting esophageal varices in patients with compensated liver cirrhosis," *Journal of Ultrasound in Medicine*, vol. 35, no. 7, pp. 1373–1381, 2016.

[8] A. Karatzas, C. Triantos, M. Kalafateli et al., "Multidetector computed tomography versus platelet/spleen diameter ratio as methods for the detection of gastroesophageal varices," *Annals of Gastroenterology*, vol. 29, no. 1, pp. 71–78, 2016.

[9] D. Zhao, H. Mao, C.-C. Huang, and S.-H. Zhang, "Study on noninvasive prediction indicators for incidence of esophageal varices of patients with liver cirrhosis caused by hepatitis B," *Journal of Shanghai Jiaotong University*, vol. 35, no. 3, pp. 386–390, 2015.

[10] G. Valero and G. Olympia, "A retrospective study on non-invasive predictors of esophageal varices in patients with liver cirrhosis, a Makati Medical Center experience," *Journal of Gastroenterology and Hepatology (Australia)*, vol. 30, article 358, 2015.

[11] H. Stefanescu, C. Radu, B. Procopet et al., "Non-invasive ménage à trois for the prediction of high-risk varices: stepwise algorithm using lok score, liver and spleen stiffness," *Liver International*, vol. 35, no. 2, pp. 317–325, 2015.

[12] E. J. Cho, M. Y. Kim, J.-H. Lee et al., "Diagnostic and prognostic values of noninvasive predictors of portal hypertension in patients with alcoholic cirrhosis," *PLoS ONE*, vol. 10, no. 7, Article ID e0133935, 2015.

[13] A. M. Albreedy, "Platelet count to spleen diameter ratio and to spleen area ratio as predictors for esopha-geal varices in chronic hepatitis C patients with liver cirrhosis," *Journal of the Egyptian Society of Parasitology*, vol. 45, no. 3, pp. 485–492, 2015.

[14] S. Zafar and M. M. Latif, "Diagnostic accuracy of platelet count/spleen diameter ratio for detection of esophageal varices in cirrhotic patients taking endoscopy as gold standard," *Pakistan Journal of Medical and Health Sciences*, vol. 8, no. 4, pp. 951–954, 2014.

[15] L. Wang, J. Hu, S. Dong et al., "Noninvasive prediction of large esophageal varices in liver cirrhosis patients," *Clinical and Investigative Medicine*, vol. 37, no. 1, pp. E38–E46, 2014.

[16] A. González-Ojeda, G. Cervantes-Guevara, M. Chávez-Sánchez et al., "Platelet count/spleen diameter ratio to predict

esophageal varices in Mexican patients with hepatic cirrhosis," *World Journal of Gastroenterology*, vol. 20, no. 8, pp. 2079–2084, 2014.

[17] D. Chiodi, N. Hernández, G. Saona et al., "Noninvasive diagnosis of esophageal varices in cirrhotic patients," *Acta Gastroenterologica Latinoamericana*, vol. 44, no. 2, pp. 108–113, 2014.

[18] P. Sharma, V. Kirnake, P. Tyagi et al., "Spleen stiffness in patients with cirrhosis in predicting esophageal varices," *American Journal of Gastroenterology*, vol. 108, no. 7, pp. 1101–1107, 2013.

[19] Y. Saad, M. Said, M. O. Idris, A. Rabee, and Z. Salama, "Liver stiffness measurement by fibroscan predicts the presence and size of esophageal varices in egyptian patients with HCV related liver cirrhosis," *Journal of Clinical and Diagnostic Research*, vol. 7, no. 10, pp. 2253–2257, 2013.

[20] P. A. Rajendran, A. Philip, D. Krishnadas, K. C. George, Jayaprakash, and S. Devi, "Platelet count to spleen size ratio—a simple noninvasive tool to identify small varices from large varices in patients having cirrohsis and portal hypertension," *Journal of Clinical and Experimental Hepatology*, vol. 3, no. 1, p. S93, 2013.

[21] A. R. Masjedizadeh, E. Hajiani, P. A. Nejad, J. Hashemi, A. A. Shayesteh, and Z. Yasin, "Efficacy platelet/spleen diameter ratio for detection of esophageal varices in cirrhotic patients," *Journal of Gastroenterology and Hepatology Research*, vol. 2, no. 5, pp. 590–592, 2013.

[22] V. Calvaruso, F. Bronte, E. Conte, F. Simone, A. Craxì, and V. Di Marco, "Modified spleen stiffness measurement by transient elastography is associated with presence of large oesophageal varices in patients with compensated hepatitis C virus cirrhosis," *Journal of Viral Hepatitis*, vol. 20, no. 12, pp. 867–874, 2013.

[23] S. Nisar, S. Nazir, A. Butt, A. Hussain, and K. R. Yousaf, "Validity of platelet count/spleen diameter ratio for the noninvasive diagnosis of esophageal varices in cirrhotic patients," *Pakistan Journal of Medical and Health Sciences*, vol. 6, no. 1, pp. 269–274, 2012.

[24] M. Mangone, A. Moretti, F. Alivernini et al., "Platelet count/spleen diameter ratio for non-invasive diagnosis of oesophageal varices: is it useful in compensated cirrhosis?" *Digestive and Liver Disease*, vol. 44, no. 6, pp. 504–507, 2012.

[25] A. K. Mahassadi, F. Y. Bathaix, C. Assi et al., "Usefulness of noninvasive predictors of oesophageal varices in black african cirrhotic patients in Cte d'Ivoire (West Africa)," *Gastroenterology Research and Practice*, vol. 2012, Article ID 216390, 10 pages, 2012.

[26] A. Colecchia, L. Montrone, E. Scaioli et al., "Measurement of spleen stiffness to evaluate portal hypertension and the presence of esophageal varices in patients with HCV-related cirrhosis," *Gastroenterology*, vol. 143, no. 3, pp. 646–654, 2012.

[27] M. Al-Dahshan, "Clinical application of transient elastography in prediction of portal hypertension related complication in patients with chronic liver diseases," *Journal of the Egyptian Society of Parasitology*, vol. 42, no. 1, pp. 79–88, 2012.

[28] H. Stefanescu, M. Grigorescu, M. Lupsor, B. Procopet, A. Maniu, and R. Badea, "Spleen stiffness measurement using fibroscan for the noninvasive assessment of esophageal varices in liver cirrhosis patients," *Journal of Gastroenterology and Hepatology (Australia)*, vol. 26, no. 1, pp. 164–170, 2011.

[29] J. R. Mosqueira, J. B. Montiel, D. Rodríguez, and E. Monge, "Evaluation of the diagnostic test of index platelet counts/size spleen, as a predictor of the presence of esophageal varices in cirrhosis," *Revista de Gastroenterología del Perú*, vol. 31, no. 1, pp. 11–16, 2011.

[30] S. Esmat and L. Rashid, "A comparative study between three noninvasive predictors of oesophageal varices in post hepatitis C virus liver cirrhosis in Egypt," *Acta Gastro-Enterologica Belgica*, vol. 74, no. 4, pp. 497–502, 2011.

[31] J. V. Cherian, N. Deepak, R. P. Ponnusamy, A. Somasundaram, and V. Jayanthi, "Non-invasive predictors of esophageal varices," *Saudi Journal of Gastroenterology*, vol. 17, no. 1, pp. 64–68, 2011.

[32] A. Agha, M. Abdulhadi, S. Marenco et al., "Use of the platelet count/spleen diameter ratio for the noninvasive diagnosis of esophageal varices in patients with schistosomiasis," *Saudi Journal of Gastroenterology*, vol. 17, no. 5, pp. 307–311, 2011.

[33] M. A. Abu El Makarem, M. E. Shatat, Y. Shaker et al., "Platelet count/bipolar spleen diameter ratio for the prediction of esophageal varices: the special Egyptian situation: noninvasive prediction of esophageal varices," *Hepatitis Monthly*, vol. 11, no. 4, pp. 278–284, 2011.

[34] E. Schwarzenberger, T. Meyer, V. Golla, N. P. Sahdala, and A. D. Min, "Utilization of platelet count spleen diameter ratio in predicting the presence of esophageal varices in patients with cirrhosis," *Journal of Clinical Gastroenterology*, vol. 44, no. 2, pp. 146–150, 2010.

[35] A. Sarangapani, C. Shanmugam, M. Kalyanasundaram, B. Rangachari, P. Thangavelu, and J. K. Subbarayan, "Noninvasive prediction of large esophageal varices in chronic liver disease patients," *Saudi Journal of Gastroenterology*, vol. 16, no. 1, pp. 38–42, 2010.

[36] E. H. Nashaat, H. Abd-Elaziz, M. Sabry, and A. A. Ibrahim, "Non-endoscopic predictors of esophageal varices and portal hypertensive gastropathy," *Nature and Science*, vol. 8, no. 6, pp. 43–50, 2010.

[37] Â. Z. De Mattos, A. A. De Mattos, F. F. Vianna, M. I. Musskopf, J. C. Pereira-Lima, and A. C. Maciel, "Platelet count/spleen diameter ratio: analysis of its capacity as a predictor of the existence of esophageal varices," *Arquivos de Gastroenterologia*, vol. 47, no. 3, pp. 275–278, 2010.

[38] R. Barikbin, A. Hekmatnia, N. Omidifar, M. Farghadani, and P. Adibi, "Prediction severity of esophageal varices: a new cutoff point for Platelet count/spleen diameter ratio," *Minerva Gastroenterologica e Dietologica*, vol. 56, no. 1, pp. 1–6, 2010.

[39] M. A. Sharif, R. Firdous, T. A. Khan, T. H. Rizvi, M. Shani, and M. M. Elahi, "Platelet count/splenic size ratio: a parameter to predict the presence of oesophageal varices in cirrhotics," in *Proceedings of the Asia Pacific Microwave Conference*, vol. 3, pp. 23–26, 2009.

[40] C. Cammà, S. Petta, V. Di Marco et al., "Insulin resistance is a risk factor for esophageal varices in hepatitis C virus cirrhosis," *Hepatology*, vol. 49, no. 1, pp. 195–203, 2009.

[41] F. Barrera, A. Riquelme, A. Soza et al., "Platelet count/spleen diameter ratio for non-invasive prediction of high risk esophageal varices in cirrhotic patients," *Annals of Hepatology*, vol. 8, no. 4, pp. 325–330, 2009.

[42] A. Agha, E. Anwar, K. Bashir, V. Savarino, and E. G. Giannini, "External validation of the pPlatelet count/spleen diameter ratio for the diagnosis of esophageal varices in hepatitis C virus-related cirrhosis," *Digestive Diseases and Sciences*, vol. 54, no. 3, pp. 654–660, 2009.

[43] J. Y. Yu, X. N. Liu, D. Wang, and J. J. Cui, "Non-invasive predictive factors of esophageal varices in patients with post-hepatitis B cirrhosis," *Journal of Binzhou Medical University*, vol. 31, no. 5, pp. 345–349, 2008 (Chinese).

[44] W. Tao, S. Q. Yang, X. C. Lv, and L. Yang, "Value of the platelet count/spleen diameter ratio on diagnosis of esophageal varices

in patients with cirrhosis," *Journal of Ningxia Medical College*, vol. 30, no. 3, pp. 349–350, 2008 (Chinese).

[45] A. Parrino, V. Di Gesaro, A. Terranova et al., "Non-invasive diagnosis of esophageal varices in cirrhotic patients: endoscopic vs ultrasonographic findings," *Acta Medica Mediterranea*, vol. 24, no. 1, pp. 11–18, 2008.

[46] W. W. Baig, M. V. Nagaraja, M. Varma, and R. Prabhu, "Platelet count to spleen diameter ratio for the diagnosis of esophageal varices: is it feasible?" *Canadian Journal of Gastroenterology*, vol. 22, no. 10, pp. 825–828, 2008.

[47] J. B. Lei and T. Z. Huang, "Value of the platelet count/spleen diameter ratio on predicting esophageal varices of liver cirrhosis," *Practical Clinical Medicine*, vol. 8, no. 10, pp. 25–27, 2007 (Chinese).

[48] G. H. Sethar, R. Ahmed, S. K. Rathi, and N. A. Shaikh, "Platelet count/splenic size ratio: a parameter to predict the presence of esophageal varices in cirrhotics," *Journal of the College of Physicians and Surgeons Pakistan*, vol. 16, no. 3, pp. 183–186, 2006.

[49] G. M. Legasto, J. Sevilla, A. Balay et al., "Platelet count/spleen diameter ratio: a noninvasive parameter to predict the presence of esophageal varices," *Phillippine Journal of Gastroenterology*, vol. 2, pp. 33–38, 2006.

[50] E. G. Giannini, A. Zaman, A. Kreil et al., "Platelet count/spleen diameter ratio for the noninvasive diagnosis of esophageal varices: results of a multicenter, prospective, validation study," *American Journal of Gastroenterology*, vol. 101, no. 11, pp. 2511–2519, 2006.

[51] S. Pleština, R. Pulanić, M. Kralik, S. Pleština, and M. Samaržija, "Color Doppler ultrasonography is reliable in assessing the risk of esophageal variceal bleeding in patients with liver cirrhosis," *Wiener Klinische Wochenschrift*, vol. 117, no. 19-20, pp. 711–717, 2005.

[52] E. G. Giannini, F. Botta, P. Borro et al., "Application of the platelet count/spleen diameter ratio to rule out the presence of oesophageal varices in patients with cirrhosis: a validation study based on follow-up," *Digestive and Liver Disease*, vol. 37, no. 10, pp. 779–785, 2005.

[53] X. Qi, H. Li, J. Chen et al., "Serum liver fibrosis markers for predicting the presence of gastroesophageal varices in liver cirrhosis: a retrospective cross-sectional study," *Gastroenterology Research and Practice*, vol. 2015, Article ID 274534, 6 pages, 2015.

[54] H. Deng, X. Qi, Y. Peng et al., "Diagnostic accuracy of APRI, AAR, FIB-4, FI, and king scores for diagnosis of esophageal varices in liver cirrhosis: A Retrospective Study," *Medical Science Monitor*, vol. 21, pp. 3961–3977, 2015.

[55] H. Deng, X. Qi, and X. Guo, "Diagnostic accuracy of APRI, AAR, FIB-4, FI, king, lok, forns, and fibroindex scores in predicting the presence of esophageal varices in liver cirrhosis: a systematic review and meta-analysis," *Medicine*, vol. 94, no. 42, Article ID e1795, 2015.

[56] Y.-J. Tseng, X.-Q. Zeng, J. Chen, N. Li, P.-J. Xu, and S.-Y. Chen, "Computed tomography in evaluating gastroesophageal varices in patients with portal hypertension: a meta-analysis," *Digestive and Liver Disease*, vol. 48, no. 7, pp. 695–702, 2016.

[57] S. Singh, J. E. Eaton, M. H. Murad, H. Tanaka, H. Iijima, and J. A. Talwalkar, "Accuracy of spleen stiffness measurement in detection of esophageal varices in patients with chronic liver disease: systematic review and meta-analysis," *Clinical Gastroenterology and Hepatology*, vol. 12, no. 6, pp. 935–945.e4, 2014.

[58] K.-Q. Shi, Y.-C. Fan, Z.-Z. Pan et al., "Transient elastography: a meta-analysis of diagnostic accuracy in evaluation of portal hypertension in chronic liver disease," *Liver International*, vol. 33, no. 1, pp. 62–71, 2013.

[59] A. Colli, J. C. R. Gana, D. Turner et al., "Capsule endoscopy for the diagnosis of oesophageal varices in people with chronic liver disease or portal vein thrombosis," *The Cochrane database of systematic reviews*, vol. 10, Article ID CD008760, 2014.

[60] R. Chakrabarti, D. Sen, and V. Khanna, "Is non-invasive diagnosis of esophageal varices in patients with compensated hepatic cirrhosis possible by duplex Doppler ultrasonography?" *Indian Journal of Gastroenterology*, vol. 35, no. 1, pp. 60–66, 2016.

[61] H. S. Mahmoud, E. F. Mostafa, and M. A. W. Mohammed, "Role of portal haemodynamic parameters in prediction of oesophageal varices in cirrhotic patients," *Arab Journal of Gastroenterology*, vol. 15, no. 3-4, pp. 130–134, 2014.

10

TFCP2 Genetic Polymorphism Is Associated with Predisposition to and Transplant Prognosis of Hepatocellular Carcinoma

Zhikun Liu,[1,2] **Feng Gao,**[1,2] **Zhou Shao,**[1,2] **Haiyang Xie,**[2,3] **Lin Zhou,**[2,3] **Xiao Xu,**[1,2,3] **and Shusen Zheng**[1,2,3]

[1]*Division of Hepatobiliary and Pancreatic Surgery, First Affiliated Hospital, Zhejiang University School of Medicine, Hangzhou, China*
[2]*Key Lab of Combined Multi-Organ Transplantation, Ministry of Public Health, Hangzhou, China*
[3]*Collaborative Innovation Center for Diagnosis and Treatment of Infectious Diseases, Hangzhou, China*

Correspondence should be addressed to Xiao Xu; zjxu@zju.edu.cn and Shusen Zheng; zyzss@zju.edu.cn

Academic Editor: Haruhiko Sugimura

TFCP2 is an oncogene and plays crucial roles in the incidence and progression of hepatocellular carcinoma (HCC). However, no reports are available on the impact of TFCP2 genetic polymorphism on the susceptibility to and the transplant prognosis of HCC. Here, we genotyped 7 SNPs of TFCP2 in a case-control study of 119 patients with HCC and 200 patients with chronic liver disease. Of the 7 SNPs in TFCP2, rs7959378 distributed differentially between patients with versus patients without HCC. The patients with the CA (OR = 0.58, 95% CI = 0.35–0.96), the CC (OR = 0.39, 95% CI = 0.20–0.76), and the CA/CC (OR = 0.52, 95% CI = 0.32–0.83) genotypes had significantly decreased risk for HCC compared with those carrying the rs7959378 AA genotype. After adjusting for confounding factors, rs7959378 still conferred significant risk for HCC. Furthermore, the patients who carried rs7959378 AC/CC had a higher overall survival and lower relapse-free survival than those with the rs7959378 AA genotype. Similar results were found in the multivariate analysis adjusted by AFP, tumor size and tumor number, and differentiation. These findings indicate that rs7959378 is associated with the risk of HCC in patient with chronic liver disease and prognosis of HCC patients after liver transplantation.

1. Introduction

Hepatocellular carcinoma (HCC) is a worldwide prevalent and deadly neoplasia [1]. HCC occurs usually in the background of chronic liver diseases, such as hepatitis virus infection and liver cirrhosis [2, 3]. The prevalence of hepatitis B virus (HBV) carriage is reported to be 350 million people worldwide [4]. In China, chronic HBV infection has a high prevalence with approximately 93 million individuals (National Health and Family Planning Commission of the PRC). In addition to HBV, chronic infection with the hepatitis C virus, excessive alcohol consumption, and heavy aflatoxin exposure have also been proposed as risk factors for HCC [5–7]. Some genetic markers have also been reported to be HCC risk and prognostic factors [8]. Despite those advances, as a multifactorial and complex process, the exact pathogenesis of HCC is still unclear.

The transcription factor CP2 (TFCP2) has been shown to regulate diverse cellular and viral promoters and plays roles in cell cycle progression and cell survival [9–12]. Yoo et al. [13] firstly reported that TFCP2 overexpression is detected in more than 90% of cases of human HCC patients compared to normal liver and is associated with the stage and grade of the disease. There are increasing evidences that TFCP2 is a key factor for hepatocarcinogenesis and prognosis. Additionally, TFCP2 contributes to 5-fluorouracil resistance [14]. To understand the mechanisms of TFCP2 involved in HCC development and progression, our colleagues and other groups have found that TFCP2

TFCP2 Genetic Polymorphism Is Associated with Predisposition to and Transplant Prognosis...

83

could enhance invasion and angiogenesis of HCC via regulating osteopontin, fibronectin 1, and matrix metalloproteinase-9, respectively [13, 15, 16]. The pivotal role of TFCP2 in hepatocarcinogenesis is alternatively confirmed by the fact that TFCP2 suppression by FQI1, a specific small molecule inhibitor of TFCP2 binding to DNA, is an effective therapeutic approach for treating HCC [17].

Genetic factors may also play critical roles in the development and prognosis of HCC. Previous studies have demonstrated that genetic variant mainly in the form of single nucleotide polymorphism (SNP) plays an important role in carcinomagenesis, tumor recurrence, and prognosis of HCC patients [18, 19]. Although a close association between TFCP2 protein and HCC has been established, the genetic polymorphism of TFCP2 gene and HCC remains unknown. Seven gene polymorphisms at different loci have been identified for TFCP2 gene, including rs10876135, rs11169735, rs1056897, rs10099, rs12820966, rs7959378, and rs11169736. In this study, we enrolled chronic liver disease with or without HCC patients to study whether the above-mentioned TFCP2 polymorphisms can affect the risk and transplant prognosis of HCC.

2. Material and Methods

2.1. Subjects. The present study included 200 patients with chronic liver diseases as control and 119 patients with primary HCC who underwent liver transplantation (LT) between January 2008 and December 2012 at the First Affiliated Hospital, Zhejiang University School of Medicine, China. The diagnosis was confirmed by pathological examination and the recurrence by AFP elevation (>400 ng/ml) and/or imaging examination (MRI/CT). The subjects' recruitment was approved by the Institutional Review Board of the First Affiliated Hospital, Zhejiang University, according to the Declaration of Helsinki. Written informed consents were obtained. Data were analyzed anonymously.

All patients received LT as the initial therapy. The transarterial chemoembolization (TACE) and radiofrequency ablation (RFA) procedure were performed as the postoperative therapy in the patients with HCC relapse, if indicated. Complete follow-up data were obtained from all HCC patients (range, 1 month–66 months; median, 26 months). Primary study end points were overall survival (OS) and relapse-free survival (RFS). OS and RFS were defined as the time from the date of surgery to the date of death from HCC or to the date of local recurrence or detection of distant metastasis, respectively.

2.2. SNP Selection and Genotyping. Genomic DNA was isolated from EDTA-anticoagulated whole blood of recipients using the QIAamp DNA Blood mini kit (QIAGEN, Hilden, Germany). The potential functional SNPs of TFCP2 with minor allele frequency (MAF) of greater than 0.20 for the Han Chinese were selected from the entire gene region according to the HapMap database. Seven SNPs were found, namely, rs7959378 (5' flanking), rs11169736 (exon1), rs1056897 (exon1 (5'-UTR)), rs11169735 (exon1 (5'-UTR)), rs12820966 (exon15 (3'-UTR)), rs10876135 (exon15 (3'-

TABLE 1: Clinical data for the non-HCC and HCC groups.

Variable	Non-HCC (n = 200)	HCC (n = 119)	P value
Age (years), n (%)			0.155
≤50	128 (64)	66 (56)	
>50	72 (36)	53 (44)	
Gender			*0.008*
Male, n (%)	163 (82)	110 (92)	
Female, n (%)	37 (19)	9 (8)	
BMI (kg/m^2)*	23.2 ± 6.4	24.2 ± 8.5	0.299
Etiology of liver diseases, n (%)			0.164
HBV	151 (76)	98 (82)	
Others	49 (24)	21 (18)	
Child score*	9.5 ± 2.1	7.5 ± 2.1	*<0.001*
MELD score*	21.2 ± 11.8	12.1 ± 5.7	*<0.001*

BMI, body mass index; HBV, hepatitis B virus; HCC, hepatocellular carcinoma; MELD, model for end-stage liver disease. *The data were presented as mean ± SD. Values in italics indicate significance.

UTR)), and rs10099 (exon15 (3'-UTR)). The selected SNPs were detected in chronic liver disease patients with or without HCC using Applied Biosystems SNaPshot and TaqMan technology.

2.3. Statistical Analysis. The Hardy-Weinberg equilibrium was evaluated using Pearson's χ^2 test separately for HCC subjects and controls. The TFCP2 genotype distributions and allele frequencies were compared by using χ^2 analysis or Fisher's exact test. The multivariate logistic regression analysis was conducted to determine the association of TFCP2 polymorphism and HCC susceptibility, with the adjustment with several noncomparable factors, such as gender, MELD score, and Child score at enrollment. For survival comparison, we performed the Kaplan-Meier analyses stratified by the TFCP2 genotypes. The significance of the differences in survival among different genotype carriers was evaluated with the log-rank test. The univariate and multivariate Cox proportional hazard models were conducted to determine the prognostic values of TFCP2 genotype in HCC patients. The hazard ratio (HR) and the 95% confidence interval (95% CI) were calculated. All these above-mentioned statistical analyses were performed by using the SPSS software package (version 18.0; SPSS Inc., Chicago, Illinois). A P value less than 0.05 was considered to be statistically significant.

3. Results

3.1. Clinical Characteristics of the Study Population. A total of 319 patients were included and grouped into non-HCC group (n = 200) and HCC group (n = 119). The basic parameters of the two groups are summarized in Table 1. HBV constituted the majority of the etiology in both the non-HCC and the HCC group, and the proportion of HBV was similar between the two groups (76% versus 82%, P = 0.164). Compared to the non-HCC group, the HCC patients were predominantly men (P = 0.008) and had significantly lower

TABLE 2: Genotype distributions of the 7 SNPs in non-HCC and HCC groups.

	Genotype	Non-HCC	HCC	OR	P	OR*	P*
rs7959378	AA	60 (30)	54 (45)	1 (ref)		1 (ref)	
	AC	94 (47)	49 (41)	0.58 (0.35–0.96)	0.034	0.64 (0.36–1.16)	0.141
	CC	46 (23)	16 (14)	0.39 (0.20–0.76)	0.006	0.43 (0.20–0.92)	0.030
	AC + CC	140 (70)	65 (55)	0.52 (0.32–0.83)	0.006	0.57 (0.33–0.98)	0.044
	A allele	214 (53)	157 (66)	1 (ref)		1 (ref)	
	C allele	186 (47)	81 (34)	0.59 (0.43–0.83)	0.002	0.63 (0.43–0.93)	0.018
rs11169736	GG	127 (63)	76 (64)	1 (ref)		1 (ref)	
	GT	66 (33)	41 (34)	1.04 (0.64–1.68)	0.879	0.98 (0.56–1.72)	0.954
	TT	7 (4)	2 (2)	0.48 (0.10–2.36)	0.364	0.25 (0.05–1.35)	0.108
	GT + TT	73 (37)	43 (36)	0.98 (0.61–1.58)	0.948	0.88 (0.51–1.51)	0.643
	G allele	320 (80)	193 (81)	1 (ref)		1 (ref)	
	T allele	80 (20)	45 (19)	0.93 (0.62–1.40)	0.737	0.80 (0.51–1.27)	0.351
rs1056897	AA	8 (4)	2 (2)	1 (ref)		1 (ref)	
	AG	69 (35)	39 (33)	2.26 (0.46–11.2)	0.317	3.79 (0.71–20.3)	0.121
	GG	123 (61)	78 (65)	2.54 (0.53–12.3)	0.247	4.49 (0.85–23.6)	0.076
	AA + AG	192 (96)	117 (98)	2.44 (0.51–11.7)	0.265	4.20 (0.81–21.8)	0.087
	A allele	85 (21)	43 (18)	1 (ref)		1 (ref)	
	G allele	315 (79)	195 (82)	1.22 (0.81–1.84)	0.332	1.40 (0.89–2.23)	0.147
rs11169735	CC	115 (58)	78 (65)	1 (ref)		1 (ref)	
	CT	70 (35)	38 (32)	0.80 (0.49–1.30)	0.372	0.94 (0.54–1.64)	0.822
	TT	15 (7)	3 (3)	0.30 (0.08–1.05)	0.060	0.63 (0.16–2.51)	0.514
	CT + TT	85 (42)	41 (35)	0.71 (0.44–1.14)	0.156	0.90 (0.52–1.54)	0.698
	C allele	300 (75)	194 (81)	1 (ref)		1 (ref)	
	T allele	100 (25)	44 (19)	0.68 (0.46–1.01)	0.058	0.88 (0.56–1.39)	0.584
rs12820966	AA	130 (65)	79 (66)	1 (ref)		1 (ref)	
	AC	62 (31)	38 (32)	1.01 (0.62–1.65)	0.973	0.95 (0.54–1.68)	0.864
	CC	8 (4)	2 (2)	0.41 (0.09–1.99)	0.269	0.25 (0.05–1.31)	0.101
	AC + CC	70 (35)	40 (34)	0.94 (0.58–1.52)	0.801	0.84 (0.49–1.46)	0.542
	A allele	322 (80)	196 (82)	1 (ref)		1 (ref)	
	C allele	78 (20)	42 (18)	0.89 (0.58–1.34)	0.563	0.77 (0.48–1.23)	0.273
rs10876135	GG	129 (64)	91 (76)	1 (ref)		1 (ref)	
	GA	66 (33)	27 (23)	0.28 (0.03–2.47)	0.254	0.53 (0.05–5.42)	0.591
	AA	5 (3)	1 (1)	0.58 (0.34–0.97)	0.041	0.69 (0.39–1.25)	0.223
	GA + AA	71 (36)	28 (24)	0.56 (0.34–0.93)	0.026	0.69 (0.38–1.22)	0.199
	G allele	324 (81)	209 (88)	1 (ref)		1 (ref)	
	A allele	76 (19)	29 (12)	0.59 (0.37–0.94)	0.026	0.72 (0.43–1.21)	0.214
rs10099	CC	78 (39)	56 (47)	1 (ref)		1 (ref)	
	CT	87 (44)	51 (43)	0.82 (0.50–1.33)	0.415	1.0 (0.56–1.76)	0.986
	TT	35 (17)	12 (10)	0.48 (0.23–1.00)	0.050	0.49 (0.22–1.10)	0.083
	CT + TT	122 (61)	63 (53)	0.72 (0.46–1.14)	0.159	0.83 (0.49–1.40)	0.479
	C allele	243 (61)	163 (68)	1 (ref)		1 (ref)	
	T allele	157 (39)	75 (32)	0.71 (0.51–1.0)	0.050	0.74 (0.51–1.10)	0.132

*P value or odds ratio after adjusting for gender, MELD score, and Child score. OR, odds ratio. Values in italics indicate significance.

MELD and Child scores ($P < 0.001$). The genotype frequencies of all SNPs in the control groups were in the Hardy-Weinberg equilibrium (all P values > 0.05).

3.2. Association Analysis of Candidate SNPs with HCC Risk. We conducted genotyping experiments for the 7 TFCP2 polymorphisms in chronic liver disease patients without HCC ($n = 200$) and with HCC ($n = 119$). The genotype frequencies of TFCP2 gene polymorphism in HCC and controls are presented in Table 2. Of the 7 SNPs in TFCP2, rs7959378 distributed differentially between patients with and without HCC. For rs7959378 polymorphism, the HCC

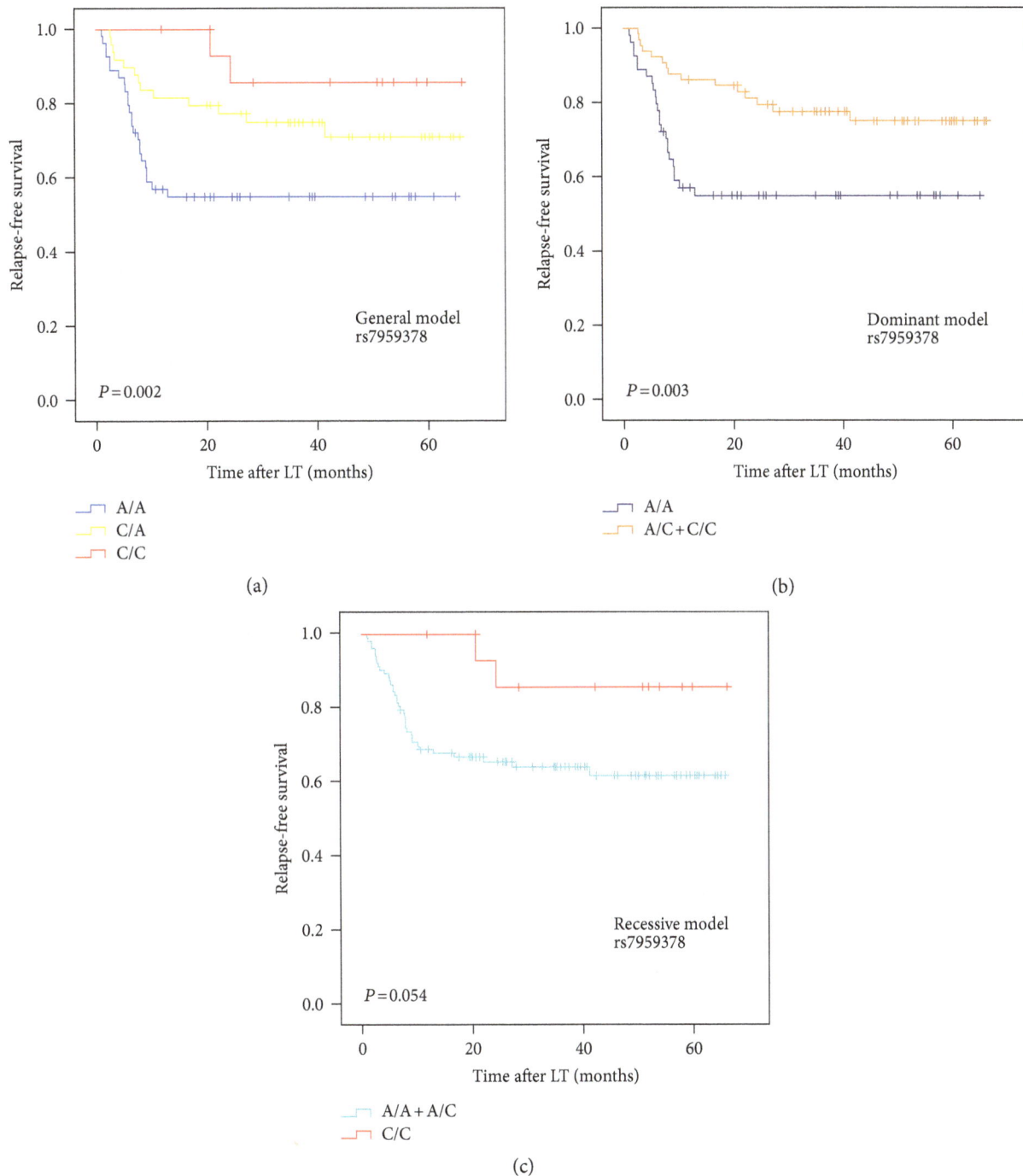

FIGURE 1: The Kaplan-Meier survival curves for relapse-free survival of the HCC patients stratified by rs7959378 genotypes under general model (a), dominant model (b), and recessive model (c).

patients had a lower prevalence of CC (14%) than the control subjects (23%, $P = 0.041$). For allele comparison, HCC subjects had lower C allele frequency (34%) than the controls (47%, $P = 0.002$). Compared with the patients carrying the rs7959378 AA genotype, those with the CC genotype had a decreased risk for HCC with an OR of 0.39 (95% CI 0.20–0.76, $P = 0.006$) and the CA/CC genotypes had a decreased risk for HCC (OR = 0.52, 95% CI 0.32–0.83, $P = 0.006$). After adjusting for gender, MELD score, and

Child score, rs7959378 also conferred significant risk for the disease (CC genotype, OR = 0.43, 95% CI 0.20–0.96, $P = 0.030$; CA/CC genotypes, OR = 0.57, 95% CI 0.33–0.98, $P = 0.044$). We further analyzed the effect of the alleles of rs7959378. With rs7959378 A allele as reference, the OR for rs7959378 C allele carriage was 0.63 (95% CI 0.43–0.93, $P = 0.018$). For the other SNPs, the genotype and allele frequencies were not associated with the HCC risk after the adjustment with the aforementioned confounding factors.

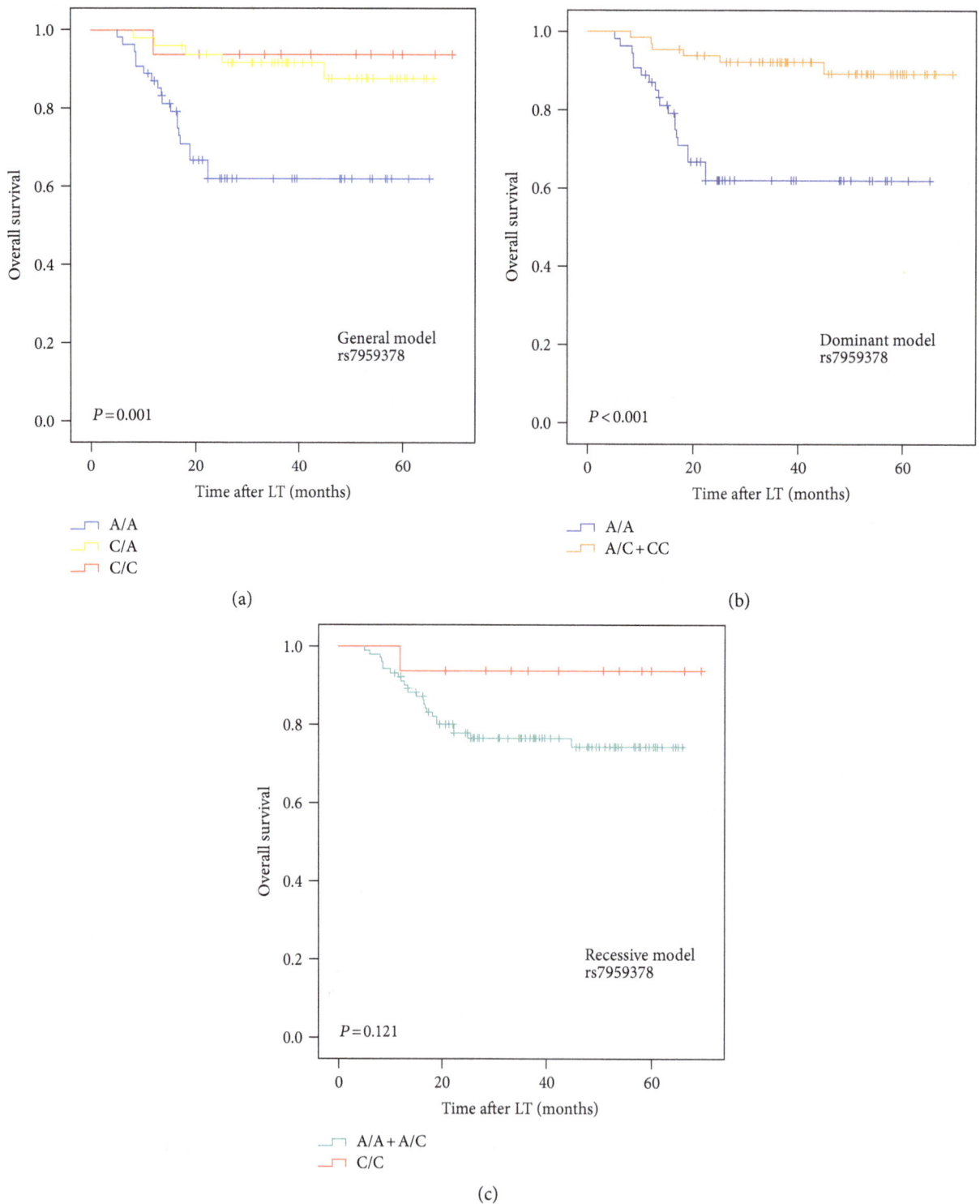

FIGURE 2: The Kaplan-Meier survival curves for overall survival of the HCC patients stratified by rs7959378 genotypes under general model (a), dominant model (b), and recessive model (c).

3.3. TFCP2 rs7959378 Was Associated with the Prognosis of HCC Patients after LT. We next analyzed the association between the TFCP2 SNPs and the prognosis of HCC after LT. We found that rs7959378 was significantly associated with RFS and OS in Kaplan-Meier analysis. The patients who carried the AC or CC genotype (general model: $P = 0.002$)

and AC+CC genotype (dominant model: $P = 0.003$) had a significantly better RFS than those with the AA genotype (Figure 1). The patients who carried the AC or CC genotype (general model: $P = 0.001$) and AC+CC genotype (dominant model: $P < 0.001$) had a significantly better OS than those with the AA genotype (Figure 2).

TABLE 3: Association between the TFCP2 rs7959378 genotype and survival in HCC patients after LT.

rs7959378	RFS				OS			
	HR	P	HR*	P^*	HR	P	HR*	P^*
General		0.014		0.041		0.003		0.021
AA	1 (ref)		1 (ref)				1 (ref)	
AC	0.46 (0.24–0.91)	0.026	0.46 (0.23–0.94)	0.033	0.22 (0.08–0.59)	0.003	0.27 (0.10–0.75)	0.012
CC	0.19 (0.05–0.81)	0.025	0.25 (0.06–1.14)	0.073	0.13 (0.02–1.00)	0.050	0.16 (0.02–1.23)	0.123
Dominant								
AA	1 (ref)		1 (ref)		1 (ref)		1 (ref)	
AC + CC	0.39 (0.20–0.75)	0.005	0.42 (0.21–0.84)	0.014	0.20 (0.08–0.50)	0.001	0.25 (0.08–0.59)	0.006
Recessive								
AA + AC	1 (ref)		1 (ref)		1 (ref)		1 (ref)	
CC	0.27 (0.07–1.13)	0.073	0.39 (0.09–1.66)	0.201	0.23 (0.03–1.73)	0.155	0.34 (0.05–2.60)	0.299

*Adjusted by AFP, tumor size and tumor number, and differentiation. RFS, relapse-free survival. OS, overall survival. HR, hazard ratio. Values in italics indicate significance.

TABLE 4: Association between the rs7959378 genotypes and the clinical features of HCC patients.

Features	rs7959378A>C genotypes n (%)			P
	AA	AC	CC	
AFP				0.474
≤400	41 (49)	33 (39)	10 (12)	
>400	13 (37)	16 (46)	6 (17)	
Tumor number				0.037
Single	27 (37)	33 (45)	13 (18)	
Multiple	27 (59)	16 (35)	3 (6)	
Tumor size				0.053
≤5 cm	32 (39)	37 (45)	14 (16)	
>5 cm	22 (61)	12 (33)	2 (6)	
Differentiation				0.622
Poor	15 (40)	18 (47)	5 (13)	
Mod./well	39 (48)	31 (38)	11 (14)	

AFP, α-fetoprotein. Value in italics indicates significance.

By the univariate Cox regression analysis, we found that patients with the AC or CC genotype (general model) and AC + CC genotype (dominant model) had a significantly better prognosis than those with the AA genotype (Table 3). Multivariate analysis according to the Cox regression hazard model adjusted by AFP, tumor size and tumor number, and differentiation was next performed to evaluate the independent predictive effect of rs7959378 polymorphism on RFS and OS (Table 3). The results showed that, compared with patients carrying the AA genotype, those with the AC genotype (adjusted $P = 0.033, 0.012$ for RFS and OS, resp.) and AC + CC genotype (adjusted $P = 0.014, 0.006$ for RFS and OS, resp.) had a significantly decreased risk of relapse and death. Taken together, these results imply that rs7959378 could be used as an independent prognostic marker for HCC after LT.

We next analyzed the association between TFCP2 rs7959378 and the clinicopathological features in all HCC subjects (Table 4). Compared with the rs7959378 AA genotype, the rs7959378 AC and CC genotypes appeared less frequently in HCC patients with a single tumor ($P = 0.037$). The rs7959378 CC genotype showed a trend toward lower frequency in larger tumors ($P = 0.053$). And no significant associations were observed between rs7959378 and other characteristics.

4. Discussions

Accumulating evidence has illustrated that host genetic factors are widely viewed as the common basis of the different outcomes of chronic liver diseases [20–22]. In this study, we examined the association of the seven SNPs from TFCP2 on the susceptibility of HCC in chronic liver disease subjects in a Chinese population and found that rs7959378 was significantly associated with the risk of HCC. Individuals carrying the rs7959378 C allele (AC or CC genotypes) have a decreased risk of HCC, compared to those with the AA genotype. In addition, our data showed that rs7959378 predicted postoperative relapse-free survival and overall survival for HCC patients after LT. To our knowledge, this is the first report of the genetic association between the TFCP2 gene and the risk of HCC.

TFCP2 overexpression is firstly detected in human HCC patients and associated with the stage and grade of the disease [13]. Then, TFCP2 was found to contribute to 5-fluorouracil resistance [14]. We found that TFCP2 could enhance the invasion of HCC via regulating fibronectin 1 [16]. Additionally, TFCP2 has also been identified as an important determinant of multiple cancers [23, 24]. Polymorphisms in genes, including exons, introns, and untranslated regions, have been shown to affect the processing of mRNAs as well as their regulatory effects and expressions, thus affecting the development and prognosis of different cancers [25, 26]. No studies have specifically addressed the role of TFCP2 polymorphisms in HCC so far. The result presented here showed that subjects with TFCP2 rs7959378 C allele and CC genotype had decreased risk of HCC compared with those with AA genotype after adjusting for noncomparable factors. And those patients with CC genotype also had less probability of multiple tumors.

Our results also indicated that TFCP2 rs7959378 was significantly associated with RFS and OS of HCC patients after LT. The patients with the CC and AC + CC genotypes had a significantly decreased risk of relapse and death compared with those carrying the AA genotype. Further multivariate analysis combined the Cox regression hazard model analysis confirmed rs7959378 as an independent prognostic factor. rs7959378 had a significant association with the number of tumor lesions. Based on our findings, TFCP2 rs7959378 might be used to predict which HCC patients are at risk of poor clinical outcomes in the future.

In conclusion, we report an association between TFCP2 rs7959378 and the risk of HCC and prognosis of HCC after LT, which is independent of other known risk factors. These data highlight the importance of understanding the roles of TFCP2 genetic polymorphisms in HCC pathogenesis, at least in a Chinese population. These findings suggest that TFCP2 rs7959378 could potentially be included in a multifactorial risk assessment and also used as a prognostic predictor for HCC patients who underwent LT.

Competing Interests

The authors declare that there are no ethical/legal conflicts involved in the article.

Acknowledgments

This study was supported by the National High-Tech R&D Program of China (863 Program) (no. 2012AA020204), the National Science and Technology major projects (no. 2012ZX10002010-001-005), and the "Program for New Century Excellent Talents in University" of the Ministry of Education of China.

References

[1] J. Ferlay, I. Soerjomataram, R. Dikshit et al., "Cancer incidence and mortality worldwide: sources, methods and major patterns in GLOBOCAN 2012," *International Journal of Cancer*, vol. 136, no. 5, pp. E359–E386, 2015.

[2] J. Gao, Y. Xiong, Y. Wang, G. Zheng, and H. Xu, "Hepatitis B virus X protein activates Notch signaling by its effects on Notch1 and Notch4 in human hepatocellular carcinoma," *International Journal of Oncology*, vol. 48, no. 1, pp. 329–337, 2016.

[3] T. Kapitanov, U. P. Neumann, and M. Schmeding, "Hepatocellular carcinoma in liver cirrhosis: surgical resection versus transarterial chemoembolization—a meta-analysis," *Gastroenterology Research and Practice*, vol. 2015, Article ID 696120, 2015.

[4] European Association For The Study Of The Liver, "EASL clinical practice guidelines: management of chronic hepatitis B virus infection," *Journal of Hepatology*, vol. 57, no. 1, pp. 167–185, 2012.

[5] T. A. Dragani, "Risk of HCC: genetic heterogeneity and complex genetics," *Journal of Hepatology*, vol. 52, no. 2, pp. 252–257, 2010.

[6] N. B. Ha, A. Ahmed, W. Ayoub et al., "Risk factors for hepatocellular carcinoma in patients with chronic liver disease: a case-control study," *Cancer Causes & Control*, vol. 23, no. 3, pp. 455–462, 2012.

[7] A. B. Hafeez Bhatti, F. S. Dar, A. Waheed, K. Shafique, F. Sultan, and N. H. Shah, "Hepatocellular carcinoma in Pakistan: national trends and global perspective," *Gastroenterology Research and Practice*, vol. 2016, Article ID 5942306, 2016.

[8] R. A. Varier and M. Vermeulen, "Epigenetics and the prognosis of hepatocellular carcinoma," *Epigenomics*, vol. 4, no. 4, 368 pages, 2012.

[9] C. H. Kim, C. Heath, A. Bertuch, and U. Hansen, "Specific stimulation of simian virus 40 late transcription in vitro by a cellular factor binding the simian virus 40 21-base-pair repeat promoter element," *Proceedings of the National Academy of Sciences of the United States of America*, vol. 84, no. 17, pp. 6025–6029, 1987.

[10] J. Veljkovic and U. Hansen, "Lineage-specific and ubiquitous biological roles of the mammalian transcription factor LSF," *Gene*, vol. 343, no. 1, pp. 23–40, 2004.

[11] U. Hansen, L. Owens, and U. H. Saxena, "Transcription factors LSF and E2Fs: tandem cyclists driving G0 to S?" *Cell Cycle*, vol. 8, no. 14, pp. 2146–2151, 2009.

[12] U. H. Saxena, C. M. Powell, J. K. Fecko et al., "Phosphorylation by cyclin C/cyclin-dependent kinase 2 following mitogenic stimulation of murine fibroblasts inhibits transcriptional activity of LSF during G1 progression," *Molecular and Cellular Biology*, vol. 29, no. 9, pp. 2335–2345, 2009.

[13] B. K. Yoo, L. Emdad, R. Gredler et al., "Transcription factor late SV40 factor (LSF) functions as an oncogene in hepatocellular carcinoma," *Proceedings of the National Academy of Sciences of the United States of America*, vol. 107, no. 18, pp. 8357–8362, 2010.

[14] B. K. Yoo, R. Gredler, N. Vozhilla et al., "Identification of genes conferring resistance to 5-fluorouracil," *Proceedings of the National Academy of Sciences of the United States of America*, vol. 106, no. 31, pp. 12938–12943, 2009.

[15] P. K. Santhekadur, R. Gredler, D. Chen et al., "Late SV40 factor (LSF) enhances angiogenesis by transcriptionally up-regulating matrix metalloproteinase-9 (MMP-9)," *The Journal of Biological Chemistry*, vol. 287, no. 5, pp. 3425–3432, 2012.

[16] X. Xu, Z. Liu, L. Zhou et al., "Characterization of genome-wide TFCP2 targets in hepatocellular carcinoma: implication of targets FN1 and TJP1 in metastasis," *Journal of Experimental & Clinical Cancer Research*, vol. 34, 6 pages, 2015.

[17] T. J. Grant, J. A. Bishop, L. M. Christadore et al., "Antiproliferative small-molecule inhibitors of transcription factor LSF reveal oncogene addiction to LSF in hepatocellular carcinoma," *Proceedings of the National Academy of Sciences of the United States of America*, vol. 109, no. 12, pp. 4503–4508, 2012.

[18] C. Peng, Z. Guo, X. Wu, and X. L. Zhang, "A polymorphism at the microRNA binding site in the 3′ untranslated region of RYR3 is associated with outcome in hepatocellular carcinoma," *Onco Targets and Therapy*, vol. 8, pp. 2075–2079, 2015.

[19] X. Guo, D. Li, Y. Chen et al., "SNP rs2057482 in HIF1A gene predicts clinical outcome of aggressive hepatocellular carcinoma patients after surgery," *Scientific Reports*, vol. 5, article 11846, 2015.

[20] S. S. Kim, H. J. Cho, H. Y. Lee et al., "Genetic polymorphisms in the Wnt/beta-catenin pathway genes as predictors of tumor development and survival in patients with hepatitis B virus-associated hepatocellular carcinoma," *Clinical Biochemistry*, vol. 49, no. 10-11, pp. 792–801, 2016.

[21] X. Lao, S. Ren, Y. Lu, D. Yang, X. Qin, and S. Li, "Genetic polymorphisms of C-reactive protein increase susceptibility to HBV-related hepatocellular carcinoma in a Guangxi male population," *International Journal of Clinical and Experimental Pathology*, vol. 8, no. 12, pp. 16055–16063, 2015.

[22] D. K. Jiang, X. P. Ma, X. Wu et al., "Genetic variations in STAT4, C2, HLA-DRB1 and HLA-DQ associated with risk of hepatitis B virus-related liver cirrhosis," *Scientific Reports*, vol. 5, article 16278, 2015.

[23] Y. Goto, I. Yajima, M. Kumasaka et al., "Transcription factor LSF (TFCP2) inhibits melanoma growth," *Oncotarget*, vol. 7, no. 3, pp. 2379–2390, 2016.

[24] H. Jiang, J. Du, J. Jin, X. Qi, Y. Pu, and B. Fei, "LSF expression and its prognostic implication in colorectal cancer," *International Journal of Clinical and Experimental Pathology*, vol. 7, no. 9, pp. 6024–6031, 2014.

[25] S. Fransson, M. Ostensson, A. Djos, N. Javanmardi, P. Kogner, and T. Martinsson, "Estimation of copy number aberrations: comparison of exome sequencing data with SNP microarrays identifies homozygous deletions of 19q13.2 and CIC in neuroblastoma," *International Journal of Oncology*, vol. 48, no. 3, pp. 1103–1116, 2016.

[26] S. Chiba, N. Tsuchiya, Y. Horikawa et al., "Functional mononucleotide repeat polymorphism in the promoter region of HGF is associated with risk and malignant aggressiveness of bladder cancer," *International Journal of Oncology*, vol. 44, no. 3, pp. 678–684, 2014.

11

Primary Care Provider Perceptions of Colorectal Cancer Screening Barriers: Implications for Designing Quality Improvement Interventions

Jennifer M. Weiss,[1,2,3] **Perry J. Pickhardt,**[4] **Jessica R. Schumacher,**[5] **Aaron Potvien,**[6]
David H. Kim,[4] **Patrick R. Pfau,**[1,2] **Elizabeth A. Jacobs,**[2] **and Maureen A. Smith**[3,5,6,7]

[1]*Division of Gastroenterology and Hepatology, University of Wisconsin School of Medicine and Public Health, Madison, WI, USA*
[2]*Department of Medicine, University of Wisconsin School of Medicine and Public Health, Madison, WI, USA*
[3]*University of Wisconsin Carbone Cancer Center, Madison, WI, USA*
[4]*Department of Radiology, University of Wisconsin School of Medicine and Public Health, Madison, WI, USA*
[5]*Department of Surgery, University of Wisconsin School of Medicine and Public Health, Madison, WI, USA*
[6]*Department of Population Health Sciences, University of Wisconsin School of Medicine and Public Health, Madison, WI, USA*
[7]*Department of Family Medicine, University of Wisconsin School of Medicine and Public Health, Madison, WI, USA*

Correspondence should be addressed to Jennifer M. Weiss; jmw@medicine.wisc.edu

Academic Editor: Leticia Moreira

Aims. Colorectal cancer (CRC) screening is underutilized. Increasing CRC screening rates requires interventions targeting multiple barriers at each level of the healthcare organization (patient, provider, and system). We examined groups of primary care providers (PCPs) based on perceptions of screening barriers and the relationship to CRC screening rates to inform approaches for conducting barrier assessments prior to designing and implementing quality improvement interventions. *Methods.* We conducted a retrospective cohort study linking EHR and survey data. PCPs with complete survey responses for questions addressing CRC screening barriers were included (N = 166 PCPs; 39,430 patients eligible for CRC screening). Cluster analysis identified groups of PCPs. Multivariate logistic regression estimated odds ratios and 95% confidence intervals for predictors of membership in one of the PCP groups. *Results.* We found two distinct groups: (1) PCPs identifying multiple barriers to CRC screening at patient, provider, and system levels (N = 75) and (2) PCPs identifying no major barriers to screening (N = 91). PCPs in the top half of CRC screening performance were more likely to identify multiple barriers than the bottom performers (OR, 4.14; 95% CI, 2.43–7.08). *Conclusions.* High-performing PCPs can more effectively identify CRC screening barriers. Targeting high-performers when conducting a barrier assessment is a novel approach to assist in designing quality improvement interventions for CRC screening.

1. Introduction

Despite recent improvements in colorectal cancer (CRC) incidence and mortality, CRC remains the second leading cause of cancer-related death for men and women in the United States [1]. If screening modalities were optimally employed, CRC mortality would be largely preventable [2–9]. Although CRC screening is strongly endorsed by multiple professional societies and achievable using a variety of

methods, national rates remain suboptimal, with only two-thirds of eligible individuals undergoing screening [10–12].

Previous efforts to improve CRC screening rates in the United States yielded an overall increase from ~50% to 65% over the past decade. However, rates have reached a plateau [13]. Evidence suggests targeting interventions to specifically identified barriers is likely to change practice [14]. This is critical to achieving further improvements in CRC screening rates, given the number and complexity of potential CRC screening barriers. However, as stated in a Cochrane review, "we do not yet know the most effective ways to identify barriers, to pick out from amongst all the barriers those that are most important to address, or how to select interventions likely to overcome them" [14].

Primary care providers (PCPs) are a logical source of information about barriers to CRC screening due to their integral role in cancer prevention. PCP recommendation is one of the strongest predictors of screening utilization, even with insurance disparities [15–19]. Yet it is not known which PCPs are best positioned to identify key CRC screening barriers in a health system. It is possible that targeting specific subgroups of PCPs (e.g., low- or high-performers) might yield the most comprehensive barrier assessment. In this study, we examine PCPs' identification of major barriers to CRC screening at each level of the healthcare system, determine if distinct groups of PCPs exist, and examine predictors of membership in these groups. Our results provide valuable information for determining which PCPs can reliably identify CRC screening barriers, with important implications for conducting barrier assessments prior to designing quality improvement interventions.

2. Materials and Methods

2.1. Study Design. The study was conducted in one of the 12 largest multispecialty physician groups in the United States. This group has approximately 1.7 million ambulatory visits per year, delivered by over 300 PCPs in more than 40 multispecialty and community-based primary care clinic sites.

A survey of CRC screening beliefs and practices was mailed to all PCPs within the physician group in February 2010. The goal was to gather data on the current landscape of CRC screening practices in the participating healthcare system prior to designing and implementing system-wide quality improvement interventions. The survey was based on the National Cancer Institute Survey of Colorectal Cancer Screening Practices, developed in collaboration with the CDC and Centers for Medicare and Medicaid Services, and has been used extensively in prior research [15, 20–22]. Survey items were divided into four sections: (1) cancer screening beliefs and practices; (2) attitudes toward CRC screening; (3) CRC screening modalities; and (4) provider characteristics. The overall survey response rate was 70% ($N = 226/322$). We present an analysis of a specific subset of survey items that assessed the importance of perceived barriers to CRC screening at the patient, provider, and system levels and restricted the sample to respondents who completed the entire subset of interest ($N = 166/226$), 73% of the survey responders. Survey responses were linked to patient panel, provider, and clinic level characteristics obtained from the electronic health record (EHR). This study was approved by the Institutional Review Board at the University of Wisconsin-Madison.

2.2. Survey Variables. Survey items assessed PCP perceptions of barriers to CRC screening at patient, provider, and system levels. Responses were dichotomized as "major barrier" or

"minor/not a barrier." *Patient-level barriers* included fear of finding cancer, belief that screening is not effective, embarrassment or anxiety about screening tests, lack of awareness of screening or perception of CRC as a nonserious health threat, fear of an invasive test, and concern about tolerating colonoscopy bowel prep. *Provider-level barriers* included the perception that PCPs do not routinely recommend screening to their patients and lack of time in clinic to discuss screening. *System-level barriers* included long wait times between ordering and scheduling a test, financial cost to patients, shortage of trained providers to conduct screening, and lack of a system for identifying patients eligible for screening. Two additional questions were included to assess provider and system-level barriers. The provider barrier question asked respondents if they had a method to identify which patients were in need of CRC screening exams. Answer choices were yes (coded as "minor/not a barrier") or no (coded as "major barrier"). The system barrier question instructed respondents to "comment on the current capacity of facilities and personnel in your organization to meet the demand for performing colonoscopy." Answer choices were "more than enough," "just about right," "inadequate," and "don't know." Responses were dichotomized with "inadequate" considered a "major barrier," and "more than enough/just about right/don't know" coded as "minor/not a barrier."

2.3. Patient, Provider, and Clinic Characteristics. Sample characteristics were obtained from the EHR. Patient variables included age, gender, race, marital status, primary language, insurance coverage, and comorbidities. A healthcare resource utilization score was calculated for each patient using Ambulatory Care Groups (ACG) based on outpatient and inpatient diagnoses from 12 months prior to survey administration [23, 24]. Provider variables included gender, specialty (Internal Medicine/Family Medicine), years in practice, CRC screening rates in 2009, and size of patient panel eligible for CRC screening. Clinic variables included clinic management and number of providers within the clinic. Clinic distance to the nearest colonoscopy facility was calculated using geographical software. Patients were assigned to PCPs using the plurality provider algorithm described by Pham et al. [25]. PCPs were assigned to clinics by the clinic at which the provider billed the majority of their Evaluation & Management (E&M) visits in 2009.

2.4. Identification of Screen-Eligible Population. We used EHR data to identify the pool of patients eligible for CRC screening in 2009 based on Healthcare Effectiveness Data and Information Set (HEDIS) metrics [26]. Adults aged 50–75 years were included if they were "currently managed" by the physician group. The definition of "currently managed" has been previously published [20]. Patients were excluded if they had a total colectomy based on ICD-9 codes and CPT codes.

2.5. Identification of CRC Screening Completion. Completion of CRC screening was defined as (a) fecal occult blood test (FOBT) in the prior 12 months, (b) flexible sigmoidoscopy, double contrast barium enema, or CT colonography in the past 5 years [11], or (c) colonoscopy in the past 10 years determined by HEDIS codes [26]. All PCPs in the physician group have access to colonoscopy and CT colonography, and most local third party payers cover CT colonography as a CRC screening option at the participating institution [27].

2.6. Statistical Analysis. Our primary goal was to determine if distinct categories of PCPs exist based on perceived CRC screening barriers. Cluster analysis was used to organize PCPs into meaningful structures based on survey responses [28]. Final identification of cluster groups was based on hierarchical cluster analysis using average linkage. Hierarchical clustering allows smaller clusters to be nested within larger ones reflecting a gradation of survey responses; average linkage allows clusters to be hierarchically related without depending on prior knowledge that the clusters resemble chains (single linkage) or are spatially compact (complete linkage) [29].

We compared the frequency of patient, provider, and clinic variables for the PCP cluster groups using χ^2 tests for categorical variables and two-way analysis of variance tests for continuous variables. Multivariate logistic regression with robust estimation of standard errors and clustering at the clinic level was performed using the logit procedure in Stata to obtain odds ratios and 95% confidence intervals for provider and clinic level predictors of membership in one of the PCP groups. Analyses were conducted with Stata 12.0 (StataCorp, College Station, TX) and SAS 9.3 (SAS Institute, Cary, NC) software. All tests of significance used two-sided p values at the $p < 0.05$ level.

3. Results

3.1. Distribution of Survey Responses. Cluster analysis identified two groups of PCPs based on perceived barriers to CRC screening at patient, provider, and system levels: (1) PCPs who perceived multiple major barriers to CRC screening ($N = 75$) and (2) PCPs who perceived no major barriers to CRC screening ($N = 91$). Figure 1 shows the percent of PCPs in each group who perceived each patient, provider, and system-level barrier as a major barrier.

3.2. Sample Characteristics. Overall, the 166 PCPs included in this analysis worked at 24 primary care clinics and cared for 39,430 patients eligible for CRC screening, according to the methodology previously described. The majority of patients were 50–60 years old, White, married, primarily English speaking, and covered by commercial insurance (Table 1). Of the 166 PCPs, 52% were female, over half practiced Internal Medicine (52%), and two-thirds had practiced >10 years. The average number of patients eligible for CRC screening in a provider's panel was 238. Two-thirds of the primary care clinics were physician-owned with an average distance of 7.6 miles to the nearest colonoscopy facility.

PCPs who perceived multiple barriers to CRC screening ($N = 75$) cared for 26,420 patients eligible for screening and worked at 14 different primary care clinics. Comparatively, PCPs who perceived no major barriers to CRC screening ($N = 91$) cared for 13,010 patients eligible for screening and worked at 10 different primary care clinics. The patients

assigned to PCPs who perceived multiple barriers were more often female (61% versus 48%, $p < 0.001$), spoke English as a primary language (92% versus 89%, $p < 0.001$), and had more commercial insurance coverage (67% versus 63%, $p < 0.001$). There was no significant difference between the percent of patients with congestive heart failure and diabetes mellitus or the average ACG resource utilization score between the patients assigned to the two groups. Providers who perceived multiple barriers were more often female (61% versus 45%, $p = 0.043$), had a higher CRC screening rate on average (66% versus 59%, $p = 0.013$), and on average had a larger patient panel eligible for CRC screening compared to the PCPs who perceived no major barriers (250 versus 91 patients, $p < 0.001$). There was no significant difference in clinic characteristics between the two groups of PCPs.

3.3. Predictors of Membership in PCP Groups. In the adjusted model with provider and clinic characteristics, the most significant predictor of membership in one of the PCP groups was provider CRC screening rate (Table 2). PCPs identifying multiple barriers were more likely to be in the top half in terms of CRC screening performance (OR, 4.14; 95% CI, 2.43–7.08). The mean CRC screening rate for the top performers compared to the bottom performers was 75% versus 49% (data not shown). PCP gender, specialty, and years in practice were not significant predictors of membership in a PCP group.

4. Discussion

Our study identified two distinct groups of primary care providers for assistance with CRC screening barrier assessment: (1) PCPs who perceive multiple major barriers to CRC screening and (2) PCPs who perceive no major barriers. The PCPs identifying multiple barriers were four times as likely to be in the top half in terms of CRC screening performance compared to PCPs identifying no major barriers. We hypothesize that high-performers were able to identify barriers at multiple levels of the healthcare system because they are more actively engaged in the CRC screening process and therefore encounter and are attuned to more barriers. This is a critical finding, as the identification of key barriers to screening may allow for the development of targeted interventions to improve CRC screening at a time when rates have plateaued [13].

We found that the PCPs who identified more barriers to CRC screening accurately assessed the climate of our healthcare system at the time of the survey. At the time of survey administration there was a shortage of gastroenterologists in our healthcare system to perform colonoscopies, inadequate capacity to meet the demand for colonoscopies, and very long wait times (>1 year) between ordering and scheduling the exam. These PCPs also identified lack of a system for identifying patients eligible for screening as a major barrier. Although all clinics and PCPs used the same EHR, there was no standard alert at the time of the survey. In response to the survey data, more gastroenterologists were hired to address these issues, significant changes were made to the scheduling process, and the wait time was successfully decreased to <3

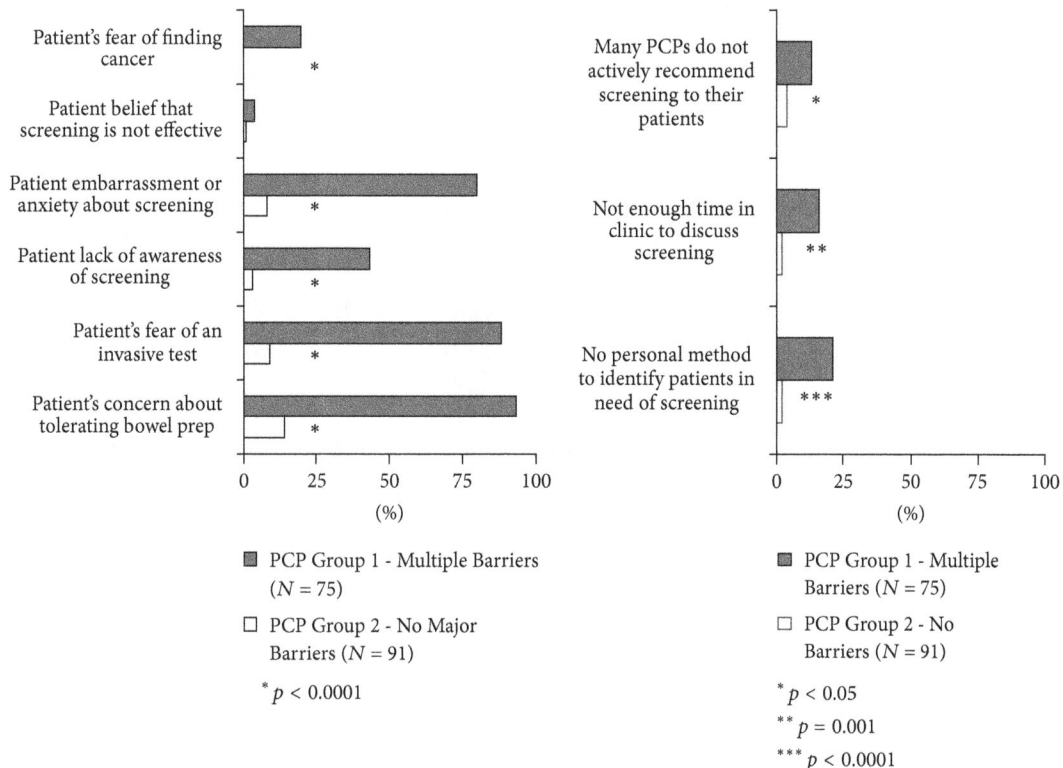

(a) Patient-level barriers

(b) Provider-level barriers

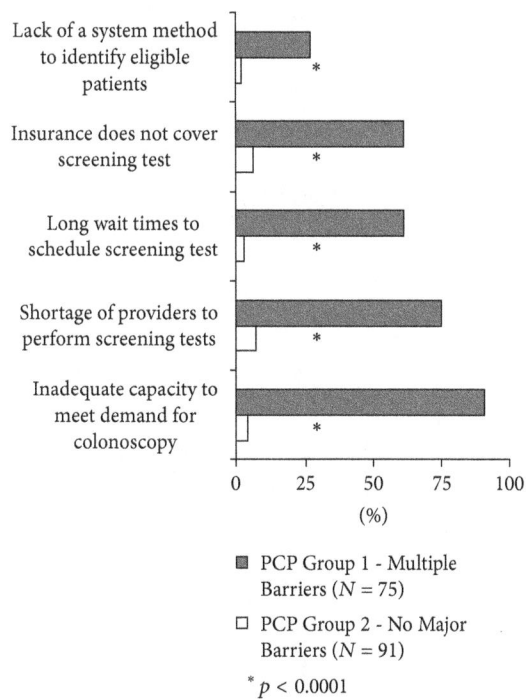

(c) System-level barriers

FIGURE 1: Distribution of survey responses across the two groups of providers for (a) perceived patient-level barriers, (b) perceived provider-level barriers, and (c) perceived system-level barriers.

TABLE 1: Sample characteristics of patients, providers, and clinics (overall and by provider perceptions of barriers).

	Overall	Multiple perceived barriers to CRC screening	No perceived barriers to CRC screening	p value
Patient characteristics	$N = 39{,}430$	$N = 26{,}420$	$N = 13{,}010$	
Age, %				
50–54	27	27	27	
55–59	27	27	26	<0.001
60–64	21	21	21	
65–69	14	14	14	
70–75	11	11	12	
Gender, %				<0.001
Female	56	61	48	
Race, %				0.046
White	93	93	92	
Marital status, %				0.004
Married	71	70	72	
Language, %				
English (as primary language)	91	92	89	<0.001
Primarily non-English	1	1	1	
Unknown	8	7	10	
Insurance, %				
Commercial	66	67	63	
Medicare	24	24	25	<0.001
Medicaid or uninsured	2	2	2	
Missing	9	8	10	
Comorbidities, %				
Congestive heart failure	1	1	1	0.835
Diabetes mellitus	9	9	10	0.437
Hypertension	36	36	35	0.005
ACG resource utilization score (mean, SD)	0.58 (0.42)	0.58 (0.42)	0.58 (0.43)	0.537
Primary care provider characteristics	$N = 166$	$N = 75$	$N = 91$	
Age, %				
30–39	24	20	27	
40–49	26	29	23	0.470
50–59	25	28	22	
60–69	9	11	8	
Missing	16	12	20	
Gender, %				0.043
Female	52	61	45	
Specialty, %				0.133
Internal medicine	52	53	52	
Family medicine	48	47	48	
Years in practice, %				
<10 yrs	18	15	21	
10–20 yrs	31	33	30	0.358
>20 yrs	35	40	31	
Missing	16	12	18	
Average CRC screening rate (%) in the year prior to survey administration (mean, SD)	62 (17.5)	66 (15.7)	59 (18.4)	0.013
Number of patients eligible for CRC screening in a provider's panel (mean, SD)	238 (232)	250 (182)	91 (128)	<0.001

TABLE 1: Continued.

	Overall	Multiple perceived barriers to CRC screening	No perceived barriers to CRC screening	p value
Primary care clinic characteristics	N = 24	N = 14	N = 10	
Clinic management, %				
Physician-owned	67	64	70	0.77
Hospital-owned	33	36	30	
Distance to nearest colonoscopy center in miles, (mean, SD)	7.6 (5.6)	7.1 (3.8)	8.5 (7.7)	0.564
Number of providers within the clinic, (mean, SD)	6.9 (4.9)	8.4 (5.5)	4.8 (3.0)	0.074

SD = standard deviation, ACG = ambulatory care group, and CRC = colorectal cancer.

TABLE 2: Adjusted odds ratios and 95% confidence intervals for provider and clinic predictors of membership in PCP group perceiving multiple barriers (N = 166).

	OR	95% CI	p value
Primary care provider characteristics			
Gender			
Male	(ref)		
Female	2.13	0.88, 5.13	0.090
Specialty			
Family medicine	(ref)		
Internal medicine	0.69	0.19, 2.37	0.552
Years in practice			
<10 yrs	(ref)		
10–20 yrs	1.12	0.53, 2.35	0.764
>20 yrs	1.24	0.52, 2.92	0.626
Missing	0.69	0.24, 2.00	0.498
CRC screening rate			
Bottom half	(ref)		
Top half	4.14	2.43, 7.08	<0.0001
Primary care clinic characteristics			
Clinic management			
Hospital-owned	(ref)		
Physician-owned	0.53	0.18, 1.57	0.253
Distance to nearest colonoscopy center in miles	0.97	0.87, 1.07	0.520
Number of providers within the clinic	0.95	0.90, 0.99	0.044

OR = odds ratio, CI = confidence interval, ACG = ambulatory care group, and CRC = colorectal cancer.

months. In addition, a system-wide health maintenance alert was developed for patients overdue for CRC screening and was implemented for all clinics and PCPs through the EHR.

Interestingly, few PCPs in both groups felt that PCPs not actively recommending screening to their patients was a major barrier. This is despite the fact that the large majority of patients who are not current with CRC screening, 94% of those are over 50 years old [16] and 84% of those over 65 years old [17], list no physician recommendation as a major reason. This may be due to the fact that PCPs are not aware of their degree of influence on a patient's decision to be screened or they think that the majority of PCPs are recommending CRC screening to all eligible patients. Also of interest is that PCP years in practice did not predict membership in a PCP group. This is contrary to some studies that suggest that providers

who have been in practice longer may be less likely to deliver high-quality care, possibly due to out of date information or rapidly changing guidelines [30, 31].

There is significant evidence that interventions tailored to specific barriers can improve care delivery. In a large meta-analysis, Baker et al. [14] compared interventions designed to improve receipt of preventive care that were either tailored or not tailored to address identified barriers and compared these groups to a no-intervention control group. They concluded that interventions tailored to prospectively identified barriers are more likely to improve practice. Tailoring interventions to increase CRC screening is critical, due to the complexity of barriers that results from multiple available CRC screening modalities, the number of providers required for the process, and the various locations where screening can be performed.

Baker et al. [14] also noted that the methods used to identify barriers varied widely between the studies; therefore, the best methods for identifying barriers require further research. It is common practice to call upon high-performing providers and healthcare systems to share their "best practices" so that lower-performers can learn how to improve their CRC screening rates [32]. In addition, we often see low-performing providers interviewed or surveyed about the barriers that are preventing them from being a "high-performer." Our results suggest that lower-performing providers are less likely to identify barriers at different levels within the healthcare system. The results also suggest that initial barrier assessments should target high-performing providers to identify pertinent barriers and possible facilitators to assist in the design and implementation of interventions to improve CRC screening rates.

There are limitations to this study. First, we report findings from a large academic physician group, which could impact generalizability. However, large multispecialty systems are quickly becoming a preferred way to provide high-quality health care and are therefore critical to the understanding of modern health care delivery [33]. Second, our nearly all-white patient population may limit potential generalizability to healthcare systems with a more diverse patient population. Third, the survey reports perceptions of barriers to CRC screening in our healthcare system in 2009-2010. While this was more than five years ago, there is no reason to believe that perceptions of barriers have fundamentally shifted since that time. In addition, our study shows that high-performers are able to more accurately identify CRC screening barriers within a healthcare system and this same concept can be applied to other systems where the exact details of the barriers may be different. Fourth, there are inherent selection biases when relying on survey data, such as nonresponse bias [34–36]. This impact is likely minimal due to our high response rate. Typical survey response rates for healthcare providers are well below 50% [37]. Our overall response rate was 70%; the sample for this study included providers with complete responses to the questions of interest which is 51% of the overall sample. Fifth, a number of our variables rely on the EHR, which could result in missing data and possible misclassification of a completed screening test. However, this is unlikely to result in a systematic bias across clinical settings since all clinics used a fully integrated EHR that has been populated with all data since 1991 (including scanned documents that were manually reviewed to assess completion of CRC screening outside the system). Finally, our cluster analysis used dichotomized survey responses (major barrier versus minor/not a barrier) which results in a loss of some of the finer details in the survey data. However, this was necessary due to the sample size.

5. Conclusions

Multiple healthcare organizations across the country have signed the American Cancer Society call for screening 80% of eligible patients for colorectal cancer by 2018. In order to reach this goal, large initiatives will be formed. In this study, we identified two groups of PCPs: (1) PCPs who perceive multiple major barriers to CRC screening and (2) PCPs who perceive no major barriers. PCPs identifying multiple barriers were more likely to be in the top half in terms of CRC screening performance, suggesting that high-performers of quality metrics of interest should be targeted as the source for effective barrier identification prior to the design and implementation of interventions. Future research will involve determining if the impact and sustainability of these interventions are enhanced for providers who identified the barriers or if the impact is the same for all PCPs.

Disclosure

The funding sources had no role in the design and conduct of the study; collection, management, analysis, and interpretation of the data; preparation, review, or approval of the manuscript; or the decision to submit this manuscript for publication.

Competing Interests

Perry J. Pickhardt, M.D., is a cofounder of VirtuoCTC and shareholder in SHINE and Cellectar. David H. Kim, M.D., is a cofounder of VirtuoCTC, consultant for Viatronix, on the Medical Advisory Board for Digitalartforms, and shareholder in Cellectar and Elucent. Patrick R. Pfau, M.D., serves on the Scientific Advisory Board of EXACT Sciences. Jennifer M. Weiss, M.D., M.S.; Jessica R. Schumacher, Ph.D.; Aaron Potvien, M.S.; Elizabeth A. Jacobs, M.D., MAPP; and Maureen A. Smith, M.D., Ph.D., MPH, declare that they have no competing interests.

Authors' Contributions

All of the authors certify that they warrant authorship by their contribution to the (1) conception/design of the study and/or analysis/interpretation of the data, (2) writing of the manuscript, and (3) approval of the final version. The corresponding author (Jennifer M. Weiss) certifies that she had full access to all of the data in the study and takes responsibility for the integrity of the data and the accuracy of the data analysis. Jennifer M. Weiss, Jessica R. Schumacher, Maureen A. Smith, and Perry J. Pickhardt conceived the study and participated in its design and coordination. Jennifer M. Weiss, Jessica R. Schumacher, Aaron Potvien, and Maureen A. Smith performed the acquisition, analysis, and interpretation of data. Jennifer M. Weiss and Maureen A. Smith drafted the manuscript. All authors contributed to a critical revision of the manuscript for important intellectual content. Jennifer M. Weiss, Jessica R. Schumacher, Aaron Potvien, and Maureen A. Smith performed statistical analysis. All authors read and approved the final manuscript.

Acknowledgments

This work was supported by Grants R01 CA144835 and P30 CA014520 from the National Cancer Institute; Grant UL1TR000427 from the National Center for Advancing

Translational Sciences (NCATS); Grant MRSG-13-144-01-CPHPS a Mentored Research Scholar Grant in Applied and Clinical Research from the American Cancer Society; and the University of Wisconsin Health Innovation Program.

References

[1] R. Siegel, D. Naishadham, and A. Jemal, "Cancer statistics, 2013," *CA Cancer Journal for Clinicians*, vol. 63, no. 1, pp. 11–30, 2013.

[2] S. Winawer, R. Fletcher, D. Rex et al., "Colorectal cancer screening and surveillance: clinical guidelines and rationale—update based on new evidence," *Gastroenterology*, vol. 124, no. 2, pp. 544–560, 2003.

[3] O. Kronborg, C. Fenger, J. Olsen, O. D. Jørgensen, and O. Søndergaard, "Randomised study of screening for colorectal cancer with faecal-occult-blood test," *The Lancet*, vol. 348, no. 9040, pp. 1467–1471, 1996.

[4] J. S. Mandel, T. R. Church, F. Ederer, and J. H. Bond, "Colorectal cancer mortality: effectiveness of biennial screening for fecal occult blood," *Journal of the National Cancer Institute*, vol. 91, no. 5, pp. 434–437, 1999.

[5] J. D. Hardcastle, J. O. Chamberlain, M. H. E. Robinson et al., "Randomised controlled trial of faecal-occult-blood screening for colorectal cancer," *The Lancet*, vol. 348, no. 9040, pp. 1472–1477, 1996.

[6] P. A. Newcomb, R. G. Norfleet, B. E. Storer, T. S. Surawicz, and P. M. Marcus, "Screening sigmoidoscopy and colorectal cancer mortality," *Journal of the National Cancer Institute*, vol. 84, no. 20, pp. 1572–1575, 1992.

[7] J. V. Selby, G. D. Friedman, C. P. Quesenberry Jr., and N. S. Weiss, "A case-control study of screening sigmoidoscopy and mortality from colorectal cancer," *The New England Journal of Medicine*, vol. 326, no. 10, pp. 653–657, 1992.

[8] A. G. Zauber, S. J. Winawer, M. J. O'Brien et al., "Colonoscopic polypectomy and long-term prevention of colorectal-cancer deaths," *New England Journal of Medicine*, vol. 366, no. 8, pp. 687–696, 2012.

[9] R. Nishihara, K. Wu, P. Lochhead et al., "Long-term colorectal-cancer incidence and mortality after lower endoscopy," *The New England Journal of Medicine*, vol. 369, no. 12, pp. 1095–1105, 2013.

[10] United States Preventive Services Task Force, *Guide to Clinical Preventive Services*, Agency for Healthcare Research and Quality, Rockville, Md, USA, 2007.

[11] B. Levin, D. A. Lieberman, B. McFarland et al., "Screening and surveillance for the early detection of colorectal cancer and adenomatous polyps, 2008: a joint guideline from the American Cancer Society, the US Multi-Society Task Force on Colorectal Cancer, and the American College of Radiology," *CA Cancer Journal for Clinicians*, vol. 58, no. 3, pp. 130–160, 2008.

[12] J. A. Shapiro, L. C. Seeff, T. D. Thompson, M. R. Nadel, C. N. Klabunde, and S. W. Vernon, "Colorectal cancer test use from the 2005 national health interview survey," *Cancer Epidemiology Biomarkers and Prevention*, vol. 17, no. 7, pp. 1623–1630, 2008.

[13] C. N. Klabunde, D. A. Joseph, J. B. King, A. White, M. Plescia, and Centers for Disease Control and Prevention (CDC), "Vital signs: colorectal cancer screening test use—United States, 2012," *Morbidity and Mortality Weekly Report*, vol. 62, no. 44, pp. 881–888, 2013.

[14] R. Baker, J. Camosso-Stefinovic, C. Gillies et al., "Tailored interventions to overcome identified barriers to change: effects on professional practice and health care outcomes," *The Cochrane Database of Systematic Reviews*, no. 3, Article ID CD005470, 2010.

[15] C. N. Klabunde, S. W. Vernon, M. R. Nadel, N. Breen, L. C. Seeff, and M. L. Brown, "Barriers to colorectal cancer screening: a comparison of reports from primary care physicians and average-risk adults," *Medical Care*, vol. 43, no. 9, pp. 939–944, 2005.

[16] L. C. Seeff, M. R. Nadel, C. N. Klabunde et al., "Patterns and predictors of colorectal cancer test use in the adult U.S. population," *Cancer*, vol. 100, no. 10, pp. 2093–2103, 2004.

[17] Z. Berkowitz, N. A. Hawkins, L. A. Peipins, M. C. White, and M. R. Nadel, "Beliefs, risk perceptions, and gaps in knowledge as barriers to colorectal cancer screening in older adults," *Journal of the American Geriatrics Society*, vol. 56, no. 2, pp. 307–314, 2008.

[18] A. Gilbert and N. Kanarek, "Colorectal cancer screening: physician recommendation is influential advice to Marylanders," *Preventive Medicine*, vol. 41, no. 2, pp. 367–379, 2005.

[19] C. P. Cairns and K. Viswanath, "Communication and colorectal cancer screening among the uninsured: data from the health information national trends survey (United States)," *Cancer Causes and Control*, vol. 17, no. 9, pp. 1115–1125, 2006.

[20] J. M. Weiss, M. A. Smith, P. J. Pickhardt et al., "Predictors of colorectal cancer screening variation among primary-care providers and clinics," *The American Journal of Gastroenterology*, vol. 108, no. 7, pp. 1159–1167, 2013.

[21] P. A. Mysliwiec, M. L. Brown, C. N. Klabunde, and D. F. Ransohoff, "Are physicians doing too much colonoscopy? A national survey of colorectal surveillance after polypectomy," *Annals of Internal Medicine*, vol. 141, no. 4, pp. 264–271, 2004.

[22] M. R. Nadel, J. A. Shapiro, C. N. Klabunde et al., "A national survey of primary care physicians' methods for screening for fecal occult blood," *Annals of Internal Medicine*, vol. 142, no. 2, pp. 86–94, 2005.

[23] L. A. Petersen, K. Pietz, L. D. Woodard, and M. Byrne, "Comparison of the predictive validity of diagnosis-based risk adjusters for clinical outcomes," *Medical Care*, vol. 43, no. 1, pp. 61–67, 2005.

[24] A. J. Perkins, K. Kroenke, J. Unützer et al., "Common comorbidity scales were similar in their ability to predict health care costs and mortality," *Journal of Clinical Epidemiology*, vol. 57, no. 10, pp. 1040–1048, 2004.

[25] H. H. Pham, D. Schrag, A. S. O'Malley, B. Wu, and P. B. Bach, "Care patterns in medicare and their implications for pay for performance," *New England Journal of Medicine*, vol. 356, no. 11, pp. 1130–1139, 2007.

[26] National Committee for Quality Assurance, *HEDIS 2012 Summary Tables of Measures, Product Lines, and Changes*, National Committee for Quality Assurance, Washington, DC, USA, 2011.

[27] P. J. Pickhardt, A. J. Taylor, D. H. Kim, M. Reichelderfer, D. V. Gopal, and P. R. Pfau, "Screening for colorectal neoplasia with CT colonography: initial experience from the 1st year of coverage by third-party payers," *Radiology*, vol. 241, no. 2, pp. 417–425, 2006.

[28] A. D. Gordon, *Classification*, Chapman & Hall/CRC, Boca Raton, Fla, USA, 1999.

[29] L. Kaufman and P. Rousseeuw, *Finding Groups in Data*, Wiley, New York, NY, USA, 1990.

[30] S.-O. Rhee, "Factors determining the quality of physician performance in patient care," *Medical Care*, vol. 14, no. 9, pp. 733–750, 1976.

[31] N. K. Choudhry, R. H. Fletcher, and S. B. Soumerai, "Systematic review: the relationship between clinical experience and quality of health care," *Annals of Internal Medicine*, vol. 142, no. 4, pp. 260–273, 2005.

[32] C. O'Dell and C. J. Grayson, "If only we knew what we know: identification and transfer of internal best practices," *California Management Review*, vol. 40, no. 3, pp. 154–174, 1998.

[33] F. J. Crosson, "The delivery system matters," *Health Affairs*, vol. 24, no. 6, pp. 1543–1548, 2005.

[34] J. C. Whitehead, P. A. Groothuis, and G. C. Blomquist, "Testing for non-response and sample selection bias in contingent valuation: analysis of a combination phone/mail survey," *Economics Letters*, vol. 41, no. 2, pp. 215–220, 1993.

[35] J.-F. Etter and T. V. Perneger, "Analysis of non-response bias in a mailed health survey," *Journal of Clinical Epidemiology*, vol. 50, no. 10, pp. 1123–1128, 1997.

[36] S. Barclay, C. Todd, I. Finlay, G. Grande, and P. Wyatt, "Not another questionnaire! Maximizing the response rate, predicting non-response and assessing non-response bias in postal questionnaire studies of GPs," *Family Practice*, vol. 19, no. 1, pp. 105–111, 2002.

[37] S. E. Kellerman and J. Herold, "Physician response to surveys: a review of the literature," *American Journal of Preventive Medicine*, vol. 20, no. 1, pp. 61–67, 2001.

12

Genetic Background and Clinical Characters of Pediatric Chronic Pancreatitis: Data and Implications from the East

Muyun Liu, Tian Xia, Di Zhang, Lianghao Hu, Zhuan Liao, Chang Sun, and Zhaoshen Li

Department of Gastroenterology, Changhai Hospital, Second Military Medical University, Shanghai, China

Correspondence should be addressed to Chang Sun; xxxyyy@sina.com and Zhaoshen Li; zhaoshen-li@hotmail.com

Academic Editor: Michel Kahaleh

Background. The clinical pattern and genetic background of juvenile idiopathic chronic pancreatitis (ICP) are yet unclear. *Methods.* A retrospective study of 73 Chinese juvenile ICP patients was performed, and genetic tests were carried out to detect relevant mutations using direct sequencing technique and high-resolution melting technique. Subjects without pancreatitis served as controls. *Results.* The SPINK1 c.194+2T>C variant was present in 56.16% and 42.00% of juvenile and adult ICP patients, respectively ($p = 0.020$), but was not present in any of the control subjects. Thirty-four (46.58%) of the 73 juvenile ICP patients were male, and a significantly higher ratio of male patients in the adult group was identified (46.58% versus 64.00%, $p = 0.022$). Although most of the juvenile patients presented with abdominal pain (70/73, 95.89%), the patterns of pain attack are significantly different in patients with or without SPINK1 c.194+2T>C mutation. Patients carrying the mutation are more likely to present with recurrent acute pancreatitis (70.70%). *Conclusions.* The main symptom of pediatric ICP was abdominal pain. SPINK1 c.194+2T>C mutation had a higher occurrence in juvenile ICP patients than in adult group and typically presented with recurrent acute pancreatitis. There may be unidentified factors that lead to a greater incidence rate of ICP in adult male population.

1. Introduction

Chronic pancreatitis (CP) is defined as a progressive fibro-inflammatory disease characterized by the irreversible damage of the pancreas, associated with chronic or recurrent abdominal pain and impairment of exocrine and endocrine function, occasionally associated with pancreatic lump, jaundice, and ascites [1–3]. Genetic variations have been recognized as a major etiology factor for this disease [4, 5]. CP is a rare disorder in children and adolescents, which will result in excessive number of missed school days and reduction in activities, even addiction to pain medication. Frequent visit to the hospital also causes psychological impairment and self-abasement in underage patients. Researches in the last decade have proven an increasing incidence of CP in children [6].

Environmental factors such as alcoholic consumption, cigarette addiction, and diet immoderation play a smaller role in the onset of chronic pancreatitis than found in adults; thus, the etiology of juvenile CP can be distinct from adult patients [7]. The most common etiological factors of juvenile CP were idiopathic, anatomical anomalies, hyperlipidemia, and trauma. In Chinese population, 73.8% among all pediatric CP patients are idiopathic chronic pancreatitis (ICP) [6, 8] and the main symptom is multiple episodes of mild to moderate abdominal pain [9].

Childhood-onset chronic pancreatitis has distinct features in etiologies, diagnosis, and treatment methods from adult population [10, 11]. Recently, an international multicenter INSPPIRE (International Study Group of Pediatric Pancreatitis: In Search for a Cure) consortium has taken a great step forward to reveal the epidemiology, clinical characteristics, and genetic background of pediatric CP in western population [6, 12]. By investigating 146 pediatric patients from U.S., Canada, and Australia who were diagnosed with CP, they draw the conclusion that relevant pathogenic gene mutations were found in 73% of pediatric CP patients which confirmed the role of genetic variation in adolescent CP patients on the basis of a vast western population. Notably, this study reported a tight connection between serine protease inhibitor Kazal type 1 (SPINK1, OMIM 167790) c.101A>G mutation and the onset of pediatric CP.

Protease serine 1 (PRSS1, OMIM 276000), cystic fibrosis transmembrane conductance regulator (CFTR, OMIM 602421), chymotrypsin C (CTRC, OMIM 601405), and SPINK1 exonic mutation are the most frequently detected gene mutations in Caucasian population [13]. Among more than 100 reported SPINK1 variants, the SPINK1 c.101A>G mutation is most frequently detected in Caucasian population while SPINK1 c.194+2T>C has often been reported in Asian populations. Among the limited investigation concerning SPINK1 c.194+2T>C mutation in western populations, Rosendahl et al. found 2.1% CP patients from Germany who carried SPINK1 c.194+2T>C mutation in comparison to 16.2% patients who carried c.101A>G mutation [14]. However, the situation is completely different in Asian countries. SPINK1 c.101A>G mutation is less frequently found in Asian pediatric CP patients while c.194+2T>C was found in 9.37% to 31.25% of patients according to studies from Japan and Korea [15, 16]. Studies among Chinese population reveal that SPINK1 c.194+2T>C mutation is most frequently seen in Chinese CP patients [17, 18].

In order to further elucidate the diversity in genetic background and clinical characters between Asian and Caucasian pediatric CP patients as well as to address whether the genetic heterogeneity results in different clinical patterns, we performed this retrospective analysis. In this study, we only included pediatric ICP (idiopathic chronic pancreatitis) patients ruling out those with a specific pathogenesis such as pancreatic injury and anatomic abnormality to avoid complication.

2. Materials and Methods

2.1. Subjects. This was a retrospective study, and all consecutive patients with ICP that received treatment from July 2011 to March 2016 at the Department of Gastroenterology at Changhai Hospital of the Second Military Medical University were included in the study. Our endoscopic center introduced the first extracorporeal shock wave lithotripsy machine targeting pancreatic stones and is well known as the largest ERCP training center in China. So pediatric CP patients are also hospitalized in our department.

The diagnosis of CP was made in the appropriate clinical setting if there was evidence of pancreatic duct dilatation and irregularity and/or pancreatic calcification found in imaging studies [2]. Idiopathic chronic pancreatitis was diagnosed if preexisting disorders likely to cause chronic pancreatitis (hypertriglyceridemia, primary hyperparathyroidism, abdominal trauma, and pancreatic duct stenosis caused by operation), hereditary chronic pancreatitis (HCP) (as determined by family history), and excessive alcohol consumption were absolutely ruled out [19]. Juvenile idiopathic chronic pancreatitis was diagnosed with the age at the first onset of symptoms being 18.0 years or younger [9].

Among all the CP patients, a total of 103 had disease onset age younger than eighteen. Sixteen of them had anatomical anomalies in pancreas and/or pancreatic duct that can be proved by computed tomography (CT) and/or magnetic resonance imaging (MRI). Family history was recorded and six pediatric patients were excluded with a clear diagnosis of HCP. Three patients were excluded with a pancreatic injury history. Notably, one patient was finally diagnosed with cyst fibrosis thus excluded from this study. A total of 77 pediatric onset CP patients were included. All 77 families were informed about the peripheral blood and genetic analysis. Two of the families refused to participate in further analysis. Among the 77 peripheral blood samples we collected, two samples degraded and failed for PCR analysis due to inappropriate storage method (Figure 1).

To compare clinical characters and genetic backgrounds of pediatric ICP patients and adult ICP patients, we randomly took 100 adult ICP patients from our database with complete chronic pancreatitis-relevant genetic background information.

The controls were healthy individuals from blood donors. "Healthy" was defined as the absence of any type of infection or known medical condition at the time of the study. We obtained 5 ml of peripheral blood from every healthy control and patient, and the samples were stored at −80°C after anticoagulation treatment with EDTA.

For deidentification, all of the samples were coded with a number to protect the privacy of the individuals during the study. All of the participants gave written informed consent to participate in this study, and the samples were processed under the approval of the Changhai Hospital Ethics Committee.

2.2. Genomic Analysis. As previously described, Qiagen DNeasy blood and tissue kit was used to extract genomic DNA from the blood sample. Direct sequencing was used to analyze mutations of SPINK1 gene (OMIM 167790) exon 3 and intron from polymerase chain reaction (PCR) products [18]. In brief, a primer pair was designed to amplify regions of the SPINK1 exon 3 and intron. PCR products were analyzed using direct sequencing (ABI Prism Automated DNA Sequencer model 3100, PE Applied Biosystems, USA). Analysis of exons 2 and 3 of PRSS1 gene (OMIM 602421) mutations was performed by direct sequencing of PCR products. Primer pairs were designed to detect PRSS1 gene exon 2 and exon 3.

A HRM (high-resolution melting) technique provided by the Shanghai Healo-Tech Corp was used to scan mutations of the CFTR (cystic fibrosis transmembrane conductance regulator, MIM 602421) gene as previously described [18]. All sequences were compared to the reference sequences available in GenBank of the National Center for Biotechnology Information database (https://www.ncbi.nlm.nih.gov).

2.3. Clinical Characters. Disease onset age was recorded according to the occurrence of disease related symptoms including acute pancreatitis, recurrent abdominal pain, chronic pancreatic pain, or radiological findings. Disease related pain patterns were defined as recurrent acute pancreatitis (RAP), recurrent abdominal pain (RP) without significant increase in serum amylase, recurrent acute pancreatitis or

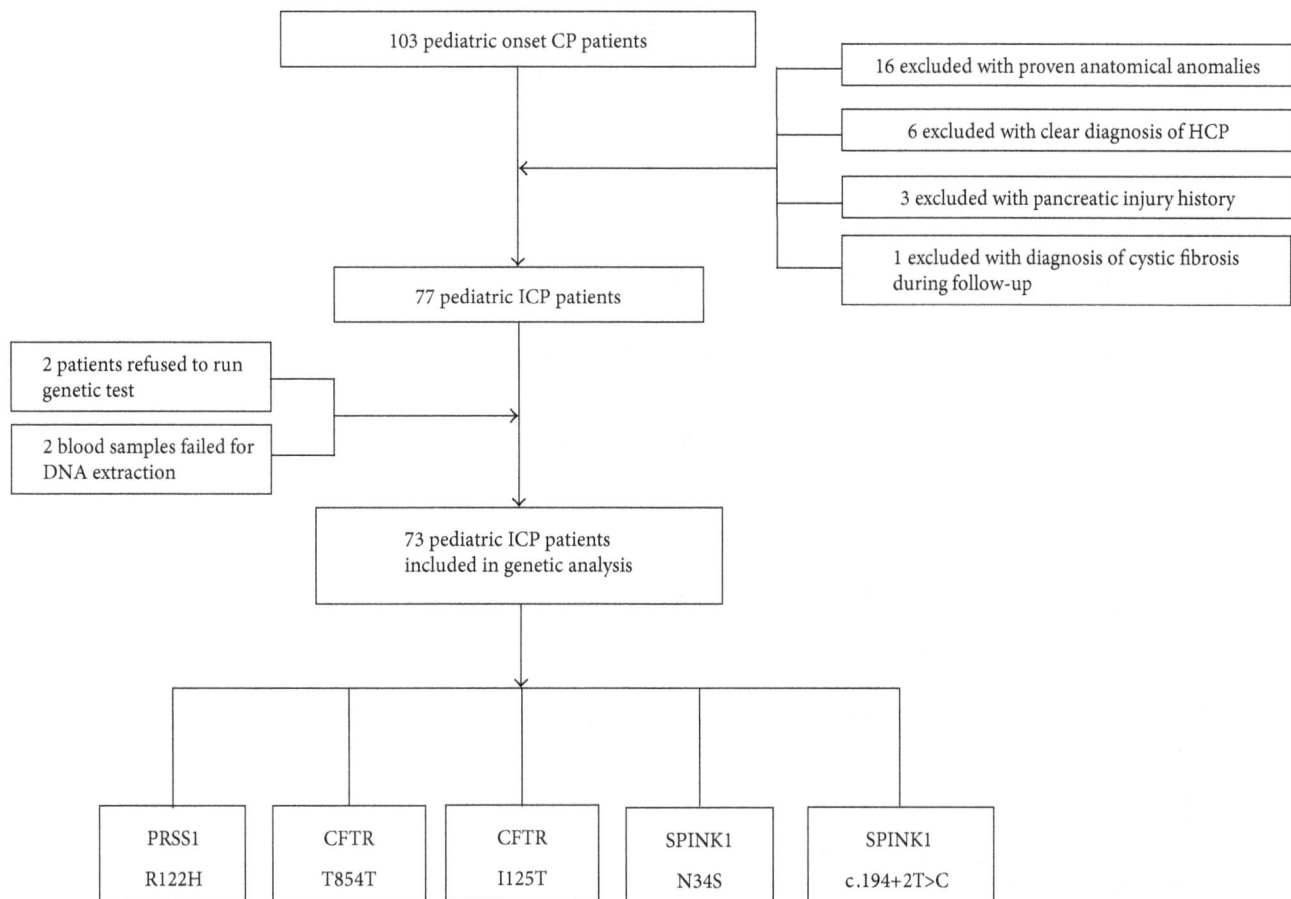

FIGURE 1: Of all the 103 pediatric ICP patients, a total of 26 patients were excluded for clear pathogenic factors such as anatomic abnormalities and pancreatic injuries.

abdominal pain (RAP/P) without significant increase in serum amylase, chronic pancreatic pain (CPP), or no pain attack. Pancreatic calcifications include both pancreatic stones located in the main or branch pancreatic ducts and calcifications found in pancreatic parenchyma. Diabetes was diagnosed with fasting glucose level over 7.0 mmol per liter and glycated hemoglobin level over 6.5% [20]. Clinical patterns and complications were recorded when patients were first included in this study.

2.4. Statistical Analysis. The data are presented as means and SDs. The unpaired t-test for comparing quantitative data and the χ^2 test for qualitative data were used when appropriate. A p value of 0.05 was used as the cutoff for statistical significance. Graphpad Prism (version 7) was used for the statistical analyses.

3. Results

3.1. General Information. A total of 73 pediatric chronic pancreatitis patients were included in the final analysis as shown in Figure 1. General information of the included pediatric ICP patients was analyzed. Of the 73 juvenile ICP patients, 34 (46.58%) were male (Table 1). In comparison with the sex distribution of juvenile and adult ICP patients

TABLE 1: Clinical characters of juvenile ICP patients.

	Children and adolescent CP patients ($n = 73$)
Age at onset	10.37 ± 3.42
Male	34 (46.58%)
Body mass index (Kg/m^2)	19.55 ± 2.36
Pain	70 (95.89%)
Jaundice	1 (1.37%)
Lump	0 (0.00%)
Pancreatic calcification	58 (79.45%)
Complications	
Ascites and/or pleural effusion	2 (2.74%)
Portal hypertension	0 (0.00%)
Pseudocyst	7 (9.59%)
Diabetes mellitus	4 (5.48%)
Steatorrhea	0 (0.00%)

ICP, idiopathic chronic pancreatitis; CP, chronic pancreatitis.

($n = 100$, data from published paper) among which 64% patients were male, there were significantly more male patients in adult population ($p = 0.022$). Body mass index

TABLE 2: Genetic characteristics of patients with idiopathic chronic pancreatitis and controls.

	Pediatric ICP patients ($n = 73$)	Adult ICP patients (%) ($n = 100$)	Healthy controls (%) ($n = 100$)
PRSS1 c.365G>A	14/73 (19.18%[#])	12/100 (12.00%)	0 (0%)
CFTR c.2562T>G	2/73 (2.74%)	2/100 (2.00%)	0 (0%)
SPINK1 c.101A>G	0/73 (0%)	0/100 (0.00%)	0 (0%)
c.194+2T>C*	41/73 (56.16%)	42/100 (42.00%)	0 (0%)

ICP: idiopathic chronic pancreatitis; PRSS1, protease serine 1; CFTR, cystic fibrosis transmembrane conductance regulator; SPINK1: serine protease inhibitor Kazal type 1; [#]the percentage refers to the proportion of patients within each group. *$p = 0.02$ juvenile ICP versus adult ICP.

was 19.55 ± 2.36 in pediatric ICP patients at the time of enrollment (Table 1).

3.2. Clinical Features. Nearly all of the 70 (95.89%) juvenile ICP patients presented with abdominal pain. Only 1 out of 73 (1.37%) pediatric ICP patients presented with jaundice. Imaging methods including CT, magnetic resonance imaging (MRI), B-ultrasound, and X-ray suggested pancreatic calcification in 58 (79.54%) pediatric ICP patients. Notably, one of these patients had negative pancreatic stone which has been proven by pancreatic duct obstruction presented in magnetic resonance cholangiopancreatography (MRCP) images and proven in endoscopic retrograde cholangiopancreatography (ERCP) (Table 1).

3.3. Complications. Pseudocyst was the most common complication and was noted in 9.59% (7/73) juvenile ICP patients. Ascites or pleural effusion was also relatively common in juvenile ICP patients as 2 patients (2.74%) presented with these symptoms. Both patients were hospitalized during episode of acute pancreatitis (Table 1). Diabetes on presentation was noted in 4 out of the 73 (5.48%) juvenile ICP patients at the time of enrollment. So far, none of the patients with diabetes had microvascular or macrovascular complications on presentation. One out of the four patients relied on insulin treatment. During our follow-up, another patient had endocrine function deterioration and finally started insulin treatment to steadily control blood glucose. None of the 73 pediatric ICP patients had steatorrhea at enrollment or during follow-up. Continuous supplement of pancreatic enzymes for some of the patient may have interfered with the observation of exocrine function deterioration.

3.4. Genetic Profile. Among the 73 pediatric ICP patients, 14 (19.18%) carried PRSS1 C.365G>A gene mutation compared to 12 (12%) in adult ICP patients; all of these patients carried PRSS1 C.365G>A heterozygous mutation. No significant difference was observed between adult and pediatric populations. Heterozygous CFTR C.2562T>G mutation was observed in 2.74% (2/73) pediatric patients compared to 2.00% (2/100) in adult patients, and no statistical difference was noticed.

Neither juvenile nor adult ICP patients had SPINK1 C.101A>G mutation. Of the 73 juvenile ICP patients, 41 (56.16%) patients had c.194+2T>C mutation as compared with 42 (42.00%) of 100 adult patients suggesting a higher mutation rate in the juvenile group ($p = 0.002$) (Table 2). Among the 41 pediatric chronic pancreatitis patients, 8 carried homozygous SPINK1 c.194+2T>C mutation and

33 carried heterozygous c.194+2T>C mutation. In addition, none of the healthy controls was found to carry any relative mutations; thus, significant differences were detected between juvenile ICP patients and healthy controls as well as between adult ICP patients and healthy controls ($p < 0.001$) (Table 2).

3.5. Comparison of Pediatric CP Patients with or without SPINK1 c.194+2T>C Mutations. To address the clinical features and translational implications of SPINK1 c.194+2T>C mutation, we compared the two groups of pediatric ICP patients with or without SPINK1 c.194+2T>C mutation. No difference in CP onset age or gender distribution was noticed ($p = 0.674$; $p = 0.170$, resp.). However, the onset pattern was distinctively different among these two groups of patients. Among all 41 pediatric CP patients carrying the SPINK1 intronic mutation, 29 (70.7%) presented with RAP. The rest of pediatric patients who were carrying SPINK1 c.194+2T>C mutation presented with RP (6, 14.6%), RAP/P (1, 2.4%), CPP (3, 7.3%), and no pain attack (2, 4.9%). On the other hand, among the 32 patients without SPINK1 c.194+2T>C mutation, 10 (31.3%) presented with RAP, 2 (6.3%) presented with RP, 11 (34.4%) presented with RAP/P, 8 (25.0%) presented with CPP, and 1 (3.1%) did not present with abdominal pain. Significant difference between groups was confirmed by χ^2 test ($p < 0.001$) (Table 3).

Notably, all of the four patients with diabetes carried SPINK1 c.194+2T>C. But no statistical significance was shown due to the limited diabetes onset chances in children and adolescent patients.

4. Discussion

In the current study, we draw a picture of the clinical features and genetic backgrounds of pediatric ICP in China. In addition, we made comparison between adult and pediatric ICP patients to dig into the heterogeneity of ICP in these two patient populations. Results in our study showed that the sex distribution of juvenile and adult patients differed significantly. The percentage of male patients was higher than that in pediatric patients. According to a multicenter study initiated by the Chinese Chronic Pancreatitis Study Group to determine the nature and magnitude of CP in China, 64.99% among the 2008 patients included were male and 35.01% were female [3]. Notably, this study included chronic patients of all different etiologies. Data from Japan and western countries demonstrated elevated ICP onset rate in male population [21, 22]. Obvious difference of sex distribution between CP patients in these age groups

TABLE 3: Comparison of juvenile ICP patients with or without the SPINK1 c.194+2T>C mutations.

	Juvenile patients carrying the mutation ($n = 41$)	Juvenile patients without the mutation ($n = 32$)	p value
Age at onset (years, mean ± SD)	10.22 ± 2.91	10.56 ± 4.02	0.674
Female	19 (46.3%)	20 (65.2)	0.170
Clinical features			
Type of pain attack			<0.001
RAP	29 (70.7%)	10 (31.3%)	
RP	6 (14.6%)	2 (6.3%)	
RAP/P	1 (2.4%)	11 (34.4%)	
CPP	3 (7.3%)	8 (25.0%)	
No pain attack	2 (4.9%)	1 (3.1%)	
Jaundice	1 (2.4%)	0 (0.0%)	0.307
Pancreatic calcification	32 (78.0%)	26 (81.3%)	0.737
Complications			
Pseudocyst	4 (9.8%)	3 (9.4%)	0.956
Diabetes mellitus	4 (9.8%)	0 (0%)	0.069
Steatorrhea	0 (0.00%)	0 (0.00%)	na

SPINK1, serine protease inhibitor Kazal type 1; SD, standard deviation; RAP, recurrent acute pancreatitis; RP, recurrent abdominal pain; RAP/P, recurrent acute pancreatitis or abdominal pain without significant increasing in serum amylase; CPP, chronic pancreatic pain.

suggested that male population is more likely to be exposed to environmental factors such as smoking, unhealthy lifestyle, and a higher BMI as well as some unknown risk factors. According to previous studies, alcohol consumption at lower levels (<50 g/day) was suggested to play a modifying role in disease development and these patients were believed to represent a subset of late-onset idiopathic CP [23]. Also, previous researches confirmed the association between smoking and CP and demonstrated that this effect is dose dependent [24–27].

In our present study, we found that almost all pediatric ICP patients had abdominal pain (95.89%). Patients with early-onset idiopathic and alcoholic chronic pancreatitis are more likely to have clinical symptoms mostly presented with abdominal pain when compared with subjects with late-onset idiopathic CP [28]. Furthermore, the presence of pain in juvenile CP was 100% according to the research data in another study [2]. On the other hand, only 1.37% patients presented with jaundice and 9.59% patients presented with pancreatic pseudocyst. On this basis, the disease related pain as well as acute pancreatitis onset should be listed as the primary factor that we need to consider in clinical treatment plans.

Genetic mutations related to pancreatitis have been studied in a wide range of populations all over the world [4]. The functions of typical mutations in genes such as PRSS1 and CFTR have been elucidated, and their prevalence has been well addressed in Caucasian populations [29–31]. Gomez-Lira et al. found that the c.194+2T>C intronic alteration could abolish SPINK1 expression at the mRNA level [32]. Studies in Chinese population these years revealed that unlike in Caucasian populations, SPINK1 c.194+2T>C was the most common mutation of SPINK1 gene in Chinese CP patients [17, 18]. This has also been proven in our present

study as both juvenile and adult ICP patients were detected with a SPINK1 c.194+2T>C mutation while none of the healthy controls presented with any mutation of SPINK1. In addition, we found that the percentage of the patients carrying SPINK1 c.194+2T>C mutation was even higher in pediatric ICP patients than in adult ICP patients. This result indicates that genetic factors play a more important role in childhood ICP rather than that in adult ICP, suggesting other factors such as environment, diet, sexuality, and lifestyle may impact adult ICP patients to a greater extent with time effect. Furthermore, as c.194+2T>C mutation was not seen in any of the healthy controls, there lies a possibility that the test for c.194+2T>C mutation can serve as diagnostic criteria or even as an antenatal diagnosis method. Notably, genetic analysis of the 73 pediatric ICP patients detected PRSS1 C.365G>A mutation. According to previous studies, PRSS1 gene mutations are considered a typical feature for hereditary chronic pancreatitis [33]. However, as far as we are concerned, SPINK1 mutations have also been recognized as closely related to familial pancreatitis [33, 34]. So we analyzed the characters of all the 73 pediatric ICP patients.

The high frequency of SPINK1 c.194+2T>C mutation inspired us to dig into its clinical implications. Surprisingly, we found that the pain pattern at disease onset is distinctly different in pediatric ICP patients with or without SPINK1 c.194+2T>C mutation. The most common type of pain attack in pediatric patients carrying the intronic mutation is recurrent acute pancreatitis which is found in 70.7% of all cases. However, the pattern of pain attack in patients without SPINK1 c.194+2T>C mutation can be characterized as RAP, RP, RAP/P, and CPP in a decentralized fashion. This result gives us a hint that, for pediatric patients suffering from RAP attack, an examination of related gene mutation should be recommended. Whether this finding can serve as an implication of the genetic connection between RAP and CP is quite fascinating. Our group has initiated a screening of genetic mutations in Chinese recurrent pancreatitis patients and hopefully this study could further reveal the whole picture.

Due to the limited time of disease progression, very few pediatric ICP patients presented with endocrine and exocrine function impairment. However, all of the 4 patients with diabetes mellitus carried SPINK1 c.194+2T>C mutation. In the previous studies from our group, we found that SPINK1 c.194+2T>C mutation is a predisposing factor for the earlier onset of pancreatic diabetes [18] which is consistent with this result.

According to a recent publication from Korea, pancreatic duct stones occurred more frequently in patients with the c.194+2T>C pathogenic variant [35]. It gives us a hint to look into this situation from another clinical prospective. As a majority of chronic pancreatitis patients came to our treatment center hoping to undergo interventional treatments including ESWL and ERCP to resolve pancreatic ductal obstruction, the occurrence of pancreatic stone might be higher. We are undergoing further analysis to elucidate this discovery.

According to the 2012 American Community Survey, Asian American comprises 15.5 million out of the whole population in the United States. Moreover, Asian population has been growing in North America, Austria, and New Zealand. Thus, gene diversity should be considered for a better coverage of different races. As the frequency of SPINK1 c.194+2T>C is rather in Chinese chronic patients and distinct clinical features have been addressed, we propose that this intronic variant should arouse more attention in researchers and clinicians all over the world to better facilitate the practice of precision medicine.

5. Conclusion

By comparing different groups of ICP patients, we concluded that SPINK1 c.194+2T>C mutation had a higher occurrence in juvenile ICP patients than in the adult group. There are more male patients in adult ICP population than in pediatric patients. More patients carrying SPINK1 c.194+2T>C presented with recurrent acute pancreatitis at disease onset. We should pay more attention to pathogenic intronic variants in relevant studies among different races and generations.

Abbreviations

ICP: Idiopathic chronic pancreatitis
SPINK1: Serine protease inhibitor Kazal type 1.

Competing Interests

The authors indicated no potential conflicts of interest.

Authors' Contributions

Zhaoshen Li, Chang Sun, and Zhuan Liao participated in the conception and design of the study. Muyun Liu, Chang Sun,

Tian Xia, Di Zhang, and Lianghao Hu participated in the generation, collection, assembly, analysis, and/or interpretation of data. Muyun Liu, Zhuan Liao, Chang Sun, and Zhaoshen Li participated in the drafting or revision of the manuscript. Muyun Liu, Tian Xia, Lianghao Hu, Zhuan Liao, Chang Sun, and Zhaoshen Li participated in the approval of the final version of the manuscript.

Acknowledgments

This work was supported by Grants 81101832 and 81470885 from the National Natural Science Foundation of China. The authors thank Dr. Weiqin Lu from the Division of Gastroenterology and Hepatology, Department of Medicine, Stony Brook University, Stony Brook, NY, USA, for her kind advice for this study.

References

[1] S. Majumder and S. T. Chari, "Chronic pancreatitis," *The Lancet*, vol. 387, no. 10031, pp. 1957–1966, 2016.

[2] R. K. Tandon, N. Sato, and P. K. Garg, "Chronic pancreatitis: Asia-Pacific consensus report," *Journal of Gastroenterology and Hepatology*, vol. 17, no. 4, pp. 508–518, 2002.

[3] L. W. Wang, Z. S. Li, S. D. Li, Z. D. Jin, D. W. Zou, and F. Chen, "Prevalence and clinical features of chronic pancreatitis in China: a retrospective multicenter analysis over 10 years," *Pancreas*, vol. 38, no. 3, pp. 248–254, 2009.

[4] M. N. B. Sahin-Tóth, *Genetic Risk Factors in Chronic Pancreatitis*, 2015, http://www.pancreasgenetics.org/.

[5] D. C. Whitcomb, "Genetic risk factors for pancreatic disorders," *Gastroenterology*, vol. 144, no. 6, pp. 1292–1302, 2013.

[6] V. D. Morinville, S. Z. Husain, H. Bai et al., "Definitions of pediatric pancreatitis and survey of present clinical practices," *Journal of Pediatric Gastroenterology and Nutrition*, vol. 55, no. 3, pp. 261–265, 2012.

[7] D. Yadav, A. Slivka, S. Sherman et al., "Smoking is underrecognized as a risk factor for chronic pancreatitis," *Pancreatology*, vol. 10, no. 6, pp. 713–719, 2010.

[8] W. Wang, Z. Liao, Z. S. Li et al., "Chronic pancreatitis in Chinese children: etiology, clinical presentation and imaging diagnosis," *Journal of Gastroenterology and Hepatology*, vol. 24, no. 12, pp. 1862–1868, 2009.

[9] Z. S. Li, W. Wang, Z. Liao et al., "A long-term follow-up study on endoscopic management of children and adolescents with chronic pancreatitis," *The American Journal of Gastroenterology*, vol. 105, no. 8, pp. 1884–1892, 2010.

[10] M. Sathiyasekaran, V. Biradar, G. Ramaswamy et al., "Pancreatitis in children," *Indian Journal of Pediatrics*, vol. 83, no. 12–13, pp. 1459–1472, 2016.

[11] E. Kolodziejczyk, E. Jurkiewicz, J. Pertkiewicz et al., "MRCP versus ERCP in the evaluation of chronic pancreatitis in children: which is the better choice?" *Pancreas*, vol. 45, no. 8, pp. 1115–1119, 2016.

[12] S. Kumar, C. Y. Ooi, S. Werlin et al., "Risk factors associated with pediatric acute recurrent and chronic pancreatitis: lessons from INSPPIRE," *JAMA Pediatrics*, vol. 170, no. 6, pp. 562–569, 2016.

[13] E. Masson, J. M. Chen, M. P. Audrezet, D. N. Cooper, and C. Ferec, "A conservative assessment of the major genetic causes of idiopathic chronic pancreatitis: data from a

comprehensive analysis of PRSS1, SPINK1, CTRC and CFTR genes in 253 young French patients," *PLoS One*, vol. 8, no. 8, article e73522, 2013.

[14] J. Rosendahl, O. Landt, J. Bernadova et al., "CFTR, SPINK1, CTRC and PRSS1 variants in chronic pancreatitis: is the role of mutated CFTR overestimated?" *Gut*, vol. 62, no. 4, pp. 582–592, 2013.

[15] N. Saito, M. Suzuki, Y. Sakurai et al., "Genetic analysis of Japanese children with acute recurrent and chronic pancreatitis," *Journal of Pediatric Gastroenterology and Nutrition*, vol. 63, no. 4, pp. 431–436, 2016.

[16] Y. J. Lee, K. M. Kim, J. H. Choi, B. H. Lee, G. H. Kim, and H. W. Yoo, "High incidence of PRSS1 and SPINK1 mutations in Korean children with acute recurrent and chronic pancreatitis," *Journal of Pediatric Gastroenterology and Nutrition*, vol. 52, no. 4, pp. 478–481, 2011.

[17] Y. T. Chang, S. C. Wei, P. C. L et al., "Association and differential role of PRSS1 and SPINK1 mutation in early-onset and late-onset idiopathic chronic pancreatitis in Chinese subjects," *Gut*, vol. 58, no. 6, article 885, 2009.

[18] C. Sun, Z. Liao, L. Jiang et al., "The contribution of the SPINK1 c.194+2T>C mutation to the clinical course of idiopathic chronic pancreatitis in Chinese patients," *Digestive and Liver Disease*, vol. 45, no. 1, pp. 38–42, 2013.

[19] D. K. Bhasin, G. Singh, S. S. Rana et al., "Clinical profile of idiopathic chronic pancreatitis in north India," *Clinical Gastroenterology and Hepatology*, vol. 7, no. 5, pp. 594–599, 2009.

[20] D. L. Cahen, D. J. Gouma, Y. Nio et al., "Endoscopic versus surgical drainage of the pancreatic duct in chronic pancreatitis," *The New England Journal of Medicine*, vol. 356, no. 7, pp. 676–684, 2007.

[21] M. Hirota, T. Shimosegawa, A. Masamune et al., "The sixth nationwide epidemiological survey of chronic pancreatitis in Japan," *Pancreatology*, vol. 12, no. 2, pp. 79–84, 2012.

[22] D. Yadav, L. Timmons, J. T. Benson, R. A. Dierkhising, and S. T. Chari, "Incidence, prevalence, and survival of chronic pancreatitis: a population-based study," *The American Journal of Gastroenterology*, vol. 106, no. 12, pp. 2192–2199, 2011.

[23] M. R. Lankisch, M. Imoto, P. Layer, and E. P. DiMagno, "The effect of small amounts of alcohol on the clinical course of chronic pancreatitis," *Mayo Clinic Proceedings*, vol. 76, no. 3, pp. 242–251, 2001.

[24] D. Yadav, R. H. Hawes, R. E. Brand et al., "Alcohol consumption, cigarette smoking, and the risk of recurrent acute and chronic pancreatitis," *Archives of Internal Medicine*, vol. 169, no. 11, pp. 1035–1045, 2009.

[25] G. Talamini, C. Bassi, M. Falconi et al., "Alcohol and smoking as risk factors in chronic pancreatitis and pancreatic cancer," *Digestive Diseases and Sciences*, vol. 44, no. 7, pp. 1303–1311, 1999.

[26] M. Imoto and E. P. DiMagno, "Cigarette smoking increases the risk of pancreatic calcification in late-onset but not early-onset idiopathic chronic pancreatitis," *Pancreas*, vol. 21, no. 2, pp. 115–119, 2000.

[27] Y. Lin, A. Tamakoshi, T. Hayakawa, M. Ogawa, and Y. Ohno, "Cigarette smoking as a risk factor for chronic pancreatitis: a case–control study in Japan. Research Committee on Intractable Pancreatic Diseases," *Pancreas*, vol. 21, no. 2, pp. 109–114, 2000.

[28] P. Layer, H. Yamamoto, L. Kalthoff, J. E. Clain, L. J. Bakken, and E. P. DiMagno, "The different courses of early- and

late-onset idiopathic and alcoholic chronic pancreatitis," *Gastroenterology*, vol. 107, no. 5, pp. 1481–1487, 1994.

[29] H. Witt, S. Beer, J. Rosendahl et al., "Variants in CPA1 are strongly associated with early onset chronic pancreatitis," *Nature Genetics*, vol. 45, no. 10, pp. 1216–1220, 2013.

[30] M. C. Gorry, D. Gabbaizedeh, W. Furey et al., "Mutations in the cationic trypsinogen gene are associated with recurrent acute and chronic pancreatitis," *Gastroenterology*, vol. 113, no. 4, pp. 1063–1068, 1997.

[31] J. Rosendahl, H. Witt, R. Szmola et al., "Chymotrypsin C (CTRC) variants that diminish activity or secretion are associated with chronic pancreatitis," *Nature Genetics*, vol. 40, no. 1, pp. 78–82, 2008.

[32] M. Gomez-Lira, D. Bonamini, C. Castellani et al., "Mutations in the SPINK1 gene in idiopathic pancreatitis Italian patients," *European Journal of Human Genetics*, vol. 11, no. 7, pp. 543–546, 2003.

[33] N. Teich and J. Mössner, "Hereditary chronic pancreatitis," *Best Practice & Research Clinical Gastroenterology*, vol. 22, no. 1, pp. 115–130, 2008.

[34] G. R. Chandak, M. M. Idris, D. N. Reddy et al., "Absence of PRSS1 mutations and association of SPINK1 trypsin inhibitor mutations in hereditary and non-hereditary chronic pancreatitis," *Gut*, vol. 53, no. 5, pp. 723–728, 2004.

[35] S. M. Cho, S. Shin, and K. A. Lee, "PRSS1, SPINK1, CFTR, and CTRC pathogenic variants in Korean patients with idiopathic pancreatitis," *Annals of Laboratory Medicine*, vol. 36, no. 6, pp. 555–560, 2016.

13

Tumor Budding, uPA, and PAI-1 in Colorectal Cancer: Update of a Prospective Study

Bruno Märkl,[1] **Jochen Hardt,**[2] **Simon Franz,**[1] **Tina Schaller,**[1] **Gerhard Schenkirsch,**[3]
Bernadette Kriening,[4] **Reinhard Hoffmann,**[2] **and Stefan Rüth**[4]

[1]*Institute of Pathology, Klinikum Augsburg, Augsburg, Germany*
[2]*Institute of Laboratory Medicine and Microbiology, Klinikum Augsburg, Augsburg, Germany*
[3]*Clinical and Population-Based Cancer Registry Augsburg, Augsburg, Germany*
[4]*Department of Visceral Surgery, Klinikum Augsburg, Augsburg, Germany*

Correspondence should be addressed to Bruno Märkl; bruno.maerkl@klinikum-augsburg.de

Academic Editor: Mitsuro Kanda

Aims. The prognostic role of the proteases uPA and PAI-1, as well as tumor budding, in colon cancer, has been investigated previously. *Methods.* We provide 6-year follow-up data and results of the validation set. The initial test set and validation set consisted of 55 colon cancers and 68 colorectal cancers, respectively. Tissue samples were analyzed for uPA and PAI-1 using a commercially available Enzyme-Linked Immunosorbent Assay (ELISA). Tumor budding was analyzed on cytokeratin-stained slides. Survival analyses were performed using cut-offs that were determined previously. *Results.* uPA was not prognostic for outcome. PAI-1 showed a trend towards reduced cancer specific survival in PAI-1 high-grade cases (68 versus 83 months; $P = 0.091$). The combination of high-grade PAI-1 and tumor budding was associated with significantly reduced cancer specific survival (60 versus 83 months; $P = 0.021$). After pooling the data from both sets, multivariate analyses revealed that the factors pN-stage, V-stage, and a combination of tumor budding and PAI-1 were independently prognostic for the association with distant metastases. *Conclusions.* A synergistic adverse effect of PAI-1 and tumor budding in uni- and multivariable analyses was found. PAI-1 could serve as a target for anticancer therapy.

1. Introduction

The role of the microenvironment in cancer has recently gained growing attention. Different conditions can inhibit or enhance tumor growth and dissemination. For example, tumor-associated inflammatory reactions can induce tumor inhibition or promotion. Bioactive molecules released from inflammatory cells to the microenvironment support different hallmark capabilities, including proliferation, cell death limitation, angiogenesis, and matrix modification [1]. Because of its central role in tumor progression, different elements of the microenvironment, such as angiogenesis and the t-cell response, have been identified as interesting targets for anticancer therapy [2]. These general concepts are also valid for colorectal cancer, which is the third leading cause

of cancer in the US, with an estimated incidence of approximately 132,000 cases in 2016 [3]. The plasmin/plasminogen system plays an important role in the interaction between the tumor and its matrix. This system consists of the urokinase plasminogen activator (uPA), cell surface receptor urokinase plasminogen activator (uPAR), and its inhibitors plasminogen activator inhibitors 1 and 2 (PAI-1 and PAI-2). UPA and PAI-1 are known to be predictors of aggressive behavior in breast cancer and have been recommended for the diagnosis of node negative breast cancers since 2007. Between 2007 and 2008 our group investigated the potential prognostic value of an ELISA-based uPA and PAI-1 evaluation in colon cancer. Moreover, we assumed that tumor budding, as the histomorphological correlate of epithelial-mesenchymal-transition (EMT), was also associated with the activity of the plasmin/plasminogen system. In this previous study, we found a strong association between elevated uPA levels and tumor budding, as well as high-grade histology. PAI-1 was predictive of distant metastases [4]. We now provide a 6-year follow-up. Additionally, we evaluated another set of cases to validate the findings from the previous study. A subset of rectal cancers was included to estimate whether the findings in these locations were similar to those in colon cancer.

2. Materials and Methods

2.1. Patients and Specimen Preparation. The test set has been described before. In brief, it consists of 59 colon specimens with 55 cancer lesions that were collected between August 2007 and September 2008. Follow-up data were provided by the clinical and population-based cancer registry of Augsburg, Augsburg, Germany. Additional information was retrieved from the files of the Institute of Pathology and the clinic information system. The physicians that were responsible for further care were contacted to gain information, especially concerning disease control or progression. This study was approved by the ethical committee of the Landesärztekammer Bayern. Informed and written consent was obtained from all patients.

The 68 colorectal cancer cases of the validation set were collected between April and November 2014. This study was approved by the internal review board of the Klinikum Augsburg on the basis of the recommendation by the ethical committee of Landesärztekammer Bayern regarding the previous study. The inclusion criteria for this study were established or suspected colorectal cancer and an elective oncological resection. Emergency surgery or noncurative intentions were criteria for exclusion.

The specimen preparation has been described before. In brief, a $1 \, cm^3$ tissue block was cut from the invasive tumor region in the fresh tissue immediately after receiving the unfixed specimen. The time between resection and sample collection was less than 30 minutes. In 13 cases from the test set, samples from nonneoplastic regions were also collected. The samples were stored at $-20°C$ for a maximum of 14 days before performing ELISA. Malignancy and the estimation of proportion of the neoplastic cells in 10% steps were confirmed by H&E histology in all samples for the ELISA.

2.2. Laboratory Assay. A commercially available ELISA kit for uPA and PAI-1 that is certified for usage in breast cancer was used (Femtelle Test (EF 899), Sekisui Diagnostics, Stamford, CT). The test was conducted according to the protocol recommended by the manufacturer and has been described before [4]. In brief, frozen tissue samples were disrupted by mechanical force under permanent cooling. Tri-Buffer, supplemented with the nonionic detergent Triton X-100, was used to extract the tumor cell cytosol. The suspensions were centrifuged to separate the soluble fractions from the cell debris. The total protein concentrations of the cytosolic fractions were measured. On day 2, a diluted tissue extract was added to antibody-coated microwells and incubated overnight. On day 3, detection antibodies were added and incubated. After another incubation step with the

enzyme conjugates, the reactions were stopped with 0.5 M H_2SO_4 and the absorption of the solution was measured using a microwell reader at 450 nm. The levels of uPA and PAI-1 were expressed in nanograms per milligram (ng/mg) of tumor protein. Based on the evaluation of the test set [4] the cut-off values for uPA and PAI-1 were $\geq 4 \, ng/mg$ and $\geq 40 \, ng/mg$, respectively, to discriminate between low and high-grade levels.

2.3. Tumor Budding and Immunohistochemistry. Tumor budding was defined as isolated tumor cells or clusters of up to four cells at the invasion front according to Ueno et al. Because of the usage of a microscope with an eyepiece with a field number of 25, the cut-off for high-grade budding was adjusted to ≥ 30 buds/20-fold magnification in comparison to the original publication [15]. The evaluation was performed on slides that were immunohistochemically stained for pan-cytokeratin to enhance the detectability of single cells. All reactions were performed using a Ventana Benchmark Ultra system. Cell Conditioning Solution (CC1) (Ventana - Roche Diagnostics, Mannheim Germany) was used at the pretreatment step during the processing of all sections. The diagnostic antibody against keratin KL1 (mouse, monoclonal, 1 : 100) was provided by Medac, Wedel, Germany. Independent evaluations were performed by two pathologists (Bruno Märkl and Tina Schaller). In cases of a discrepancy concerning the discrimination between no/low tumor budding and high-grade tumor budding, a consensus decision was made using a double-headed microscope.

Immunohistochemistry for the mismatch repair proteins PMS2 and MSH6 was performed to determine the mismatch repair status in the cases of the validation set where evaluations concerning microsatellite instability (MSI) and/or mismatch repair deficiency (MMRd) have not been performed in the frame of the routine diagnostic. The following diagnostic antibodies were used: PMS2 (Clone EP51, ready to use,) (Clone EP49, ready to use). All reactions were developed using the Ventana Ultravision detection system (Roche Diagnostics, Mannheim, Germany).

2.4. Statistical Analysis. The Mann–Whitney Rank Sum test was used to compare numeric values. Correlations were calculated with Pearson Product Correlation. Tabulated data were compared using the χ^2 test or Fisher's Exact test depending on the number of observations. Backward stepwise logistic regression analysis was used to identify independent predictors of metastatic disease. For the survival analysis, Kaplan-Meier Curves were calculated and differences were analyzed with the Log-Rank test. The mean survival times were calculated because the median survival was not reached in most analyses. For the determination of the median follow-up time, the method of Schemper and Smith was used. The Cox regression proportional hazards model was used for the multivariate analysis of cancer specific analysis. The Cohens-Kappa value was calculated to evaluate the interobserver variability during the tumor budding evaluation. All calculations were performed using the Sigma Plot 13.0 software package (Systat, Richmond, VA, USA). P values < 0.05 were considered significant.

Table 1: Clinicopathologic data: test set.

	Malignant ($n = 55$)	Nonmalignant ($n = 4$)
Mean age ± SD	71 ± 13	68 ± 8
Gender (m : f)	0.57 : 1	0.33 : 1
Right colon	19	3
Left colon	36	1
Conventional histological type	48	/
Mucinous type	4	/
Medullary type	1	/
Micropapillary type	2	/
Infiltrative invasion type*	4	/
pT 1/2	16	/
pT 3/4	39	/
Low/moderate grade	39	/
High grade	16	/
Node positive	21	/
Lymphatic invasion	4	/
Venous invasion	6	/
Perineural invasion	3	/
Strong chronic inflammation	11	/
Metastatic disease	7	/
Mean LN, number ± SD	33 ± 18	19 ± 6

*Infiltrative type according to Jass. SD, standard deviation; LN, lymph nodes.

3. Results

3.1. Test Set: Patients and Follow-Up. The test set consists of 55 colon cancer cases. Forty-seven of these cases met the criteria for survival analysis. The basic clinicopathological data have been described before and are briefly given in Table 1. The mean and median follow-up times were 75 and 80 months (95% CI: 76.9–83.1).

3.2. Test Set: Cancer Specific Survival (CSS). Cancer specific survival was not different in cases with low and high uPA levels with a mean CSS time of 80 months (95% CI: 70–91) versus 76 months (95% CI: 59–94) ($P = 0.735$), respectively. However, a clear trend towards adverse outcome was found for PAI-1. Cases with high PAI-1 levels showed a mean CSS time of 68 months (95% CI: 47–89) compared to low PAI-1 level cases with a CSS time of 83 months (95% CI: 74–93) ($P = 0.091$). High-grade tumor budding was also associated with impaired survival, with a mean CSS time of 71 months (95% CI: 53–89) versus 83 months for low-grade tumor budding (95% CI: 73–33) ($P = 0.187$). Although this difference was not statistically significant, the Kaplan-Meier curves showed a clear discrimination between the two groups. After combining the parameters *tumor budding* and *PAI-1,* the cases with no or only a single positive revealed a significantly higher CCS in comparison to cases that were positive for both. The mean times for negative/single positive versus double positive cases were 83 months (95% CI: 74–91) and 60 months (95% CI: 29–91), respectively ($P = 0.021$). The

Kaplan-Meier curves are shown in Figure 1. After performing multivariate analysis including the factors *N-stage, vascular invasion, PAI-1, tumor budding,* and the *combination of PAI1 and tumor budding,* only N-stage was found to be independently prognostic. However, the *combination of PAI-1 and tumor budding* just failed independence, with a P-for-Enter of 0.057.

3.3. Validation Set: Patients and Correlations between uPA, PAI-1, and Tumor Budding. The validation set consists of 68 colorectal cancer cases. The clinicopathological data are summarized in Table 2. The two investigators of tumor budding reached a moderate interobserver agreement with a κ-value of 0.48.

All samples contained neoplastic cells. The mean percentage of the vital tumor was 640.207 ± 22% (Range 5–90%). There was a weak nonsignificant association between the tumor amount and the level of uPA and no association with PAI-1 ($R = 0.207$, $P = 0.093$; $R = 0.0594$, $P = 633$).

The mean uPA and PAI-1 levels were 4.0 ± 2.2 and 38.1 ± 33.7 ng/mg protein. Both parameters showed a strong correlation ($R = 0.709$; $P < 0.001$) with each other. However, in this set, tumor budding did not correlate significantly with uPA or PAI-1 ($R = 0.08$ and $R = 0.218$) (Figure 2).

3.4. Validation Set: Proteinase Levels and Tumor Budding according to Other Histopathological Factors. There was no difference in the uPA and PAI-1 levels when comparing cases with and without vascular invasion. Additionally, no difference was found between the uPA levels in node negative or node positive cases (Figure 3(c)). However, there was a significant difference between these subgroups regarding the PAI-1 levels with a median level of 35.5 versus 16.5 ng/mg protein ($P = 0.043$) (Figure 3(d)). The association between nonconventional histological type and high uPA and PAI-1 values is remarkable, in this context ($P = 0.002$; $P < 0.001$). Further significant differences were found for uPA and PAI-1 between the different pT-stages ($P = 0.007$; $P < 0.001$) (Figures 3(a) and 3(b)) and grading ($P < 0.001$; $P = 0.007$) (Figures 3(e) and 3(f)). Additionally, a nonsignificant trend towards higher PAI-1 levels was found in metastatic disease ($P = 0.153$) (Figure 3(h)), whereas the uPA levels showed no significant differences between localized and metastatic disease (Figure 3(g)).

The clinicopathological data, stratified according to the cut-off values for uPA and PAI-1 that were determined during the first evaluation of the test set, are given along with the data for tumor budding in Table 2. In brief, there was a clear trend towards a higher rate of locally advanced cancers (68% versus 89%; $P = 0.07$) and a significantly higher rate of high-grade tumors in the uPA-high group (10% versus 39%; $P = 0.01$). Both parameters were also significantly differentially distributed in the PAI-1 low versus high groups (63% versus 100%; $P = 0.002$ and 50% versus 67%; $P = 0.01$, resp.).

High-grade tumor budding was more highly associated with male gender ($P = 0.05$) and node positivity (50% versus 76%; $P = 0.091$). It was also significantly associated with a left side location (49% versus 65%; $P = 0.029$), venous invasion (10% versus 65%; $P = 0.022$), and metastatic disease (10% versus 47%; $P = 0.002$).

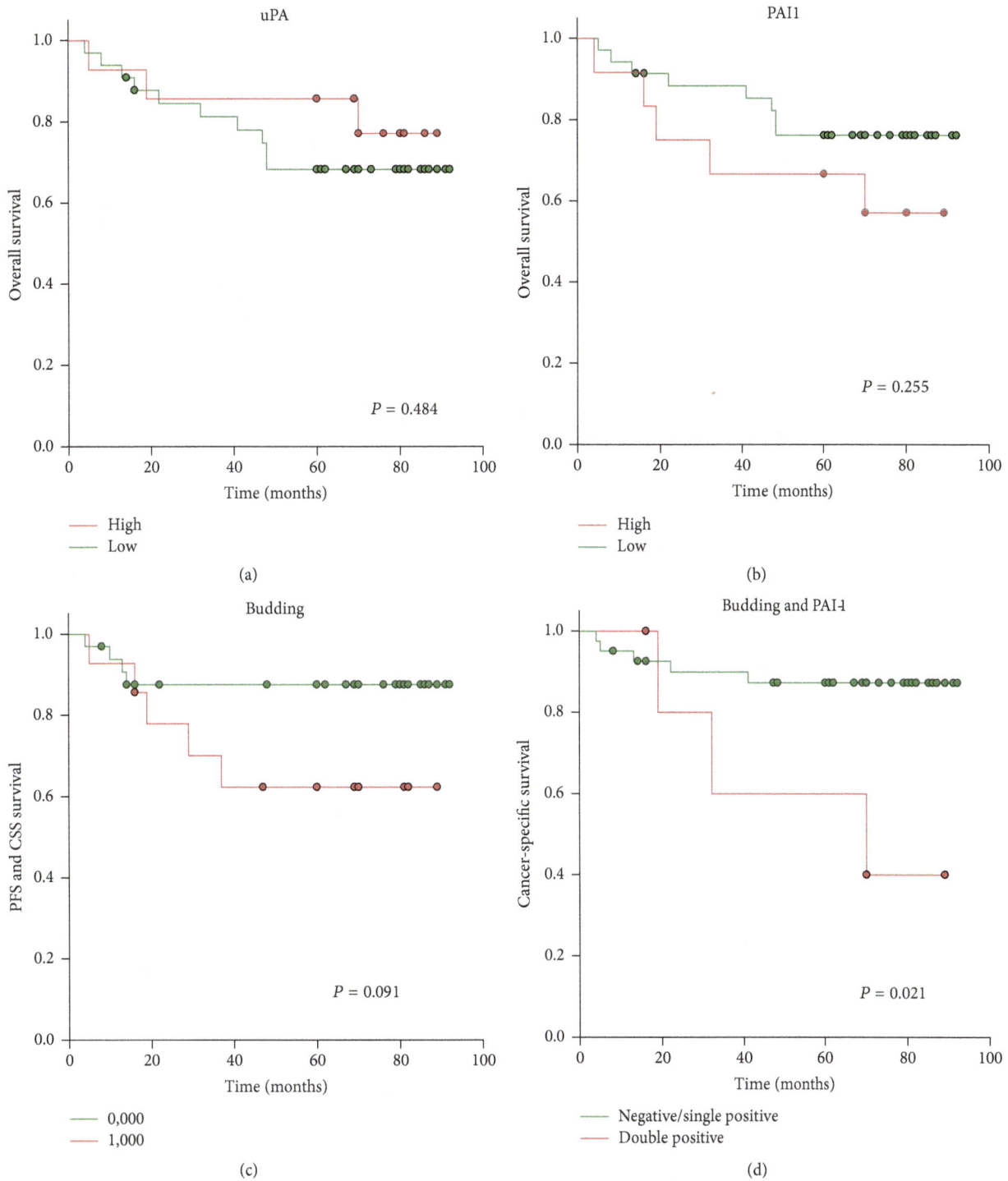

FIGURE 1: Test set: cancer specific survival of (a) uPA, (b) PAI-1, (c) tumor budding, and (d) a combination of tumor budding and PAI-1 (no or one positive versus double positive). Cut-offs: uPA ≥ 4.0 ng/mg protein; PAI-1 ≥ 40 ng/mg protein; tumor budding ≥ 30 buds/20-fold magnification.

3.5. Pooled Data. After pooling the data from the test and the validation set, the risk for the occurrence of distant metastases was calculated for pT-stage, pN-stage, venous invasion, grading, uPA, PAI-1, tumor budding, and the combination of tumor budding and PAI-1 (Figure 4). Significant prognostic effects were found for pT-stage, pN-stage, venous invasion, PAI-1, tumor budding, and the combination of tumor budding and PAI-1. The corresponding odds ratios were inf., 30.8, 21.3, 4.1, 6.7 and 13.5, respectively. UPA just failed to meet significance with $P = 0.051$ (OR: 3.5).

TABLE 2: Clinicopathological data: validation set.

	Complete collection (n = 68)	uPA low (n = 40)	uPA high (n = 28)	P value	PAI-1 low (n = 44)	PAI-1 high (n = 24)	P value	Budding low (n = 51)	Budding high (n = 17)	P value
Mean age ± SD	68 ± 11	68 ± 10	67 ± 12	1.0	68 ± 11	67 ± 12	0.753	69 ± 11	64 ± 11	0.091
Gender m : f	1:0.9	1:0.74	1:1.15	0.514	1:0.7	1:1.4	0.262	1:1.2	1:0.3	0.05
Right colon	32 (47%)	17 (43%)	15 (54%)		21 (48%)	11 (46%)		26 (51%)	6 (35%)	
Left colon	18 (26%)	11 (28%)	7 (25%)		9 (20%)	9 (38%)		16 (31%)	2 (12%)	
Total colon	3 (4%)	1 (3%)	2 (7%)	0.462*	1 (2%)	2 (8%)	0.103*	1 (2%)	2 (12%)	0.029*
Rectum	15 (22%)	11 (28%)	4 (14%)	0.319#	13 (30%)	2 (8%)	0.087#	8 (16%)	7 (41%)	0.043#
Conventional histological type	56 (82%)	38 (95%)	18 (64%)		42 (95%)	14 (58%)		42 (82%)	14 (82%)	
Mucinous type	8 (12%)	1 (3%)	7 (25%)		1 (2%)	7 (29%)		6 (12%)	2 (12%)	
Medullary type	1 (1%)	0 (0%)	1 (4%)		0 (0%)	1 (4%)		1 (2%)	0 (0%)	
Micropapillary type	3 (4%)	1 (3%)	2 (7%)	0.002**	1 (2%)	2 (8%)	<0.001**	2 (4%)	1 (6%)	1.0**
Infiltrative type‡	6 (9%)	6 (15%)	0 (0%)	0.164	6 (14%)	0 (0%)	0.083	3 (6%)	3 (18%)	0.160
pT 1/2	16 (24%)	13 (33%)	3 (11%)		16 (36%)	0 (0%)		14 (27%)	2 (12%)	
pT 3/4	52 (76%)	27 (68%)	25 (89%)	0.073	28 (64%)	24 (100%)	0.002	37 (73%)	15 (88%)	0.322
Grading: low grade	53 (78%)	36 (90%)	17 (61%)	0.01	39 (89%)	14 (58%)	0.01	41 (80%)	12 (71%)	0.501
Grading: high grade	15 (22%)	4 (10%)	11 (39%)		5 (11%)	10 (42%)		10 (20%)	5 (29%)	
Node positive	38 (56%)	21 (53%)	17 (61%)	0.404	22 (50%)	16 (67%)	0.286	25 (49%)	13 (76%)	0.091
Lymphatic invasion	15 (22%)	10 (25%)	5 (18%)	0.563	9 (20%)	6 (25%)	0.762	8 (16%)	7 (41%)	0.043
Venous invasion	11 (16%)	6 (15%)	5 (18%)	0.319	6 (14%)	5 (21%)	0.500	5 (10%)	6 (35%)	0.022
Perineural invasion	10 (15%)	5 (13%)	5 (18%)	0.730	7 (16%)	3 (13%)	1.000	6 (12%)	4 (24%)	0.254
Strong chronic inflammation	13 (19%)	6 (15%)	7 (25%)	0.357	10 (23%)	3 (13%)	0.355	13 (25%)	0 (0%)	0.028
MSI/MMRd	9 (13%)	3 (8%)	6 (21%)	0.146	5 (11%)	4 (17%)	0.710	9 (18%)	0 (0%)	0.099
Metastatic disease	13 (19%)	5 (13%)	8 (29%)	0.124	6 (14%)	7 (29%)	0.195	5 (10%)	8 (47%)	0.002
Mean LN, number ± SD	43 ± 17	44 ± 20	42 ± 12	0.837	42 ± 19	45 ± 13	0.068	43 ± 18	42 ± 16	0.949
Neoadjuvant therapy	7 (47%)†	4 (36%)	3 (75%)	0.282†	6 (46%)	1 (50%)	1.000†	3 (38%)	4 (57%)	0.619†

SD, standard deviation; LN, lymph nodes. *Calculation includes all locations (right, left, total, and rectum). **Conventional versus group of nonconventional types. #Rectal versus nonrectal cancers. ‡According to Jass [5]. †Basis is the number of rectal cancers.

TABLE 3: Comparison of the results: test set versus validation set.

	uPA			PAI-1			Budding	
	Test set mean values	Val. set mean values	Val.-set cut-off	Test set mean values	Val. set mean values	Val. set cut-off	Test set mean values	Val. set cut-off
Grading	Y	Y	Y	N	Y	Y	Y	N
T-stage	N	Y	T	N	Y	Y	N	N
N-stage	N	N	N	N	Y	N	Y	T
V-stage	N	N	N	Y	T	N	N	Y
M-stage	Y*	T	T	Y*	T	Y	Y*	Y

Y, statistically prognostic; N, not statistically prognostic; T, trend towards prognostic relevance; bold and italic fonts, concordance between test and validation set; bold italic font, discordance between test and validation set. *Evaluation according to cut-off stratification.

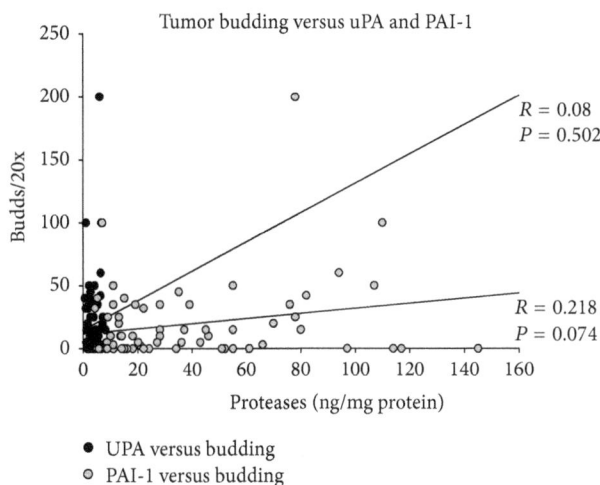

FIGURE 2: Correlation between tumor budding and uPA and PAI-1.

The multivariate analyses revealed that the factors pN-stage, venous invasion, and combination of tumor budding and PAI-1 were independently prognostic for the occurrence of distant metastases.

4. Discussion

Here, we provide follow-up data from a prospective study that was initially performed in 2007/2008 to investigate the role of the serine proteases uPA and PAI-1 in tumor budding in colon cancer [4]. Moreover, we present the initial data from a recently performed validation study. The survival analysis of the test set revealed a nonsignificant trend towards an adverse outcome for patients with high PAI-1 tissue concentrations and high-grade tumor budding. The fact that a combination of both factors leads to a significant discrimination regarding cancer specific survival can be seen as an indication that both factors interact and enhance tumor cell migration and tumor progression. Tumor budding is characterized by the loss of E-cadherin, a mesenchymal phenotype, and detachment from neoplastic glands [16–20]. Other authors have described similar connections between the function of

the plasmin system and tumor budding. Recently, Sánchez-Tilló et al. reported that ZEP1 regulates uPA and PAI and is expressed in dedifferentiated cells at the invasion front that have lost E-cadherin [13]. Minoo et al. found that immunohistochemical overexpression of uPA and the loss of E-cadherin and APAF-1 are predictive of the infiltrating tumor border [7]. Hiendlmeyer et al. found that β-catenin upregulates uPA expression. The evaluation of our test set revealed strong correlations between tumor budding and uPA and PAI-1 levels [22]. However, in our validation set, we only found a weak correlation between budding and PAI-1 with marginal significance. The median PAI-1 and uPA levels were evaluated in cases with high-grade budding. An interesting finding is that uPA and PAI-1 levels were strongly associated with the histological type in the validation set. Specifically, the mucinous type was significantly more often found in the uPA- and PAI-1-high groups. Reevaluating the test set revealed a trend ($P = 0.167$) in this direction.

In our initial study, we showed an association between the tissue levels of uPA and PAI-1 and aggressive histopathological features of colon cancers. The recently finished validation study confirmed the role of these proteases as negative prognostic markers in colon cancers. This was true when the mean values were compared and also when the collection was stratified according to previously determined cut-off values. However, it has to be stated that the combinations of factors that were associated with each other were not completely identical (Table 3), which is very likely influenced by the relatively small number of cases for these studies, including all stages of cancers, which is a clear limitation. Another limitation is that the two studies are not optimally balanced. The validation study included proportions of right sided, nodal positive cancers, as well more cases with vascular invasion and distant metastases, which may have also contributed to the instability found in the results. Nevertheless, whenever significant differences were found, they indicated an association of the proteases with aggressive behavior. This was especially true for PAI-1 and tumor budding.

A multivariable analysis performed after pooling the data from both sets revealed that pN-stage, V-stage, tumor budding, and PAI-1 were independently associated with distant metastases. The prognostic role of PAI-1 in colorectal cancers has been evaluated by several other groups, and the

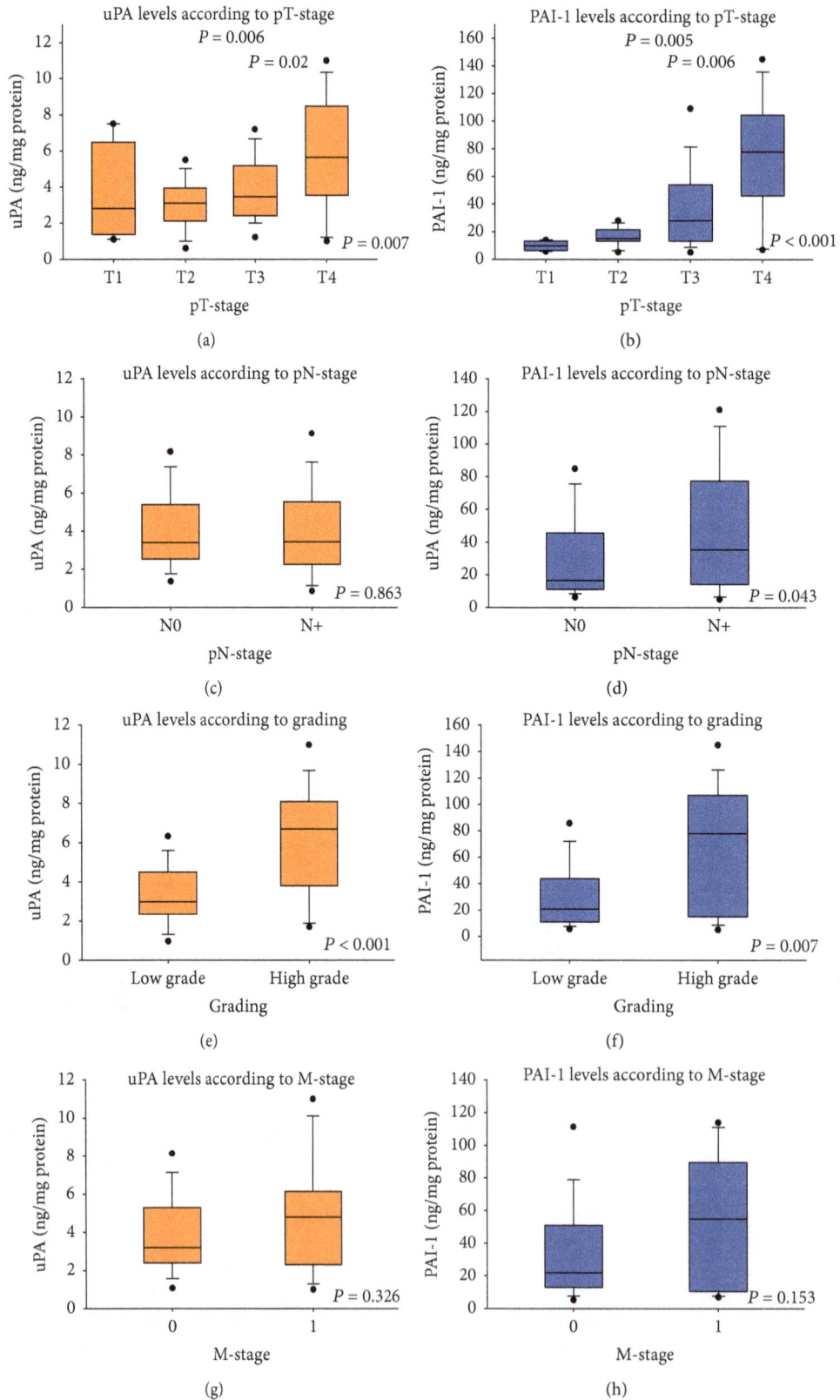

FIGURE 3: Validation set: mean tissue levels of uPA and PAI-1 according to pT-stage (a and b), pN-stage (c and d), grading (e and f), and M-stage (g and h).

TABLE 4: Previous studies investigating the prognostic role of uPA and PAI-1 in colorectal cancer.

References	Year	n	Specimen	Protease	Method	Results
Mutoh et al. [6]	2008	25	Mice experimental	PAI-1 and PAI-1 inhibitors SK116 and 215	ELISA, RT-PCR, polyp formation, tissue	PAI-1 Blockers suppress polyp formation
Minoo et al. [7]	2009	975	Colorectal	uPA, uPAR	IHC, microarray	uPA but not uPAR is independently prognostic
Yamada et al. [8]	2010	100	Colorectal	PAI-1	ELISA, plasma	Predictive of postoperative recurrence
Kushlinskii et al. [9]	2013	166	Colorectal	uPA, PAI-1, tPA	ELISA, plasma	PAI-1 prognostic but only in univariate analysis
Hogan et al. [10]	2013		Colon cancer and mesenchymal stem cells	PAI-1	Cell cultures	PAI-1 is secreted by MSC
Kim et al. [11]	2013	3136	Colorectal	PAI-1	ELISA, plasma	No independent association between PAI-1 and polyp-formation; univariable weakly significant
Iacoviello et al. [12]	2013	850	Colorectal	PAI-1	ELISA, plasma	Risk factor for colorectal cancer
Sánchez-Tilló [13]	2013		Colorectal		Cell cultures	ZEB1 regulates uPA and PAI1 and promotes invasiveness
Chen et al. [14]	2015	108	Colorectal	PAI-1	ELISA, plasma, and cell cultures	Silencing of PAI-1 suppresses CR cancer progression

ELISA, Enzyme-Linked Immunosorbent Assay; RT-PCR, reverse transcription polymerase chain reaction; IHC, immunohistochemistry; MSC, mesenchymal stem cells; CR, colorectal. Note: literature from 1993–2008 is given in [4].

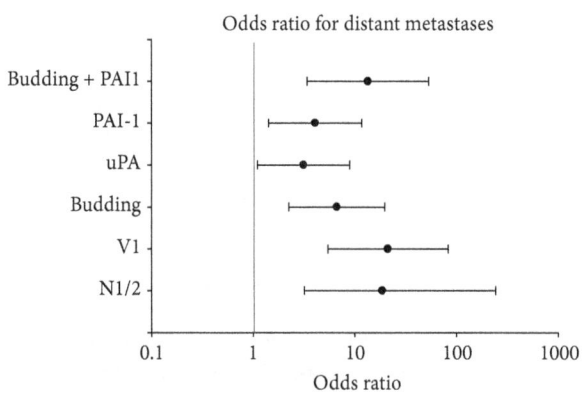

FIGURE 4: Pooled data: odds ratios of different risk factors for the association with distant metastases. Note the logarithmic scale of the X-axis.

overwhelming majority of studies confirmed that PAI-1 is an adverse factor [4]. An overview of the more recently published literature is given in Table 4 [6–14]. Wang et al. performed a meta-analysis to evaluate the influence of the PAI-1 4G/5G polymorphism. Individuals with a 4G/4G genotype have increased PAI-1 plasma levels and show an increased susceptibility to colorectal and endometrial cancer [23]. Iacoviello et al. also found increased plasma levels of PAI-1 in patients with colon cancers compared to controls in a large retrospective analysis [12]. Experimental data came from Hogan et al. and Chen et al., who show that cancer cell functions are influenced by PAI-1 [10, 14]. Moreover, Chen et al. demonstrated compromised tumor growth caused by the silencing of PAI-1.

In the analyses of the test and validation sets, UPA was found to be inferior concerning its prognostic significance in comparison to PAI-1 and tumor budding. Kushlinskii et al. also found PAI-1, but not uPA, to be prognostic in colorectal cancer [9]. However, this result is in contrast to those of other studies that reported strong correlations with aggressive behaviors, including impaired survival rates [7, 24–29]. Most of these studies were performed using immuno-histochemistry, which could be a technical explanation for this discrepancy. Ganesh et al. and Herszènyi et al. used ELISA and also reported impressive survival differences [25, 30]. The main difference between their investigations and ours is that they used a different ELISA. However, it seems unlikely that this can fully explain this strong discrepancy. It remains unclear why we could not confirm the data of these authors.

Tumor budding is gaining recognition as a promising and robust prognostic factor in colorectal cancer. It is especially interesting for the evaluation of malignant polyps in the preoperative setting and in stage II cancers [31]. Its prognostic relevance in the whole gastrointestinal tract has been investigated in a large number of studies [31, 32]. However, there are still two main issues with these factors that remain unsolved. The most important of these issues is the fact that an accepted consensus on how tumor budding should be evaluated is lacking. The other point is the relatively weak interobserver agreement, at least in some of the publications [32]. Puppa et al. found a fair agreement between the international participants of their study. Cytokeratin immunohistochemistry improved the agreement [33]. In our study, we also achieved only moderate interobserver agreement, with a κ-value of 0.48. It is astonishing that, despite these limitations, tumor budding has been demonstrated to be a robust adverse factor many times. An increased risk for lymph node metastases in pT-1 cancers has been confirmed in systematic reviews and meta-analyses [34–36]. Several authors and societies recommend the evaluation of tumor budding [37–40], which underlines its importance. In our study, we also found an association between high-grade tumor budding and other adverse factors and outcomes.

Despite investigating another set of 68 cases in addition to the initial collection, this study is still hampered by a relatively low case number. Nevertheless, the data of this study with a prospective design can serve as a basis for further investigations. We found a synergistic adverse effect of PAI-1 and tumor budding in uni- and multivariable analyses. This supports the thesis that stromal degradation facilitates the migration of detached tumor cells. Because of the association with the histological type further investigations should focus on this by comparing collectives with identical UICC stages, MSI status, and/or locations. Because PAI-1 inhibitors are already available, additional investigations should address the question of whether PAI-1 could serve as a target for anticancer therapy [41].

Competing Interests

The authors declare that they have no competing interests.

Acknowledgments

This work was supported by Sekisui Diagnostics, Stamford, and by the Hermann-Egger-Stiftung. The authors are grateful to Anna-Maria Bubolz, Katharina Endhardt, and Ines Lichtmannegger for collecting the fresh tissue sample for the uPA/PAI-1 analysis. The authors also thank Monika Hallabrin and Kathrin Ferstl-Blahetek for their excellent technical assistance.

References

[1] D. Hanahan and R. A. Weinberg, "Hallmarks of cancer: the next generation," *Cell*, vol. 144, no. 5, pp. 646–674, 2011.

[2] W. H. Fridman, F. Pagès, C. Sautes-Fridman, and J. Galon, "The immune contexture in human tumours: impact on clinical outcome," *Nature Reviews Cancer*, vol. 12, no. 4, pp. 298–306, 2012.

[3] American-Cancer-Society, *Cancer Facts & Figures 2016*, American Cancer Society, Atlanta, Ga, USA, 2016.

[4] B. Märkl, I. Renk, D. V. Oruzio et al., "Tumour budding, uPA and PAI-1 are associated with aggressive behaviour in colon cancer," *Journal of Surgical Oncology*, vol. 102, no. 3, pp. 235–241, 2010.

[5] J. R. Jass, Y. Ajioka, J. P. Allen et al., "Assessment of invasive growth pattern and lymphotic infiltration in colorectal cancer," *Histopathology*, vol. 28, no. 6, pp. 543–548, 1996.

[6] M. Mutoh, N. Niho, M. Komiya et al., "Plasminogen activator inhibitor-1 (Pai-1) blockers suppress intestinal polyp formation in Min mice," *Carcinogenesis*, vol. 29, no. 4, pp. 824–829, 2008.

[7] P. Minoo, K. Baker, D. Baumhoer, L. Terracciano, A. Lugli, and I. Zlobec, "Urokinase-type plasminogen activator is a marker of aggressive phenotype and an independent prognostic factor in mismatch repair-proficient colorectal cancer," *Human Pathology*, vol. 41, no. 1, pp. 70–78, 2010.

[8] Y. Yamada, T. Arao, K. Matsumoto et al., "Plasma concentrations of VCAM-1 and PAI-1: a predictive biomarker for postoperative recurrence in colorectal cancer," *Cancer Science*, vol. 101, no. 8, pp. 1886–1890, 2010.

[9] N. E. Kushlinskii, E. S. Gershtein, E. A. Korotkova, and V. V. Prorokov, "Prognostic role of tumor-associated proteases in colorectal cancer," *Bulletin of Experimental Biology and Medicine*, vol. 154, no. 3, pp. 365–369, 2013.

[10] N. M. Hogan, M. R. Joyce, J. M. Murphy et al., "Impact of Mesenchymal Stem Cell secreted PAI-1 on colon cancer cell migration and proliferation," *Biochemical and Biophysical Research Communications*, vol. 435, no. 4, pp. 574–579, 2013.

[11] E. R. Kim, M. H. Yang, Y. J. Lim et al., "Association between plasma levels of plasminogen activator inhibitor-1 and colorectal neoplasms," *Gut and Liver*, vol. 7, no. 5, pp. 519–523, 2013.

[12] L. Iacoviello, C. Agnoli, A. De Curtis et al., "Type 1 plasminogen activator inhibitor as a common risk factor for cancer and ischaemic vascular disease: The EPICOR Study," *BMJ Open*, vol. 3, no. 11, article 12, 2013.

[13] E. Sánchez-Tilló, O. De Barrios, L. Siles et al., "ZEB1 promotes invasiveness of colorectal carcinoma cells through the opposing regulation of uPA and PAI-1," *Clinical Cancer Research*, vol. 19, no. 5, pp. 1071–1082, 2013.

[14] H. Chen, H. Peng, W. Liu et al., "Silencing of plasminogen activator inhibitor-1 suppresses colorectal cancer progression and liver metastasis," *Surgery*, vol. 158, no. 6, pp. 1704–1713, 2015.

[15] H. Ueno, J. Murphy, J. R. Jass, H. Mochizuki, and I. C. Talbot, "Tumour 'budding' as an index to estimate the potential of aggressiveness in rectal cancer," *Histopathology*, vol. 40, no. 2, pp. 127–132, 2002.

[16] F. Prall, "Tumour budding in colorectal carcinoma," *Histopathology*, vol. 50, no. 1, pp. 151–162, 2007.

[17] F. Prall, V. Weirich, and C. Ostwald, "Phenotypes of invasion in sporadic colorectal carcinomas related to aberrations of the adenomatous polyposis coli (APC) gene," *Histopathology*, vol. 50, no. 3, pp. 318–330, 2007.

[18] J. R. Jass, M. Barker, L. Fraser et al., "APC mutation and tumour budding in colorectal cancer," *Journal of Clinical Pathology*, vol. 56, no. 1, pp. 69–73, 2003.

[19] J. García-Solano, P. Conesa-Zamora, J. Trujillo-Santos, D. Torres-Moreno, M. J. Mäkinen, and M. Pérez-Guillermo, "Immunohistochemical expression profile of β-catenin, E-cadherin, P-cadherin, laminin-5γ2 chain, and SMAD4 in colorectal serrated adenocarcinoma," *Human Pathology*, vol. 43, no. 7, pp. 1094–1102, 2012.

[20] T. Brabletz, F. Hlubek, S. Spaderna et al., "Invasion and metastasis in colorectal cancer: epithelial-mesenchymal transition, mesenchymal-epithelial transition, stem cells and β-catenin," *Cells Tissues Organs*, vol. 179, no. 1-2, pp. 56–65, 2005.

[21] H. J. Nielsen, I. J. Christensen, S. Sorensen, F. Moesgaard, and N. Brunner, "Preoperative plasma plasminogen activator inhibitor type-1 and serum C-reactive protein levels in patients with colorectal cancer. The RANX05 Colorectal Cancer Study Group," *Annals of Surgical Oncology*, vol. 7, no. 8, pp. 617–623, 2000.

[22] E. Hiendlmeyer, S. Regus, S. Wassermann et al., "β-catenin upregulates the expression of the urokinase plasminogen activator in human colorectal tumors," *Cancer Research*, vol. 64, no. 4, pp. 1209–1214, 2004.

[23] S. Wang, Q. Cao, X. Wang et al., "PAI-1 4G/5G polymorphism contributes to cancer susceptibility: evidence from meta-analysis," *PLoS ONE*, vol. 8, no. 2, Article ID e56797, 2013.

[24] T. Fujii, T. Obara, S. Tanno, H. Ura, and Y. Kohgo, "Urokinase-type plasminogen activator and plasminogen activator inhibitor-1 as a prognostic factor in human colorectal carcinomas," *Hepato-Gastroenterology*, vol. 46, no. 28, pp. 2299–2308, 1999.

[25] S. Ganesh, C. F. M. Sier, G. Griffioen et al., "Prognostic relevance of plasminogen activators and their inhibitors in colorectal cancer," *Cancer Research*, vol. 54, no. 15, pp. 4065–4071, 1994.

[26] H. E. Mulcahy, D. P. O'Donoghue, M. J. Duffy et al., "Urokinase-type plasminogen activator and outcome in Dukes' B colorectal cancer," *The Lancet*, vol. 344, no. 8922, pp. 583–584, 1994.

[27] T. Sato, G. Nishimura, Y. Yonemura et al., "Association of immunohistochemical detection of urokinase-type plasminogen activator with metastasis and prognosis in colorectal cancer," *Oncology*, vol. 52, no. 4, pp. 347–352, 1995.

[28] D.-Q. Seetoo, P. J. Crowe, P. J. Russell, and J.-L. Yang, "Quantitative expression of protein markers of plasminogen activation system in prognosis of colorectal cancer," *Journal of Surgical Oncology*, vol. 82, no. 3, pp. 184–193, 2003.

[29] J.-L. Yang, D.-Q. Seetoo, Y. Wang et al., "Urokinase-type plasminogen activator and its receptor in colorectal cancer: independent prognostic factors of metastasis and cancer-specific survival and potential therapeutic targets," *International Journal of Cancer*, vol. 89, no. 5, pp. 431–439, 2000.

[30] L. Herszènyi, M. Plebani, P. Carraro et al., "The role of cysteine and serine proteases in colorectal carcinoma," *Cancer*, vol. 86, no. 7, pp. 1135–1142, 1999.

[31] V. H. Koelzer, I. Zlobec, and A. Lugli, "Tumor budding in colorectal cancer—ready for diagnostic practice?" *Human Pathology*, vol. 47, no. 1, pp. 4–19, 2016.

[32] B. Märkl and H. M. Arnholdt, "Prognostic significance of tumor budding in gastrointestinal tumors," *Expert Review of Anticancer Therapy*, vol. 11, no. 10, pp. 1521–1533, 2011.

[33] G. Puppa, C. Senore, K. Sheahan et al., "Diagnostic reproducibility of tumour budding in colorectal cancer: a multicentre, multinational study using virtual microscopy," *Histopathology*, vol. 61, no. 4, pp. 562–575, 2012.

[34] C. Beaton, C. P. Twine, G. L. Williams, and A. G. Radcliffe, "Systematic review and meta-analysis of histopathological factors influencing the risk of lymph node metastasis in early colorectal cancer," *Colorectal Disease*, vol. 15, no. 7, pp. 788–797, 2013.

[35] H. Ueno, K. Hase, Y. Hashiguchi et al., "Novel risk factors for lymph node metastasis in early invasive colorectal cancer: a multi-institution pathology review," *Journal of Gastroenterology*, vol. 49, no. 9, pp. 1314–1323, 2014.

[36] S. Bosch, S. Teerenstra, J. W. De Wilt, C. Cunningham, and I. Nagtegaal, "Predicting lymph node metastasis in pT1 colorectal cancer: a systematic review of risk factors providing rationale for therapy decisions," *Endoscopy*, vol. 45, no. 10, pp. 827–834, 2013.

[37] J. R. Jass, M. J. O'Brien, R. H. Riddell, and D. C. Snover, "Recommendations for the reporting of surgically resected specimens of colorectal carcinoma," *Virchows Archiv*, vol. 450, no. 1, pp. 1–13, 2007.

[38] M. Vieth, P. Quirke, R. Lambert, L. von Karsa, and M. Risio, "International Agency for Research on C. European guidelines for quality assurance in colorectal cancer screening and diagnosis. First Edition—annotations of colorectal lesions," *Endoscopy*, vol. 44, supplement 3, pp. SE131–SE139, 2012.

[39] T. Watanabe, M. Itabashi, Y. Shimada et al., "Japanese Society for Cancer of the Colon and Rectum (JSCCR) guidelines 2010 for the treatment of colorectal cancer," *International Journal of Clinical Oncology*, vol. 17, no. 1, pp. 1–29, 2012.

[40] C. J. H. Van De Velde, P. G. Boelens, J. M. Borras et al., "EURECCA colorectal: multidisciplinary management: European consensus conference colon & rectum," *European Journal of Cancer*, vol. 50, no. 1, pp. e1–e34, 2014.

[41] V. R. Placencio, A. Ichimura, T. Miyata, and Y. A. DeClerck, "Small molecule inhibitors of plasminogen activator inhibitor-1 elicit anti-Tumorigenic and anti-Angiogenic activity," *PLoS ONE*, vol. 10, no. 7, Article ID e0133786, 2015.

14

The Role of Mast Cells in Irritable Bowel Syndrome

Kang Nyeong Lee and Oh Young Lee

Department of Internal Medicine, Hanyang University College of Medicine, Seoul, Republic of Korea

Correspondence should be addressed to Kang Nyeong Lee; leekn@hanyang.ac.kr

Academic Editor: Magdy El-Salhy

Irritable bowel syndrome (IBS) is one of the most common functional gastrointestinal disorders, but its treatment is unsatisfactory as its pathophysiology is multifactorial. The putative factors of IBS pathophysiology are visceral hypersensitivity and intestinal dysmotility, also including psychological factors, dysregulated gut-brain axis, intestinal microbiota alterations, impaired intestinal permeability, and mucosal immune alterations. Recently, mucosal immune alterations have received much attention with the role of mast cells in IBS. Mast cells are abundant in the intestines and function as intestinal gatekeepers at the interface between the luminal environment in the intestine and the internal milieu under the intestinal epithelium. As a gatekeeper at the interface, mast cells communicate with the adjacent cells such as epithelial, neuronal, and other immune cells throughout the mediators released when they themselves are activated. Many studies have suggested that mast cells play a role in the pathophysiology of IBS. This review will focus on studies of the role of mast cell in IBS and the limitations of studies and will also consider future directions.

1. Introduction

Irritable bowel syndrome (IBS) is one of the most common functional gastrointestinal (GI) disorders with a worldwide prevalence of 5–20% [1, 2]. IBS diagnosis is based on symptoms such as recurrent abdominal pain related to defecation and accompanied by a change in the frequency or form of stool [3]. However, neither diagnostic nor therapeutic approaches are satisfactory because IBS is a multifactorial disorder and its manifestation differs from patient to patient. It has traditionally been thought to result from two abnormalities: visceral hypersensitivity and intestinal dysmotility. However, recent intensive studies have revealed that low-grade inflammation of the intestines [4], as well as alterations of gut barrier function, epithelial permeability, mucosal immunity, and gut-brain axis [5–8], is also involved.

It has been suggested that intestinal mast cells are intimately involved in these pathophysiologic changes [9, 10]. Mast cells can activate adjacent cells by releasing mediators and can also be activated themselves via IgE-mediated or non-IgE-mediated pathways. They are thus closely associated both anatomically and functionally with intestinal components such as intrinsic and extrinsic nerves of the GI

tract, intestinal smooth muscles, and secretory glands [11–15]. Furthermore, symptoms of IBS are often provoked by the ingestion of food or psychological stress, which is one of the factors to activate intestinal mast cells [12].

This connection between mast cells and IBS pathophysiology and symptomatology has been supported by numerous studies. In this review, we describe the results of those studies and their limitations and consider potential future developments.

2. Mast Cells in the Regulation of GI Physiology and Pathophysiology

The many roles of mast cells depend on their ability to secrete mediators after being activated by a variety of stimuli [13]. Mast cells can be activated via either IgE-dependent or IgE-independent pathways [16, 17]. First, IgE-dependent pathways are activated, as in allergic reactions, by binding of allergen to IgEs bound to high affinity Fc epsilon receptor (FcRI) and their subsequent cross linking [16]. Second, IgE-independent pathways are activated by various receptors on mast cells to other agents, including cytokines, neurotransmitters, anaphylatoxins such as venom, and physical stimuli such as heat and pressure as well. On the other hand, mast cell mediators are grouped as stored forms and newly synthesized ones; stored forms include histamine, serotonin, and protease, whereas newly synthesized ones include leukotrienes, prostaglandins, platelet-activating factors, and tumor necrosis factor [18, 19]. In addition to secreting these mediators, mast cells can also secrete cytokines and chemokines, transmit microRNAs, and perform paracrine or autocrine functions by secreting mitochondrial DNA and exosomes [20–22].

Mast cells are granulated cells of ~20 μm size and stay alive for a few months. Mast cells develop from CD34^{+} pluripotent progenitor cells in the bone marrow, and the mast cell precursors circulate via the blood and migrate to the intestines, where they differentiate and finally acquire such organ-specific phenotypes as intestinal mast cells [41]. Mast cells mainly function as immediate hypersensitivity in the early phase of allergic inflammation, whereas basophils, although their precursor cells are the same as mast cells, largely circulate in the blood and are recruited in the late phase of allergic response [42].

The locations of intestinal mast cells are primarily tissues at the interface like blood vessels or intestinal surfaces, and their granule contents are variable depending on factors surrounding them. They are mainly located in the lamina propria and the submucosa but are also found in the intraepithelial, smooth muscle, and serosal layers of the intestine [43]. According to their granule contents, mast cells can be grouped as those containing tryptase but no chymase and those containing tryptase, chymase, and carboxypeptidase [13, 44, 45], each predominating in different locations [46]. The functions of intestinal mast cells include regulating permeability, secretion, peristalsis, nociception, innate and adaptive immunity, and angiogenesis and affecting many diverse GI diseases such as not only functional GI disorders but also organic diseases [47].

2.1. Nerve-Mast Cell Interaction. As an effector cell in the intestines, intestinal mast cells have a pivotal function by interacting with nearby nerves of intrinsic and extrinsic neurons in the GI tract. Increasing evidence indicates that intestinal mast cells are located close to nerves [48] and, furthermore, microanatomic examinations have even shown that intestinal mast cells are directly innervated by nerves [49]. Nerve boutons formations were found in close proximity to mast cells in the rat ileal mucosa [50]. It is estimated that 70% of intestinal mast cells are in direct contact with nerves and the remaining 20% are within 1-2 μm of them [48, 49, 51]. This microanatomic association can facilitate their interaction with each other in maintaining mucosal homeostasis. Nerve-mast cell interactions were demonstrated in the study showing that stimulation of spinal nerves activated mast cells, which released mediators, and these mediators in turn activated submucosal neurons in the intestine [15]. In the rat jejunum, for instance, mast cells released mediators in response to sensitized antigen and evoked secretomotor responses, which were suppressed by tetrodotoxin, indicating neural involvement [52]. In such interactions between nerves

and mast cells, the mast cells function as both sensory and effector cells.

3. Methods for Studying the Connection between Mast Cells and IBS

Studies of the role of mast cells in the intestine have been performed in humans as well as in animal models and cultured cell lines. Human studies were performed mainly utilizing mucosal biopsies and the luminal contents of the GI tract [53]. In such studies, levels of mast cell mediators such as tryptase are quantified, after luminal contents of the intestine are aspirated. Also, after mucosal biopsies were obtained during endoscopy, they were fixed in formalin to count mast cells after immunochemical staining (tryptase/c-kit staining) and to analyze gene expression. To identify the type and degree of mast cell degranulation, mucosal biopsies are fixated in glutaraldehyde, while to measure the expression of specific MC mediators the biopsies are fixed in RNA and/or protein stabilizing agents.

Mucosal biopsies can also be incubated in certain tissue culture media for some time and then their supernatants can be used to measure the concentrations of mediators or to examine their effects on neuronal activation and muscle contraction as well as on intestinal secretion and permeability in cells (in vitro) or in animals (in vivo). Functional studies can also be performed on enteric and dorsal root ganglion (DRG) neurons and intestinal muscle strips, using techniques such as neuroimaging, patch clamp recordings, multiunit afferent recordings, and examination of visceromotor reflex. Intestinal permeability regulated by tight junction proteins in intestinal epithelial cells has been evaluated by incubating mucosal biopsies in Ussing chambers and exposing Caco-2 cell monolayers to the resulting supernatants. Using these methods, investigators could examine the pharmacological activation or blockade of mast cells.

In animal studies, hypersensitivity and stress models are exploited to explore mast cell functions in the GI tract [54]. Animal models have been widely used for studying intestinal mast cell functions: food allergies and parasite infections are the two most common types of animal models in use. For models of food allergies, rats are sensitized to protein antigens such as ovalbumin (OVA), and, for models of parasite infections, they are infected with nematodes such as *Nippostrongylus brasiliensis*. Then, flat sheets of intestine are placed in Ussing chambers and intestinal permeability is assessed by measuring ion transport after adding antigens or pharmacologic agents. In vivo functional studies have been performed in mast cell-deficient rats comparing intestinal permeability with that of control rats in the presence and absence of mast cell inhibitors [54]. The results of these studies have provided evidence that mast cells are involved in intestinal function and disease.

In models of food allergy, rats are sensitized to OVA and then mast cell counts, mediator content, and ion transport alterations are assessed. In OVA-sensitized rats, intestinal ion secretion and permeability to both small molecules and macromolecules increase, along with increases in mast cell mediators and morphologic changes indicative of mast cell degranulation, and it is identified that mast cell stabilizers blocked these responses. Furthermore, increases in permeability are not observed in mast cell-deficient animal models. These findings suggest that mast cells participate in antigen-stimulated increases of intestinal permeability. Similar findings have been obtained in models of parasitic infection. In addition to parasites-induced mucosal injuries including villus atrophy and crypt hyperplasia, intestinal permeability was increased, mast cell numbers and mucosal histamine were decreased, and serum levels of mast cell mediators were elevated [55, 56].

4. The Role of Mast Cells in Mucosal Immunity and Low-Grade Inflammation

Evidence indicates that the pathophysiology of IBS is related to a variety of cells in the intestine including epithelial cells, enteroendocrine cells, neuronal cells, and immune cells. Immune cells such as lymphocytes and mast cells interact with food antigens, intestinal microbiota, and other cells in the intestine [7]. In particular, mast cell functions as both a sensor and an effector have received much attention in IBS. Mast cells are more numerous in intestinal mucosa in IBS than in healthy controls, and an increased number of mast cells have been observed in the rectum [36, 38, 57, 58], rectosigmoid [26, 59], descending colon [23, 25, 27, 35, 60], ascending colon [32, 38], cecum [31, 57, 61], terminal ileum [24, 38, 62, 63], jejunum [29, 30, 37], and duodenum [64].

In addition to the absolute increase of intestinal mast cells in IBS, it has been claimed that their activity also increases [27]. Degranulated mast cells as seen by electron microscopy were more numerous in the colons of IBS patients, and these mast cells were close to enteric nerves [25, 60]. Moreover, these enteric nerves were found to contain the mediators, 5-hydroxytryptamine (5-HT), calcitonin gene-related peptide (CGRP), and substance P (SP) [59]. Levels of the mast cell mediators tryptase [23, 25, 33, 35, 60] and histamine [40] were also elevated in the intestinal mucosa of biopsies.

It seems therefore that it may not be the absolute increase in intestinal mast cells but rather the increase in functionally active mast cells and in their proximity to sensory nerves that is important in the development of IBS. However, an increase in mast cells and their mediators has not been observed by all workers [39, 65, 66]; the discrepancies may be due to differences between regions of the intestine, subtypes of IBS, and effects of gender as well as methodological differences in each study.

5. The Role of Mast Cells in Visceral Hypersensitivity and Intestinal Dysmotility

Visceral hypersensitivity has been reported to be associated with mast cell functions [38, 60, 67, 68]. Agents that produce IBS symptoms such as foods and stress can activate mast cells, which then secrete mediators [69]. These mediators such as histamine and protease have been reported to induce hypersensitivity in the nerve terminals of pain-transmitting afferent neurons [35, 60]. This is supported by the fact, as already mentioned, that mast cells are often close to nerve terminals of many types of neurons innervating the intestine [70]. Studies demonstrating this spatial association between mast cells and nerves have used supernatants of mucosal biopsies from patients with IBS [71, 72]. When these supernatants were injected into the mesenteric vessel of rats, intestinal sensory neurons were found to be activated [73]. The mucosal supernatants from IBS colons excited capsaicin-sensitive mesenteric nerves and mobilized Ca^{2+} in rat dorsal root ganglion (DRG) neurons [60]. Moreover, neuronal activation by these supernatants was inhibited by antihistamine or protease inhibitors, indicating that histamines and/or proteases released from mast cells are responsible for this enhanced visceral hypersensitivity in IBS [60, 73]. In addition to DRG neuronal activation, submucosal neurons in human colonic biopsies were also activated by supernatants from IBS patients and these neuronal activation instances were again blocked by inhibiting histamine, serotonin, and protease [35]. Moreover, the degree of neuronal activation shown by rectal balloon dilatation was different between hypersensitive and normosensitive IBS patients; the supernatants from hypersensitive IBS patients provoked stronger responses in the DRG neurons of guinea pigs and mice [74], and colonic administration of the supernatants from hypersensitive IBS patients also caused visceral hypersensitivity in mice [73]. Interestingly, this supernatant-induced visceral hypersensitivity was not seen in protease activated receptor 2- (PAR2-) deficient mice and was abolished by inhibiting PAR2, indicating that the hypersensitivity responses in IBS may be PAR2-mediated [75].

Mast cells are also implicated in intestinal dysmotility, one of the most important features of IBS. The evidence for this is that mast cell mediators from patients with IBS caused the myenteric motor neuron-mediated contraction of intestinal muscle in the guinea pig [34] and the strength of this effect was correlated with mast cell counts in the colonic mucosa. However, the effect was not related to the histamine, protease, or serotonin signaling pathways; instead, it was associated with purinergic P2X receptors, prostanoid receptors, and capsaicin receptor (transient receptor potential vanilloid 1, TRPV1) pathways, suggesting mediation by afferent nerves.

6. The Role of Mast Cells in Intestinal Secretion and Permeability

One of the important pathophysiologies of IBS is alterations in intestinal secretion and permeability. Increased intestinal secretion was found in patients with diarrhea-predominant IBS (IBS-D), whereas decreased intestinal secretion was found in those with constipation-predominant IBS (IBS-C). These alterations in intestinal secretion can be induced by MCs [76], which have been proven in animal models of food allergy and parasitic infection. It was also found in these models that mast cell mediators were responsible for the increase in intestinal secretion [76]. MC mediators, namely, histamine, chymase, and prostaglandin D2, stimulated water and chloride secretion in intestinal epithelia [77, 78]. Also, in human intestinal epithelial cell line, secretion of chloride was increased and decreased by histamine and histamine antagonists, respectively [79, 80].

IBS patients have been reported to have increased intestinal permeability, which was associated with mast cells [29]. Increased permeability by mast cells was demonstrated in human studies where MC stabilizers inhibited the intestinal permeability provoked by MC mediators [81]. The association between increased permeability and mast cell mediators was also identified in animal models of hypersensitivity induced by antigen challenge. In the experiments, mast cell mediators were released and macromolecules were increasingly transported [82, 83]. It was also found in studies using Ussing chambers that sensitizing antigen or worm antigen evoked biphasic short circuit current (Isc) responses in the epithelial layer [84, 85]. In these experiments, histamine or serotonin receptor antagonists increased Isc, which was reproduced by exogenously administered histamine [84, 85].

The role of mast cell mediators in intestinal secretion and permeability seems to be affected by not only histamine and serotonin but also several types of receptors and cytokines related to mast cells. When colonic epithelial cell line T84 was exposed to IL-4, the resistance of intestinal barrier in T84 was attenuated and macromolecular transport increased [86]. The attenuated barrier function and increased transport were similarly observed in the HT29 cell line of human intestinal epithelium incubated with TNF-α [87, 88]. However, chloride ion secretion in a cell line of human colonic epithelium was decreased by cytokines IL-4 and IFN-γ produced by mast cells [89, 90]. It was also shown that rat mast cell protease II increased macromolecular transport in a dose-dependent manner [83]. Additionally, the Isc in ileal segments of the rabbit was increased by IL-1 and IL-3 [91]. The increase of Isc in the rat intestine was induced by a receptor activated by mast cell tryptase, PAR2.

This increased permeability seems to be attributed to degradation of proteins sealing the paracellular space of the epithelium [92, 93]. A study of IBS patients showed that the expression of tight junction proteins was low and was correlated not only with MC activation but also with their symptoms of IBS [29]. Also, low expression of tight junction proteins in the jejunal mucosa was related to increased mast cells [29, 30]. Increased intestinal permeability and the decreased expression of tight junction proteins were also reproduced even when supernatants of mucosal biopsies were applied to Caco-2 cell monolayers [94]. Furthermore, these alterations of molecular structure and ultrastructure of tight junction were associated with mast cell activation and even with IBS symptom severity [94], suggesting a disturbance of the epithelium associated with mast cell activation and symptom presentation in IBS.

In summary, the changes in intestinal secretion and permeability have been shown to correlate with the extent of MC infiltration and the quantity of tryptase in the intestine, and intestinal permeability is increased as a result of degradation of the junctional proteins between intestinal epithelia by mast cell tryptase. Furthermore, a variety of receptors and cytokines are related to the role of mast cells in IBS regarding intestinal secretion and permeability.

7. The Role of Mast Cells in Neuroimmune and Serotonin Signaling

Mast cells cause mucosal inflammation via neuronal stimulation provoked by stress. Psychological stress such as dichotomous auditory stimuli was reported to make mast cells release mediators in IBS. The mediators including histamine, serotonin, protease, cytokines, and chemokines could develop mucosal inflammatory responses. Mucosal immune cells are activated or recruited to induce epithelial barrier dysfunction and subsequently to contribute to the development of IBS symptoms. On the other hand, enhanced mucosal inflammation activates intrinsic or extrinsic nerves, thus facilitating neuronal reflex circuit activation or decreasing visceral pain threshold. Eventually, reflex circuit activation alters physiologic responses including peristalsis, secretion, and motility. Also, frequency and severity of IBS symptoms are affected by reduced threshold of pain.

Serotonin is a main signaling molecule in the GI tract. It is produced and secreted mainly by enteroendocrine cells located in the intestinal epithelial layer. Serotonin exerts its signal transmitting function via a variety of serotonin receptors on many immune and neuronal cells. Regarding serotonin signaling in IBS, mast cells might have a pivotal role. Enteroendocrine cells stimulated by food materials or variable antigens secrete serotonin, which can activate mast cells in the lamina propria of the GI tract. These activated mast cells then induce a cascade of processes involving serotonin-mast cell-neuroimmune mechanisms. The process associated with both serotonin and mast cells may contribute to the production of IBS symptoms of pain or stool changes. Consistently, medications modulating serotonin signal pathways such as 5-HT$_3$ antagonists [95, 96] and 5-HT$_4$ agonists [97, 98] have been reported to relieve symptoms in IBS. Likely, abdominal pain in IBS as well as bowel habit changes improved by serotonin reuptake inhibitors. All these effects might be mediated by serotonin-mast cell signaling pathways. However, serotonin may have an effect on the GI physiologic and pathophysiologic processes bypassing mediation of mast cells. It could directly develop neuronal stimulation or epithelial or immune cells stimulation. Therefore, it is still determined which subset of IBS patients is influenced by mast cell mediation on the pathogenesis as well as symptom generation.

8. IBS Symptom Producers Induce Mast Cell Activation

Most IBS patients report that their symptoms develop or aggravate after food intake [99–101] or stress [102–104]. The response to foods in the intestine can develop from food allergy mediated by IgE-dependent pathways [105] and from adverse food reactions via IgG-dependent pathways or serotonin-mediated reactions [101]. In particular, foods containing capsaicin such as spicy foods are known to stimulate TRPV1 receptors on nociceptive neurons [106]. These TRPV-positive neurons close to mast cells can be controlled by capsaicin, indicating that these mast cells activate nociceptive neurons and are associated with abdominal pain in IBS [26].

Stress may produce or aggravate IBS symptoms by activating mast cells. In a clinical study, stress associated with public speaking induced intestinal barrier dysfunction, which was reproduced by corticotropin-releasing hormone administration and inhibited by disodium cromoglycate [81]. In addition, cold stress stimulated the release of histamine and tryptase from mast cells in jejunal mucosa [107]. Furthermore, mast cell mediators released by mast cell stimulants such as SP and neuron growth factor induced chloride secretion, intestinal dysmotility, and symptoms like pain and diarrhea [108, 109].

Likewise, symptoms of IBS have been shown to correlate with numbers of intestinal mast cells and levels of their mediators (Table 1). There are reports that intestinal mast cell numbers are correlated with symptom scores of abdominal pain [23–27], stool frequency or consistency, and even symptom severity [25, 28–30]. Investigators have shown that tryptase levels correlate with stool frequency and consistency in IBS-D [29, 30], whereas in IBS-C increased mast cells have been observed to relate to abdominal pain but not to constipation. Although the role of mast cells is more focused on IBS-D than IBS-C, a recent study showed a significant increase of colonic mast cells in patients with severe constipation [110]. Considering the effect of nerve growth factor from mast cells, the author suggested this finding as a compensation for impaired propulsive contraction, which might implicate a therapeutic role of mast cell activation in constipation. There have been also other workers who found no correlation between mast cells and hypersensitivity in IBS [36–40].

9. Limitations of the Study Methods and Interpretations of Results

9.1. Experimental Animal and Cell Studies. Mast cells respond to various stimuli differently depending on the species and specific organs studied, because mast cells are enormously variable in forms and functions according to the mode of stimulation and the conditions of the surrounding tissues. Mast cell lines used in experimental studies have been derived from different tissues. Also, animal models of IBS do not fully mimic the effects of IBS in humans. Furthermore, different experimental studies have used different types of methodologies. All these limiting factors should be considered when interpreting the results of experimental studies using mast cells.

9.2. Human Studies. In order to measure mast cell mediators in supernatants and to assess their biological activity, mucosal biopsies are obtained by endoscopy from IBS patients. However, the processing of biopsies is not standardized among studies. The different methods of processing may affect the biologic activities of mast cell mediators. Also, supernatants of mucosal biopsies are collected and assayed at different times among studies [53].

The symptoms of IBS are affected by a number of factors including central and peripheral mechanisms, and

subjects with different phenotypes of IBS have been shown to respond differently. Moreover, there are differences between the properties of mucosal biopsies from different patients with IBS [53]. Apart from a difference in IBS subtypes, these differences may be due to the different times when the supernatants are tested in electrophysiological studies. In addition, regardless of the IBS subtype, visceral hypersensitivity may or may not be present in individual patients, and therefore studies using supernatants from mucosal biopsies could have different outcomes even in patients of the same subtype.

When assessing mast cell infiltration in the intestine, the protocols for tissue fixation and section orientation are not standardized. In terms of staining methods for identifying mast cells, antibodies to either tryptase or CD117 were used and tissue handling can cause MC degranulation which could alter counts of mast cells by tryptase staining. Another possibility is that the increases in mast cell numbers noted in IBS patients may have been caused by those suffering at that time from infectious colitis with no or minimal symptomatic difference compared with IBS. In addition, as stress may affect mast cell densities in the intestines, those under psychological stress may have yielded greater increases in mast cell numbers than those that are not.

10. Summary and Future Directions

Mast cells play a role in different aspects of GI physiology and pathophysiology, particularly in intestinal sensation, motility, secretion, permeability, and inflammation. The symptoms of IBS, abdominal pain and stool changes, could be mediated by intestinal mast cells (Figure 1). Mast cells are located close to enteric nerves so that mast cell-nerve axis is easily activated via mediators released by mast cells and also possibly via neurotransmitters by nerve terminals. Concerning abdominal pain in IBS, mast cells are located close to the intrinsic or extrinsic nerve fibers and can stimulate the adjacent nerve fibers conveying interoceptive signals to the CNS. These signals could be perceived as painful by interaction with other contributing factors including cognitive and affective function in the brain. In terms of stool changes, they are also assumed to be attributable to mediation of mast cells involved in neuroimmune and serotonin signaling as mentioned above.

Mast cells activated by serotonin secreted from enteroendocrine cells release mediators and then the mediators evoke local physiologic reflex response by intrinsic neural circuit, altering peristalsis, perfusion, and secretion which impact intestinal transit and fluid content, therefore developing diarrhea or constipation. Also, mast cells activated by serotonin or by stress-induced efferent neuronal stimulation degranulate mediators, which in this time activate other immune cells. These immune cells may be involved in mucosal permeability changes. Then, the increased permeability can make luminal contents such as food materials or antigenic products easily pass through the epithelial barrier, which causes subsequent responses like increased intestinal secretion. Furthermore, intestinal barrier dysfunction leads to mucosal inflammation

TABLE 1: Studies examining correlations between mast cells and symptoms in IBS.

Subjects number	Sex (M : F)	Age (mean)	Bowel habits	Location	Mast cells mediators	MC-associated symptoms/findings	Ref.
25 IBS 12 CTL	7 : 18 4 : 8	36 26.9	13 IBS-D 12 IBS-C	Descending colon	Inc. MC Inc. Tryp, histamine, & serotonin	Abdominal pain	[23]
21 IBS 10 CTL	10 : 11 4 : 6	11.2 9.3	13 IBS-D 8 IBS-C	Ileum, Rt & Lt colon	MC close to nerve	Abdominal pain	[24]
44 IBS 22 CTL	13 : 31 10 : 12	40.1 32.5	22 IBS-D 22 IBS-C	Descending colon	Inc. MC Inc. Tryp	Abdominal pain	[25]
23 IBS 22 CTL	3 : 20 7 : 15	53 64	8 IBS-D 8 IBS-C 7 IBS-A	Rectosigmoid colon	Inc. MC	Abdominal pain	[26]
48 IBS 24 CTL	13 : 35 9 : 15	42.7 32	27 IBS-D 21 IBS-C	Descending colon	Inc. MC	Abdominal bloating	[27]
34 IBS 15 CTL	6 : 28 9 : 6	51 54	10 IBS-C 13 IBS-D 11 IBS-M	Cecum	Inc. MC Inc. Tryp	Symptom severity; colonic permeability	[28]
25 IBS 23 CTL	6 : 19 12 : 11	35.2 31.4	IBS-D	Jejunum	Inc. MC Inc. Tryp	Stool frequency & consistency; tight junction protein	[29]
45 IBS 30 CTL	11 : 34 14 : 16	33.7 36.3	IBS-D	Jejunum	Inc. MC Inc. Tryp	Stool frequency & consistency; CLDN2 & OCLD	[30]
50 IBS 21 CTL	9 : 41 7 : 14	53.8 56.5	21 IBS-D 29 IBS-C	Cecum	Inc. MC	Fatigue & depression	[31]
55 IBS 18 CTL	39 : 16 12 : 6	43.4 43.6	IBS-D	Ileum, ascending & sigmoid colon	Inc. MC	Rectal sensitivity	[32]
16 IBS 7 CTL	6 : 10 4 : 3	54.6 49	IBS-D	Rectum	Inc. Tryp	Intestinal permeability	[33]
37 IBS 11 CTL	10 : 27 5 : 6	35.2 24.9	16 IBS-D 21 IBS-C	Descending colon	Inc. MC	Supernatant-evoked cholinergic twitch	[34]
11 IBS 4 CTL	4 : 7 2 : 2		7 IBS-D 4 IBS-C	Descending colon	Inc. MC Inc. Tryp	Supernatant-evoked spikes	[35]
22 IBS 21 CTL	12 : 10 11 : 10	50 53.4	IBS-D	Rectum	Inc. MC Inc. SP & VIP	No correlation	[36]
20 IBS 14 CTL	6 : 14 8 : 6	32.8 27.9	IBS-D	Jejunum	Inc. MC Inc. Tryp	No correlation	[37]
18 IBS 15 CTL	8 : 10 5 : 10	42.6 41.4	IBS-D	Ileum, ascending colon, & rectum	Inc. MC	No correlation	[38]
66 IBS 20 CTL	17 : 49 7 : 13	38 31	15 IBS-D 15 IBS-C 36 IBS-A	Ascending & descending colon	Dec. MC	No correlation	[39]
60 IBS 22 CTL	17 : 43 7 : 15	36.2 30	22 IBS-D 9 IBS-C 29 IBS-A	Rectum, descending colon	Dec. MC Dec. Tryp	No correlation	[40]

CLDN: claudin; CTL: control; Dec.: decreased; IBS: irritable bowel syndrome; IBS-A: alternating IBS; IBS-C: constipation predominant IBS; IBS-D: diarrhea predominant IBS; Inc.: increased; MC: mast cell; OCLD: occludin; Tryp: tryptase; SP: substance P; VIP: vasoactive intestinal peptide.

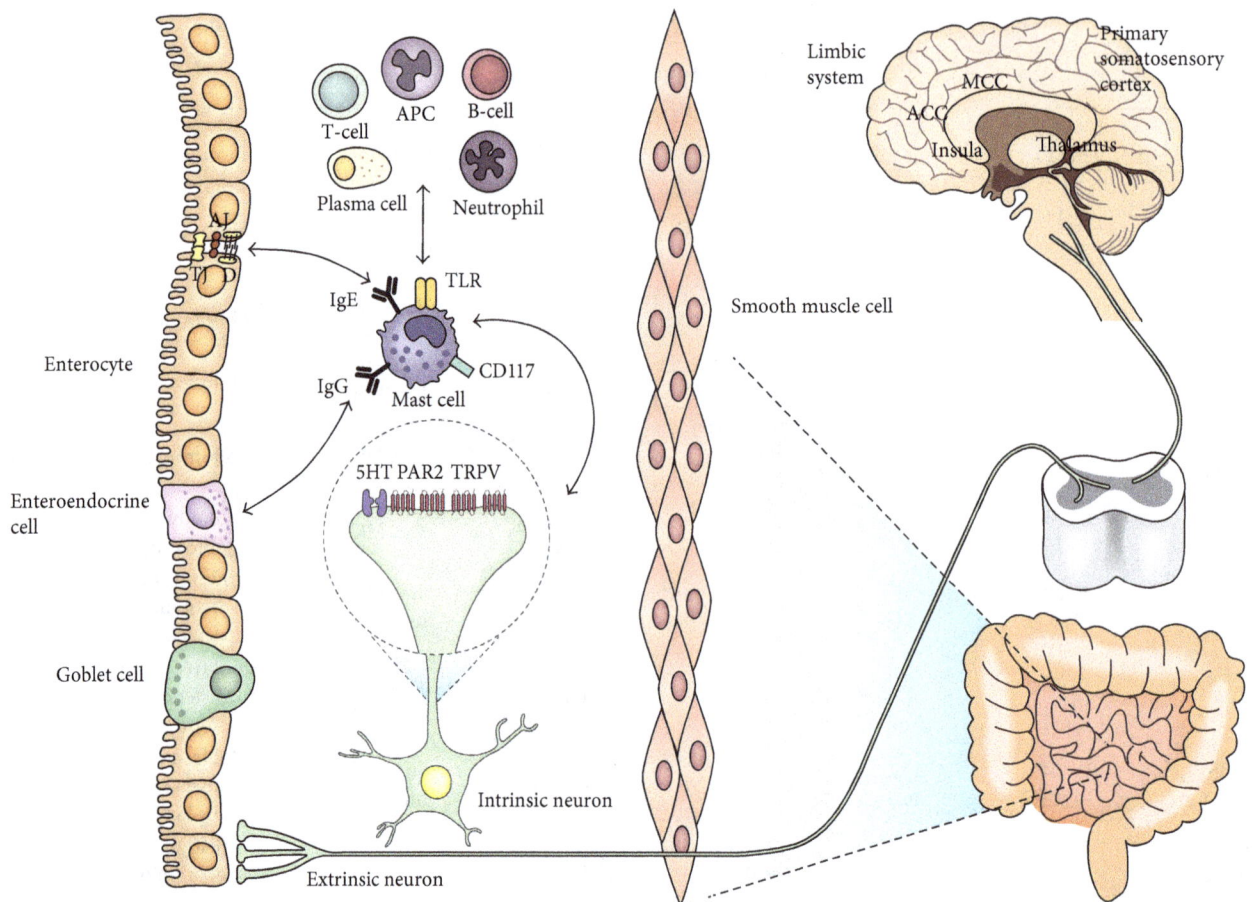

FIGURE 1: The putative role of mast cells in IBS. Both symptoms of IBS, abdominal pain and stool changes, could be mediated by intestinal mast cells. Located close to the intrinsic or extrinsic nerve fibers, mast cells can stimulate the adjacent nerve fibers conveying nociceptive signals to the CNS. These signals could be perceived as painful by interaction with other contributing factors including cognitive and affective function by cerebral cortical and subcortical regions. Mast cells activated by serotonin secreted from enteroendocrine cells release mediators and then the mediators evoke local physiologic reflex response by intrinsic and extrinsic nervous systems, altering peristalsis, perfusion, and secretion which impact intestinal transit and luminal fluid content, therefore developing diarrhea or constipation as well as abdominal pain. Also, mast cells activated by serotonin or by stress-induced efferent neuronal stimulation degranulate mediators, which in this time activate other immune cells. These immune cells may be involved in epithelial secretion or mucosal permeability changes. This intestinal barrier dysfunction may be led by mast cell-associated degradation of various epithelial gap junctional proteins.

which may contribute to further degradation of a variety of epithelial gap junctional proteins. Also, mediators seem to excite pain signaling neuronal pathways and to alter intestinal barrier function as well as intestinal motor nerves. These mast cell-mediated alterations in intestinal sensory and secretomotor function are associated with the characteristic abdominal symptoms of irritable bowel syndrome.

However, despite the intensive study results of the contribution of mast cells to IBS, the pathophysiology of IBS cannot be fully explained by the effects of mast cells. That is because IBS is a complex and heterogeneous disorder and also mast cells have an organ-specific and tissue-specific functional diversity as mentioned above. Furthermore, it is not possible for animal models to exhibit all the features of IBS in human due to multiple confounding influences of genetic, environmental, and biopsychosocial factors on the manifestations of IBS.

Future studies should as far as possible be carried out on humans, and the IBS subtypes should be more accurately defined and refined in studies on the role of mast cells. Furthermore, mast cells should be directly observed rather than using mucosal biopsies, isolated cell lines, or animal models. For this purpose, advanced imaging techniques need to be applied to living intestinal tissues. Recently, confocal endomicroscopy for intestinal diseases has offered real-time visualization of human intestines at the cellular or molecular levels [111]. This technical advance promises to yield important information on the role of MCs in IBS. Additionally, fluorescent C-kit antibody for mast cells may be used in vivo for detecting intestinal mast cells located in the lamina propria and submucous layers as in the experiment showing promising results for specific cells [112]. Further studies for the direct effect of mast cells in humans are needed, which will be helpful for developing effective methods for symptom control and eventually for complete cure of IBS.

Competing Interests

The authors declare that there are no competing interests regarding the publication of this paper.

Authors' Contributions

Kang Nyeong Lee contributed to the conception and design of the study, literature review and analysis, and drafting. Oh Young Lee contributed to critical revision and editing. Both authors approved the final version.

Acknowledgments

This work was supported by the research fund of Hanyang University (HY-2015).

References

[1] R. L. S. Soares, "Irritable bowel syndrome: a clinical review," *World Journal of Gastroenterology*, vol. 20, no. 34, pp. 12144–12160, 2014.

[2] G. F. Longstreth, W. G. Thompson, W. D. Chey, L. A. Houghton, F. Mearin, and R. C. Spiller, "Functional bowel disorders," *Gastroenterology*, vol. 130, no. 5, pp. 1480–1491, 2006.

[3] B. E. Lacy, F. Mearin, L. Chang et al., "Bowel disorders," *Gastroenterology*, vol. 150, no. 6, pp. 1393.e5–1407.e5, 2016.

[4] E. Sinagra, G. Pompei, G. Tomasello et al., "Inflammation in irritable bowel syndrome: myth or new treatment target?" *World Journal of Gastroenterology*, vol. 22, pp. 2242–2255, 2016.

[5] J. Matricon, M. Meleine, A. Gelot et al., "Review article: associations between immune activation, intestinal permeability and the irritable bowel syndrome," *Alimentary Pharmacology and Therapeutics*, vol. 36, no. 11-12, pp. 1009–1031, 2012.

[6] C. Martínez, A. González-Castro, M. Vicario, and J. Santos, "Cellular and molecular basis of intestinal barrier dysfunction in the irritable bowel syndrome," *Gut and Liver*, vol. 6, no. 3, pp. 305–315, 2012.

[7] G. Barbara, C. Cremon, G. Carini et al., "The immune system in irritable bowel syndrome," *Journal of Neurogastroenterology and Motility*, vol. 17, no. 4, pp. 349–359, 2011.

[8] Y. Tanaka, M. Kanazawa, S. Fukudo, and D. A. Drossman, "Biopsychosocial model of irritable bowel syndrome," *Journal of Neurogastroenterology and Motility*, vol. 17, no. 2, pp. 131–139, 2011.

[9] L. Zhang, J. Song, and X. Hou, "Mast cells and irritable bowel syndrome: from the bench to the bedside," *Journal of Neurogastroenterology and Motility*, vol. 22, no. 2, pp. 181–192, 2016.

[10] M. M. Wouters, M. Vicario, and J. Santos, "The role of mast cells in functional GI disorders," *Gut*, vol. 65, no. 1, pp. 155–168, 2016.

[11] D. L. Vermillion, P. B. Ernst, R. Scicchitano, and S. M. Collins, "Antigen-induced contraction of jejunal smooth muscle in the sensitized rat," *American Journal of Physiology—Gastrointestinal and Liver Physiology*, vol. 255, no. 6, pp. G701–G708, 1988.

[12] M. Gué, C. Del Rio-Lacheze, H. Eutamene, V. Théodorou, J. Fioramonti, and L. Buéno, "Stress-induced visceral hypersensitivity to rectal distension in rats: role of CRF and mast cells," *Neurogastroenterology and Motility*, vol. 9, no. 4, pp. 271–279, 1997.

[13] S. C. Bischoff, "Physiological and pathophysiological functions of intestinal mast cells," *Seminars in Immunopathology*, vol. 31, no. 2, pp. 185–205, 2009.

[14] E. Traver, R. Torres, F. De Mora, and P. Vergara, "Mucosal mast cells mediate motor response induced by chronic oral exposure to ovalbumin in the rat gastrointestinal tract," *Neurogastroenterology and Motility*, vol. 22, no. 1, pp. e34–e43, 2010.

[15] G.-D. Wang, X.-Y. Wang, S. Liu et al., "Innervation of enteric mast cells by primary spinal afferents in guinea pig and human small intestine," *American Journal of Physiology—Gastrointestinal and Liver Physiology*, vol. 307, no. 7, pp. G719–G731, 2014.

[16] J. Rivera, N. A. Fierro, A. Olivera, and R. Suzuki, "Chapter 3 new insights on mast cell activation via the high affinity receptor for IgE," *Advances in Immunology*, vol. 98, pp. 85–120, 2008.

[17] A. M. Gilfillan and J. Rivera, "The tyrosine kinase network regulating mast cell activation," *Immunological Reviews*, vol. 228, no. 1, pp. 149–169, 2009.

[18] M. B. Olszewski, A. J. Groot, J. Dastych, and E. F. Knol, "TNF trafficking to human mast cell granules: mature chain-dependent endocytosis," *The Journal of Immunology*, vol. 178, no. 9, pp. 5701–5709, 2007.

[19] J. A. Boyce, "Mast cells and eicosanoid mediators: a system of reciprocal paracrine and autocrine regulation," *Immunological Reviews*, vol. 217, no. 1, pp. 168–185, 2007.

[20] T. C. Theoharides, P. Valent, and C. Akin, "Mast cells, mastocytosis, and related disorders," *New England Journal of Medicine*, vol. 373, no. 2, pp. 163–172, 2015.

[21] B. Zhang, S. Asadi, Z. Weng, N. Sismanopoulos, and T. C. Theoharides, "Stimulated human mast cells secrete mitochondrial components that have autocrine and paracrine inflammatory actions," *PLoS ONE*, vol. 7, no. 12, Article ID e49767, 2012.

[22] D. Skokos, H. G. Botros, C. Demeure et al., "Mast cell-derived exosomes induce phenotypic and functional maturation of dendritic cells and elicit specific immune responses in vivo," *The Journal of Immunology*, vol. 170, no. 6, pp. 3037–3045, 2003.

[23] C. Cremon, G. Carini, B. Wang et al., "Intestinal serotonin release, sensory neuron activation, and abdominal pain in irritable bowel syndrome," *American Journal of Gastroenterology*, vol. 106, no. 7, pp. 1290–1298, 2011.

[24] G. Di Nardo, G. Barbara, S. Cucchiara et al., "Neuroimmune interactions at different intestinal sites are related to abdominal pain symptoms in children with IBS," *Neurogastroenterology and Motility*, vol. 26, no. 2, pp. 196–204, 2014.

[25] G. Barbara, V. Stanghellini, R. De Giorgio et al., "Activated mast cells in proximity to colonic nerves correlate with abdominal pain in irritable bowel syndrome," *Gastroenterology*, vol. 126, no. 3, pp. 693–702, 2004.

[26] A. Akbar, Y. Yiangou, P. Facer, J. R. F. Walters, P. Anand, and S. Ghosh, "Increased capsaicin receptor TRPV1-expressing sensory fibres in irritable bowel syndrome and their correlation with abdominal pain," *Gut*, vol. 57, no. 7, pp. 923–929, 2008.

[27] C. Cremon, L. Gargano, A. M. Morselli-Labate et al., "Mucosal immune activation in irritable bowel syndrome: gender-dependence and association with digestive symptoms," *The American Journal of Gastroenterology*, vol. 104, no. 2, pp. 392–400, 2009.

[28] M. Vivinus-Nébot, R. Dainese, R. Anty et al., "Combination of allergic factors can worsen diarrheic irritable bowel syndrome: role of barrier defects and mast cells," *The American Journal of Gastroenterology*, vol. 107, no. 1, pp. 75–81, 2012.

[29] C. Martínez, M. Vicario, L. Ramos et al., "The jejunum of diarrhea-predominant irritable bowel syndrome shows molecular alterations in the tight junction signaling pathway that are associated with mucosal pathobiology and clinical manifestations," *The American Journal of Gastroenterology*, vol. 107, no. 5, pp. 736–746, 2012.

[30] C. Martínez, B. Lobo, M. Pigrau et al., "Diarrhoea-predominant irritable bowel syndrome: an organic disorder with structural abnormalities in the jejunal epithelial barrier," *Gut*, vol. 62, no. 8, pp. 1160–1168, 2013.

[31] T. Piche, M. C. Saint-Paul, R. Dainese et al., "Mast cells and cellularity of the colonic mucosa correlated with fatigue and depression in irritable bowel syndrome," *Gut*, vol. 57, no. 4, pp. 468–473, 2008.

[32] J. Yang, M. Fox, Y. Cong et al., "Lactose intolerance in irritable bowel syndrome patients with diarrhoea: the roles of anxiety, activation of the innate mucosal immune system and visceral sensitivity," *Alimentary Pharmacology and Therapeutics*, vol. 39, no. 3, pp. 302–311, 2014.

[33] H. Lee, J. H. Park, D. I. Park et al., "Mucosal mast cell count is associated with intestinal permeability in patients with diarrhea predominant irritable bowel syndrome," *Journal of Neurogastroenterology and Motility*, vol. 19, no. 2, pp. 244–250, 2013.

[34] B. Balestra, R. Vicini, C. Cremon et al., "Colonic mucosal mediators from patients with irritable bowel syndrome excite enteric cholinergic motor neurons," *Neurogastroenterology and Motility*, vol. 24, no. 12, pp. 1118–e570, 2012.

[35] S. Buhner, Q. Li, S. Vignali et al., "Activation of human enteric neurons by supernatants of colonic biopsy specimens from patients with irritable bowel syndrome," *Gastroenterology*, vol. 137, no. 4, pp. 1425–1434, 2009.

[36] W. Sohn, O. Y. Lee, S. P. Lee et al., "Mast cell number, substance P and vasoactive intestinal peptide in irritable bowel syndrome with diarrhea," *Scandinavian Journal of Gastroenterology*, vol. 49, no. 1, pp. 43–51, 2014.

[37] M. Guilarte, J. Santos, I. De Torres et al., "Diarrhoea-predominant IBS patients show mast cell activation and hyperplasia in the jejunum," *Gut*, vol. 56, no. 2, pp. 203–209, 2007.

[38] J. H. Park, P.-L. Rhee, H. S. Kim et al., "Mucosal mast cell counts correlate with visceral hypersensitivity in patients with diarrhea predominant irritable bowel syndrome," *Journal of Gastroenterology and Hepatology*, vol. 21, no. 1, pp. 71–78, 2006.

[39] B. Braak, T. K. Klooker, M. M. Wouters et al., "Mucosal immune cell numbers and visceral sensitivity in patients with irritable bowel syndrome: is there any relationship?" *American Journal of Gastroenterology*, vol. 107, no. 5, pp. 715–726, 2012.

[40] T. K. Klooker, B. Braak, K. E. Koopman et al., "The mast cell stabiliser ketotifen decreases visceral hypersensitivity and improves intestinal symptoms in patients with irritable bowel syndrome," *Gut*, vol. 59, no. 9, pp. 1213–1221, 2010.

[41] L. L. Reber, R. Sibilano, K. Mukai, and S. J. Galli, "Potential effector and immunoregulatory functions of mast cells in mucosal immunity," *Mucosal Immunology*, vol. 8, no. 3, pp. 444–463, 2015.

[42] K. D. Stone, C. Prussin, and D. D. Metcalfe, "IgE, mast cells, basophils, and eosinophils," *The Journal of Allergy and Clinical Immunology*, vol. 125, no. 2, supplement 2, pp. S73–S80, 2010.

[43] S. C. Bischoff, J. Wedemeyer, A. Herrmann et al., "Quantitative assessment of intestinal eosinophils and mast cells in inflammatory bowel disease," *Histopathology*, vol. 28, no. 1, pp. 1–13, 1996.

[44] E. Z. M. da Silva, M. C. Jamur, and C. Oliver, "Mast cell function: a new vision of an old cell," *Journal of Histochemistry and Cytochemistry*, vol. 62, no. 10, pp. 698–738, 2014.

[45] S. J. Galli, M. Grimbaldeston, and M. Tsai, "Immunomodulatory mast cells: negative, as well as positive, regulators of immunity," *Nature Reviews Immunology*, vol. 8, no. 6, pp. 478–486, 2008.

[46] N. P. Hyland, M. Julio-Pieper, S. M. O'Mahony et al., "A distinct subset of submucosal mast cells undergoes hyperplasia following neonatal maternal separation: a role in visceral hypersensitivity?" *Gut*, vol. 58, no. 7, pp. 1029–1030, 2009.

[47] S. C. Bischoff, "Role of mast cells in allergic and non-allergic immune responses: comparison of human and murine data," *Nature Reviews Immunology*, vol. 7, no. 2, pp. 93–104, 2007.

[48] R. H. Stead, M. F. Dixon, N. H. Bramwell, R. H. Riddell, and J. Bienenstock, "Mast cells are closely apposed to nerves in the human gastrointestinal mucosa," *Gastroenterology*, vol. 97, no. 3, pp. 575–585, 1989.

[49] R. H. Stead, "Innervation of mucosal immune cells in the gastrointestinal tract," *Regional Immunology*, vol. 4, no. 2, pp. 91–99, 1992.

[50] B. Newson, A. Dahlström, L. Enerbäck, and H. Ahlman, "Suggestive evidence for a direct innervation of mucosal mast cells: an electron microscopic study," *Neuroscience*, vol. 10, no. 2, pp. 565–570, 1983.

[51] R. H. Stead, M. Tomioka, G. Quinonez, G. T. Simon, S. Y. Felten, and J. Bienenstock, "Intestinal mucosal mast cells in normal and nematode-infected rat intestines are in intimate contact with peptidergic nerves," *Proceedings of the National Academy of Sciences of the United States of America*, vol. 84, no. 9, pp. 2975–2979, 1987.

[52] G. A. Castro, Y. Harari, and D. Russell, "Mediators of anaphylaxis-induced ion transport changes in small intestine," *American Journal of Physiology—Gastrointestinal and Liver Physiology*, vol. 253, no. 4, pp. G540–G548, 1987.

[53] Y. Nasser, G. E. Boeckxstaens, M. M. Wouters, M. Schemann, and S. Vanner, "Using human intestinal biopsies to study the pathogenesis of irritable bowel syndrome," *Neurogastroenterology and Motility*, vol. 26, no. 4, pp. 455–469, 2014.

[54] L. C. H. Yu and M. H. Perdue, "Role of mast cells in intestinal mucosal function: studies in models of hypersensitivity and stress," *Immunological Reviews*, vol. 179, pp. 61–73, 2001.

[55] J. K. Ramage, R. H. Hunt, and M. H. Perdue, "Changes in intestinal permeability and epithelial differentiation during inflammation in the rat," *Gut*, vol. 29, no. 1, pp. 57–61, 1988.

[56] J. K. Ramage, A. Stanisz, R. Scicchitano, R. H. Hunt, and M. H. Perdue, "Effect of immunologic reactions on rat intestinal epithelium. Correlation of increased permeability to chromium 51-labeled ethylenediaminetetraacetic acid and ovalbumin during acute inflammation and anaphylaxis," *Gastroenterology*, vol. 94, no. 6, pp. 1368–1375, 1988.

[57] M. Vivinus-Nébot, R. Dainese, R. Anty et al., "Combination of allergic factors can worsen diarrheic irritable bowel syndrome: role of barrier defects and mast cells," *American Journal of Gastroenterology*, vol. 107, no. 1, pp. 75–81, 2012.

[58] S. P. Dunlop, D. Jenkins, and R. C. Spiller, "Distinctive clinical, psychological, and histological features of postinfective irritable bowel syndrome," *The American Journal of Gastroenterology*, vol. 98, no. 7, pp. 1578–1583, 2003.

[59] L.-H. Wang, X.-C. Fang, and G.-Z. Pan, "Bacillary dysentery as a causative factor of irritable bowel syndrome and its pathogenesis," *Gut*, vol. 53, no. 8, pp. 1096–1101, 2004.

[60] G. Barbara, B. Wang, V. Stanghellini et al., "Mast cell-dependent excitation of visceral-nociceptive sensory neurons in irritable bowel syndrome," *Gastroenterology*, vol. 132, no. 1, pp. 26–37, 2007.

[61] M. O'Sullivan, N. Clayton, N. P. Breslin et al., "Increased mast cells in the irritable bowel syndrome," *Neurogastroenterology & Motility*, vol. 12, no. 5, pp. 449–457, 2000.

[62] S.-H. Wang, L. Dong, J.-Y. Luo et al., "Decreased expression of serotonin in the jejunum and increased numbers of mast cells in the terminal ileum in patients with irritable bowel syndrome," *World Journal of Gastroenterology*, vol. 13, no. 45, pp. 6041–6047, 2007.

[63] A. P. Weston, W. L. Biddle, P. S. Bhatia, and P. B. Miner Jr., "Terminal ileal mucosal mast cells in irritable bowel syndrome," *Digestive Diseases and Sciences*, vol. 38, no. 9, pp. 1590–1595, 1993.

[64] M. M. Walker, N. J. Talley, M. Prabhakar et al., "Duodenal mastocytosis, eosinophilia and intraepithelial lymphocytosis as possible disease markers in the irritable bowel syndrome and functional dyspepsia," *Alimentary Pharmacology and Therapeutics*, vol. 29, no. 7, pp. 765–773, 2009.

[65] A. P. M. Kerckhoffs, J. J. M. ter Linde, L. M. A. Akkermans, and M. Samsom, "SERT and TPH-1 mRNA expression are reduced in irritable bowel syndrome patients regardless of visceral sensitivity state in large intestine," *American Journal of Physiology—Gastrointestinal and Liver Physiology*, vol. 302, no. 9, pp. G1053–G1060, 2012.

[66] V. S. Chadwick, W. Chen, D. Shu et al., "Activation of the mucosal immune system in irritable bowel syndrome," *Gastroenterology*, vol. 122, no. 7, pp. 1778–1783, 2002.

[67] J.-H. La, T.-W. Kim, T.-S. Sung, H.-J. Kim, J.-Y. Kim, and I.-S. Yang, "Role of mucosal mast cells in visceral hypersensitivity in a rat model of irritable bowel syndrome," *Journal of veterinary science*, vol. 5, no. 4, pp. 319–324, 2004.

[68] K. Ohashi, Y. Sato, H. Iwata, M. Kawai, and Y. Kurebayashi, "Colonic mast cell infiltration in rats with TNBS-induced visceral hypersensitivity," *Journal of Veterinary Medical Science*, vol. 69, no. 12, pp. 1223–1228, 2007.

[69] X.-Y. Gui, "Mast cells: a possible link between psychological stress, enteric infection, food allergy and gut hypersensitivity in the irritable bowel syndrome," *Journal of Gastroenterology and Hepatology*, vol. 13, no. 10, pp. 980–989, 1998.

[70] M. Schemann and M. Camilleri, "Functions and imaging of mast cell and neural axis of the gut," *Gastroenterology*, vol. 144, no. 4, pp. 698–704.e4, 2013.

[71] G. Barbara, C. Cremon, R. De Giorgio et al., "Mechanisms underlying visceral hypersensitivity in irritable bowel syndrome," *Current Gastroenterology Reports*, vol. 13, no. 4, pp. 308–315, 2011.

[72] M. Camilleri, K. Lasch, and W. Zhou, "Irritable bowel syndrome: methods, mechanisms, and pathophysiology. the confluence of increased permeability, inflammation, and pain in irritable bowel syndrome," *American Journal of Physiology—Gastrointestinal and Liver Physiology*, vol. 303, no. 7, pp. G775–G785, 2012.

[73] N. Cenac, C. N. Andrews, M. Holzhausen et al., "Role for protease activity in visceral pain in irritable bowel syndrome," *Journal of Clinical Investigation*, vol. 117, no. 3, pp. 636–647, 2007.

[74] S. Buhner, B. Braak, Q. Li et al., "Neuronal activation by mucosal biopsy supernatants from irritable bowel syndrome patients is linked to visceral sensitivity," *Experimental Physiology*, vol. 99, no. 10, pp. 1299–1311, 2014.

[75] E. E. Valdez-Morales, J. Overington, R. Guerrero-Alba et al., "Sensitization of peripheral sensory nerves by mediators from colonic biopsies of diarrhea-predominant irritable bowel syndrome patients: a role for PAR2," *American Journal of Gastroenterology*, vol. 108, no. 10, pp. 1634–1643, 2013.

[76] J. Santos, P.-C. Yang, J. D. Söderholm, M. Benjamin, and M. H. Perdue, "Role of mast cells in chronic stress induced colonic epithelial barrier dysfunction in the rat," *Gut*, vol. 48, no. 5, pp. 630–636, 2001.

[77] C. Alonso, M. Vicario, M. Pigrau, B. Lobo, and J. Santos, "Intestinal barrier function and the brain-gut axis," in *Advances in Experimental Medicine and Biology*, vol. 817, pp. 73–113, Springer, New York, NY, USA, 2014.

[78] K. R. Groschwitz, R. Ahrens, H. Osterfeld et al., "Mast cells regulate homeostatic intestinal epithelial migration and barrier function by a chymase/Mcpt4-dependent mechanism," *Proceedings of the National Academy of Sciences of the United States of America*, vol. 106, no. 52, pp. 22381–22386, 2009.

[79] J. A. Cohn, N. C. Dougherty, and W. F. King Jr., "Histamine stimulates calcium-mediated protein phosphorylation in a colonic epithelial cell line," *Biochemical and Biophysical Research Communications*, vol. 165, no. 2, pp. 811–816, 1989.

[80] S. I. Wasserman, K. E. Barrett, P. A. Huott, G. Beuerlein, M. F. Kagnoff, and K. Dharmsathaphorn, "Immune-related intestinal Cl- secretion. I. Effect of histamine on the T84 cell line," *American Journal of Physiology—Cell Physiology*, vol. 254, no. 1, pp. C53–C62, 1988.

[81] T. Vanuytsel, S. van Wanrooy, H. Vanheel et al., "Psychological stress and corticotropin-releasing hormone increase intestinal permeability in humans by a mast cell-dependent mechanism," *Gut*, vol. 63, no. 8, pp. 1293–1299, 2014.

[82] H. R. P. Miller, R. G. Woodbury, J. F. Huntley, and G. Newlands, "Systemic release of mucosal mast-cell protease in primed rats challenged with Nippostrongylus brasiliensis," *Immunology*, vol. 49, no. 3, pp. 471–479, 1983.

[83] C. L. Scudamore, E. M. Thornton, L. Mcmillan, G. F. J. Newlands, and H. R. P. Miller, "Release of the mucosal mast cell granule chymase, rat mast cell protease-II, during anaphylaxis is associated with the rapid development of paracellular permeability to macromolecules in rat jejunum," *Journal of Experimental Medicine*, vol. 182, no. 6, pp. 1871–1881, 1995.

[84] S. E. Crowe, P. Sestini, and M. H. Perdue, "Allergic reactions of rat jejunal mucosa. Ion transport responses to luminal antigen and inflammatory mediators," *Gastroenterology*, vol. 99, no. 1, pp. 74–82, 1990.

[85] M. H. Perdue, S. Masson, B. K. Wershil, and S. J. Galli, "Role of mast cells in ion transport abnormalities associated with intestinal anaphylaxis. Correction of the diminished secretory response in genetically mast cell-deficient W/Wv mice by bone marrow transplantation," *Journal of Clinical Investigation*, vol. 87, no. 2, pp. 687–693, 1991.

[86] S. P. Colgan, M. B. Resnick, C. A. Parkos et al., "IL-4 directly modulates function of a model human intestinal epithelium," *The Journal of Immunology*, vol. 153, no. 5, pp. 2122–2129, 1994.

[87] M. Heyman, N. Darmon, C. Dupont et al., "Mononuclear cells from infants allergic to cow's milk secrete tumor necrosis factor α, altering intestinal function," *Gastroenterology*, vol. 106, no. 6, pp. 1514–1523, 1994.

[88] L. Mahraoui, M. Heyman, O. Plique, M. T. Droy-Lefaix, and J. F. Desjeux, "Apical effect of diosmectite on damage to the intestinal barrier induced by basal tumour necrosis factor-alpha," *Gut*, vol. 40, no. 3, pp. 339–343, 1997.

[89] J. Holmgren, J. Fryklund, and H. Larsson, "Gamma-interferon-mediated down-regulation of electrolyte secretion by intestinal epithelial cells: a local immune mechanism?" *Scandinavian Journal of Immunology*, vol. 30, no. 4, pp. 499–503, 1989.

[90] G. Zünd, J. L. Madara, A. L. Dzus, C. S. Awtrey, and S. P. Colgan, "Interleukin-4 and interleukin-13 differentially regulate epithelial chloride secretion," *Journal of Biological Chemistry*, vol. 271, no. 13, pp. 7460–7464, 1996.

[91] E. B. Chang, M. W. Musch, and L. Mayer, "Interleukins 1 and 3 stimulate anion secretion in chicken intestine," *Gastroenterology*, vol. 98, no. 6, pp. 1518–1524, 1990.

[92] E. M. Wilcz-Villega, S. McClean, and M. A. O'Sullivan, "Mast cell tryptase reduces junctional adhesion molecule-A (JAM-A) expression in intestinal epithelial cells: implications for the mechanisms of barrier dysfunction in irritable bowel syndrome," *American Journal of Gastroenterology*, vol. 108, pp. 1140–1151, 2013.

[93] J. W. Lee, J. H. Park, D. I. L. Park et al., "Subjects with diarrhea-predominant IBS have increased rectal permeability responsive to tryptase," *Digestive Diseases and Sciences*, vol. 55, no. 10, pp. 2922–2928, 2010.

[94] T. Piche, G. Barbara, P. Aubert et al., "Impaired intestinal barrier integrity in the colon of patients with irritable bowel syndrome: involvement of soluble mediators," *Gut*, vol. 58, no. 2, pp. 196–201, 2009.

[95] V. Andresen, V. M. Montori, J. Keller, C. P. West, P. Layer, and M. Camilleri, "Effects of 5-hydroxytryptamine (serotonin) type 3 antagonists on symptom relief and constipation in nonconstipated irritable bowel syndrome: a systematic review and meta-analysis of randomized controlled trials," *Clinical Gastroenterology and Hepatology*, vol. 6, no. 5, pp. 545–555, 2008.

[96] R. Rahimi, S. Nikfar, and M. Abdollahi, "Efficacy and tolerability of alosetron for the treatment of irritable bowel syndrome in women and men: a meta-analysis of eight randomized, placebo-controlled, 12-week trials," *Clinical Therapeutics*, vol. 30, no. 5, pp. 884–901, 2008.

[97] B. W. Evans, W. K. Clark, D. J. Moore, and P. J. Whorwell, "Tegaserod for the treatment of irritable bowel syndrome and chronic constipation," *Cochrane database of systematic reviews*, no. 4, Article ID CD003960, 2007.

[98] L. Degen, C. Petrig, D. Studer, S. Schroller, and C. Beglinger, "Effect of tegaserod on gut transit in male and female subjects," *Neurogastroenterology and Motility*, vol. 17, no. 6, pp. 821–826, 2005.

[99] P. R. Gibson, J. Varney, S. Malakar, and J. G. Muir, "Food components and irritable bowel syndrome," *Gastroenterology*, vol. 148, no. 6, pp. 1158–1174.e4, 2015.

[100] M. Simrén, A. Månsson, A. M. Langkilde et al., "Food-related gastrointestinal symptoms in the irritable bowel syndrome," *Digestion*, vol. 63, no. 2, pp. 108–115, 2001.

[101] L. Böhn, S. Störsrud, H. Törnblom, U. Bengtsson, and M. Simrén, "Self-reported food-related gastrointestinal symptoms in IBS are common and associated with more severe symptoms and reduced quality of life," *American Journal of Gastroenterology*, vol. 108, no. 5, pp. 634–641, 2013.

[102] W. E. Whitehead, O. Palsson, and K. R. Jones, "Systematic review of the comorbidity of irritable bowel syndrome with other disorders: what are the causes and implications?" *Gastroenterology*, vol. 122, no. 4, pp. 1140–1156, 2002.

[103] D. A. Drossman, Z. Li, J. Leserman, T. C. Toomey, and Y. J. B. Hu, "Health status by gastrointestinal diagnosis and abuse history," *Gastroenterology*, vol. 110, no. 4, pp. 999–1007, 1996.

[104] A. Garakani, T. Win, S. Virk, S. Gupta, D. Kaplan, and P. S. Masand, "Comorbidity of irritable bowel syndrome in psychiatric patients: a review," *American Journal of Therapeutics*, vol. 10, no. 1, pp. 61–67, 2003.

[105] R. Cuomo, P. Andreozzi, F. P. Zito, V. Passananti, G. De Carlo, and G. Sarnelli, "Irritable bowel syndrome and food interaction," *World Journal of Gastroenterology*, vol. 20, no. 27, pp. 8837–8845, 2014.

[106] S. J. M. van Wanrooij, M. M. Wouters, L. Van Oudenhove et al., "Sensitivity testing in irritable bowel syndrome with rectal capsaicin stimulations: role of TRPV1 upregulation and sensitization in visceral hypersensitivity?" *The American Journal of Gastroenterology*, vol. 109, no. 1, pp. 99–109, 2014.

[107] C. Alonso, M. Guilarte, M. Vicario et al., "Acute experimental stress evokes a differential gender-determined increase in human intestinal macromolecular permeability," *Neurogastroenterology and Motility*, vol. 24, no. 8, pp. 740–e349, 2012.

[108] F. Barreau, C. Cartier, L. Ferrier, J. Fioramonti, and L. Bueno, "Nerve growth factor mediates alterations of colonic sensitivity and mucosal barrier induced by neonatal stress in rats," *Gastroenterology*, vol. 127, no. 2, pp. 524–534, 2004.

[109] L. Wang, A. M. Stanisz, B. K. Wershil, S. J. Galli, and M. H. Perdue, "Substance P induces ion secretion in mouse small intestine through effects on enteric nerves and mast cells," *American Journal of Physiology—Gastrointestinal and Liver Physiology*, vol. 269, no. 1, pp. G85–G92, 1995.

[110] G. Bassotti, V. Villanacci, R. Nascimbeni et al., "Colonic mast cells in controls and slow transit constipation patients," *Alimentary Pharmacology and Therapeutics*, vol. 34, no. 1, pp. 92–99, 2011.

[111] R. Kiesslich, J. Burg, M. Vieth et al., "Confocal laser endoscopy for diagnosing intraepithelial neoplasias and colorectal cancer in vivo," *Gastroenterology*, vol. 127, no. 3, pp. 706–713, 2004.

[112] R. Atreya, H. Neumann, C. Neufert et al., "In vivo imaging using fluorescent antibodies to tumor necrosis factor predicts therapeutic response in Crohn's disease," *Nature Medicine*, vol. 20, no. 3, pp. 313–318, 2014.

15

Clinical Performance of Prediction Rules and Nasogastric Lavage for the Evaluation of Upper Gastrointestinal Bleeding: A Retrospective Observational Study

Hassan K. Dakik,[1] F. Douglas Srygley,[2] Shih-Ting Chiu,[3] Shein-Chung Chow,[3] and Deborah A. Fisher[1,4]

[1]Duke Gastroenterology Division, Duke University Hospital, Durham, NC, USA
[2]Austin Gastroenterology, Austin, TX, USA
[3]Duke Biostatistics Division, Duke University Hospital, Durham, NC, USA
[4]Durham VA Health Services Research and Development Center, Durham, NC, USA

Correspondence should be addressed to Deborah A. Fisher; deborah.fisher@duke.edu

Academic Editor: Ford Bursey

Introduction. The majority of patients with acute upper gastrointestinal bleeding (UGIB) are admitted for urgent endoscopy as it can be difficult to determine who can be safely managed as an outpatient. Our objective was to compare four clinical prediction scoring systems: Glasgow Blatchford Score (GBS) and Clinical Rockall, Adamopoulos, and Tammaro scores in a sample of patients presenting to the emergency department of a large US academic center. *Methods*. We performed a retrospective cohort study of patients during 2008–2010. Our outcome was significant UGIB defined as high-risk stigmata on endoscopy, or receipt of blood transfusion or surgery, or death. *Results*. A total of 393 patients met inclusion criteria. The GBS was the most sensitive for detecting significant UGIB at 98.30% and had the highest negative predictive value (90.00%). Adding nasogastric lavage data to the GBS increased the sensitivity to 99.57%. *Conclusions*. Of all four scoring systems compared, the GBS demonstrated the highest sensitivity and negative predictive value for identifying a patient with a significant UGIB. Therefore, patients with a 0 score can be safely managed as an outpatient. Our results also suggest that performing a nasogastric lavage adds little to the diagnosis UGIB.

1. Introduction

Gastrointestinal bleeding (GIB) is a common and serious condition with an estimated 545,000 hospitalizations yearly in the United States (US) [1]. Hospitalizations for upper GIB (UGIB) have a mean length of stay of 2.7–4.4 days and a mean cost of $3,400–$13,000 [2, 3]. Currently, the majority of patients presenting with acute UGIB are admitted for an urgent esophagogastroduodenoscopy (EGD) as it can be difficult to differentiate between those patients at high risk for significant bleeding and those who can be safely managed as an outpatient [4]. Several different prognostic scoring algorithms have been proposed to facilitate clinical decision-making, specifically the determination of hospital admission versus outpatient management. These scoring systems use different combinations of clinical factors and have been evaluated to predict bleeding severity and identify those patients safe for discharge.

In initial studies, these clinical prediction rules have suggested that as many as a third of all patients presenting with an acute UGIB may be safely discharged from the emergency department (ED) to nonurgent follow-up [4]. The best studied scoring systems are the Glasgow Blatchford Score (GBS) and the Clinical Rockall score [4–9]. However, there are minimal data validating these two scoring algorithms in US populations. This may be a barrier to wider use of these scoring systems by ED providers because practices in Europe and Britain, where these scores were developed and predominantly validated, differ from US practices. In particular, the criteria for admission are notably different.

Thus, the applicability of these scores in a US health system is unclear. In addition to the GBS and Clinical Rockall scores, the Adamopoulos and Tammaro scores have been developed but only validated in a single publication each [10, 11]. To date, there have been no direct comparison studies to evaluate these four scoring systems in the same patient population to determine their head-to-head performance.

An additional issue in the management of acute UGIB is whether nasogastric (NG) lavage is needed or helpful. NG lavage is a method of attempting to obtain fluid from the stomach and, potentially, the small bowel to determine the location of a possible GIB and help determine the severity of the bleed [12]. The value of NG lavage remains controversial with conflicting results amongst studies [13–15]. Nonetheless, the practice is still common in US institutions.

Our primary goal was to determine which of the scoring systems was best able to discern patients at low risk for significant hemorrhage who could be safely managed as an outpatient. Therefore, we estimated and compared the performance characteristics of GBS, Clinical Rockall, Adamopoulos, and Tammaro scores in identifying a significant UGIB in a sample of US patients who presented to the ED with signs/symptoms consistent with an acute UGIB. Our secondary aim was to evaluate any additional value of NG lavage data when integrated into the most accurate scoring systems.

2. Methods

We performed a retrospective cohort study of patients who presented to the Duke University Hospital ED with a diagnosis of UGIB during 2008–2010. The patients were initially identified based on International Classification of Diseases Version 9 (ICD 9) codes for upper GI bleeding (e.g., upper GI bleed, hematemesis, and melena) via the Duke Enterprise Data Unified Content Explorer (DEDUCE) database which is a web-based tool allowing specific clinical data to be extracted by researchers from the electronic medical record [16]. These ICD-9 codes are listed in the following.

ICD-9 Codes for GI Bleeding

456.00 - ESOPHAGEAL VARICES WITH BLEEDING

456.20 - ESOPHAGEAL VARICES IN DISEASES CLASSIFIED ELSEWHERE WITH BLEEDING

456.80 - VARICES OF OTHER SITES

530.20 - ULCER OF ESOPHAGUS WITHOUT BLEEDING

530.21 - ULCER OF ESOPHAGUS WITH BLEEDING

530.70 - GASTROESOPHAGEAL LACERATION

531.10 - ACUTE GASTRIC ULCER WITH PERFORATION WITHOUT OBSTRUCTION

531.20 - ACUTE GASTRIC ULCER WITH HEMORRHAGE AND PERFORATION WITHOUT OBSTRUCTION

531.40 - CHRONIC OR UNSPECIFIED GASTRIC ULCER WITH HEMORRHAGE WITHOUT OBSTRUCTION

531.60 - CHRONIC OR UNSPECIFIED GASTRIC ULCER WITH HEMORRHAGE AND PERFORATION WITHOUT OBSTRUCTION

532.00 - ACUTE DUODENAL ULCER WITH HEMORRHAGE WITHOUT OBSTRUCTION

532.20 - ACUTE DUODENAL ULCER WITH HEMORRHAGE AND PERFORATION WITHOUT OBSTRUCTION

532.40 - CHRONIC OR UNSPECIFIED DUODENAL ULCER WITH HEMORRHAGE WITHOUT OBSTRUCTION

532.60 - CHRONIC OR UNSPECIFIED DUODENAL ULCER WITH HEMORRHAGE AND PERFORATION WITHOUT OBSTRUCTION

533.00 - ACUTE PEPTIC ULCER OF UNSPECIFIED SITE WITH HEMORRHAGE WITHOUT OBSTRUCTION

533.4 - CHRONIC OR UNSPECIFIED PEPTIC ULCER OF UNSPECIFIED SITE WITH HEMORRHAGE WITHOUT OBSTRUCTION

533.60 - CHRONIC OR UNSPECIFIED PEPTIC ULCER OF UNSPECIFIED SITE WITH HEMORRHAGE AND PERFORATION WITHOUT OBSTRUCTION

537.83 - ANGIODYSPLASIA OF STOMACH AND DUODENUM WITH HEMORRHAGE

537.84 - DIEULAFOY LESION (HEMORRHAGIC) OF STOMACH AND DUODENUM

578.00 - HEMATEMESIS

578.10 - BLOOD IN STOOL

578.90 - HEMORRHAGE OF GASTROINTESTINAL TRACT UNSPECIFIED

Next, the electronic medical records (EMR) for each patient were reviewed for inclusion and exclusion criteria. The EMR of eligible subjects was further abstracted using a standard protocol and data collection tool to obtain the data for each scoring algorithm (Table 1).

Inclusion criteria were all patients who presented to the ED with a primary complaint of UGIB as evidenced by hematemesis, melena, coffee ground emesis, or bright red blood per rectum in the appropriate setting (i.e., a brisk GIB as evidenced by hemodynamic changes and hemoglobin drop), from 1/1/2008 through 12/31/2010. Patients must have been seen by a physician in the ED and evaluated with a tentative diagnosis of UGIB.

Patients were excluded if there was no complaint of active bleeding (i.e., only anemia or findings consistent with occult bleeding). In addition, they were excluded if they met any of the following criteria: age <18 years old, found to have lower gastrointestinal or anal bleeding, inpatient status at the

TABLE 1: Clinical parameters used in scoring algorithms.

Scoring algorithms	Objective clinical parameters	Other clinical factors
Blatchford (GBS)	Blood urea nitrogen, hemoglobin level, systolic blood pressure, heart rate	Presentation with melena or syncope Presence of liver disease or heart failure
Clinical Rockall	Age, systolic blood pressure, heart rate	Presence of heart failure, ischemic heart disease, or any major comorbidity
Adamopoulos	Heart rate, systolic blood pressure, hemoglobin level, WBC.	Presence of fresh blood in NGT aspirate
Tamarro	Heart rate, systolic blood pressure, hemoglobin level	General condition (subjective assessment of comorbidities)

time of the onset of bleeding, or lack of sufficient information documented in the EMR to complete the scores.

The clinical factors which were abstracted included age, gender, race/ethnicity, blood urea nitrogen, hemoglobin, international normalized ratio (INR), systolic blood pressure, pulse, history of melena, history of syncope, presence of hepatic disease, history of congestive heart failure, presence of comorbidities (as described in Clinical Rockall score [17]), white blood cell count, general condition (as described by Tammaro score [10]), nasogastric lavage results (categorized as not performed, clear, bilious, coffee grounds, or red blood), use of anticoagulants, and Charleston Comorbidity Index.

The four scores were calculated as described in the literature using the above data (Table 2) [5, 10, 11, 17].

The primary clinical outcome was "significant UGIB" as defined by any of the following: the presence of high-risk stigmata on endoscopy (as defined by Forest classification [18]), receipt of blood transfusion, performance of surgery, or death while in the hospital or, if not admitted, within 30 days. If the patient was not admitted then vital status (dead, alive) or any of the above events at another hospital was investigated by examining outpatient records including clinic visits and outpatient endoscopy. For patients seen in the ED which had no subsequent records in the Duke system, we had IRB permission to contact via letter and then telephone to evaluate vital status and occurrence of any of the other events in the combined outcome.

The primary analysis was calculation of the sensitivity, specificity, positive predictive value (PPV), negative predictive value (NPV), and likelihood ratios of each scoring system to detect a significant UGIB as described above. For each scoring system we used the cutoff value described in the respective original publications.

The GBS score utilizes a combination of laboratory values and clinical parameters to calculate a cumulative numeric score. Any value greater than 0 was considered high risk as described in the original publication and subsequent validation studies [5].

The Rockall score uses similar parameters to arrive at a total numeric score. The initial manuscript described a low rebleeding and mortality rate for cumulative scores 0–2. Scores 3 or greater were noted to have higher incidence of rebleeding as well as a 5-fold increase in mortality [17].

However, this score requires the inclusion of the findings on endoscopy and associated stigmata of bleeding in the setting of peptic ulcer disease. The clinical (or preendoscopy) Rockall score utilizes only the clinical parameters available prior to endoscopic assessment and can be used as a preendoscopy predictor of bleeding risk. This score cutoff is similar to the Blatchford of ≥ 1 being considered high risk.

The Adamopoulos score utilized a simpler formula to calculate risk, which included NG lavage data. The equation was as follows:

$$
\begin{aligned}
\text{Total score} \\
= 6 \ & (\text{if fresh blood in NGT}) \\
+ 4 \ & (\text{if hemodynamically unstable}) \\
+ 4 \ & (\text{if hemoglobin less than } 8\,\text{g/dL}) \\
+ 3 \ & (\text{if WBC greater than } 12{,}000/\text{microL}) .
\end{aligned}
\tag{1}
$$

In their original cohort the authors utilized value of <7 to be consistent with low risk and greater than or equal to 11 was considered high risk. This yielded a sensitivity of 96%, specificity of 98%, and a positive predictive value of 96%. Given that our goal was to favor increased sensitivity we considered any score >7 to be consistent with a significant upper GI bleed [11].

Lastly, the Tamarro score focused on clinical predictors of significant hemorrhage such as vital signs and initial hemoglobin levels to form a basic calculation [10]. In this scoring system a higher numerical score correlated to a lower risk of hemorrhage. The authors divided their sample into three categories representing a low, intermediate, and high risk of rebleeding. However, again, as we were focusing on maximal sensitivity we combined the last 2 categories, namely, the intermediate (score 7–9) and high risk (score ≤6) into one group and considered any score < 10 to be consistent with significant GIB in our analysis.

3. Results

A total of 393 patients met our inclusion criteria for upper GIB. Characteristics of the sample are in Table 3; 247 patients were male and 146 were female with a mean age of 54.9 years.

TABLE 2: Scoring algorithms.

(a) Tamarro score

Clinical parameter	Score		
	1	2	3
General conditions	Poor	Intermediate	Good
Pulse (beats/min)	>110	90–110	<90
Systolic blood pressure (mmHg)	<90	90–110	>110
Hemoglobin level (g/dL)	≤8	9-10	>10

T-score is sum of the corresponding values for each clinical parameters.
≤6 corresponds to $T1$ (high-risk), 7–9 to $T2$ (intermediate-risk), and ≥10 to $T3$ (low-risk).

(b) Adamopoulos score

Total points = [6 (if fresh blood in NGT) + 4 (if hemodynamically unstable) + 4 (if hemoglobin < 8 g/dL) + 3 (if WBC > 12,000/μL)].
Score <7 = low risk, score ≥11 = high risk.

(c) Clinical Rockall score (before endoscopy)

Clinical parameter	Score			
	0	1	2	3
Age (years)	<60	60–79	≥80	
Shock	"No shock" SBP ≥ 100 mmHg, pulse < 100/min	"Tachycardia" SBP ≥ 100 mmHg, pulse ≥ 100/min	"Hypotension" SBP < 100 mmHg	
Comorbidity	No major comorbidities		CHF, ischemic heart disease, any major comorbidity	Renal failure, liver failure, disseminated malignancy

(d) Blatchford score

Admission risk marker	Score
Blood urea (mmol/L)	
≥6.5 <8.0	2
≥8.0 <10.0	3
≥10.0 ≤25.0	4
>25	6
Hemoglobin (g/dL) males	
≥12.0 <13.0	1
≥10.0 <12.0	3
<10.0	6
Hemoglobin (g/dL) females	
≥10.0 <12.0	1
<10.0	6
Systolic blood pressure	
100–109	1
90–99	2
<90	3
Other markers	
Pulse ≥ 100 (per min)	1
Presentation with melena	1
Presentation with syncope	2
Hepatic disease	2
Cardiac failure	2

TABLE 3: Demographics and endpoints.

		N	%
Age (mean)	54.94		
Male		247	**62.85**
Female		146	**37.15**
	White	213	**54.2**
	African American	163	**41.48**
	Asian	4	**1.02**
Race/ethnicity	Hispanic	6	**1.53**
	Native American	7	**1.78**
EGD performed		215	**54.85**
Endoscopic therapy utilized if EGD done		57	**26.51**
Blood transfusion needed		155	**39.44**
Need for surgery		1	**0.25**
Death during hospitalization		28	**7.12**

A total of 235 patients met the combined outcome of significant UGIB by either requiring blood products, having high-risk stigmata on endoscopy, needing surgery, or death. The majority of patients had follow-up available in the EMR but 16 patients were contacted because they were discharged from the ED and had no follow-up documentation available.

The results of the statistical analysis are summarized in Table 4. The GBS was the most sensitive for detecting significant UGIB at 98.30%. The specificity was expectedly lower at 22.78%. The NPV was 90.00% and the negative LR was 0.07.

Using a cutoff score of ≥ 1 as described above, the Clinical Rockall score demonstrated a high sensitivity of 92.77% with a specificity of 32.28%. The NPV was 75.00% with a negative LR of 0.22.

The Adamopoulos scoring system had the lowest sensitivity at 29.79% with a higher specificity of 92.41%. The NPV was 46.95% and the negative LR was 0.76. Modifying the cutoffs to a value ≥4 (favoring improved sensitivity) the sensitivity increased to 71.06% with a lesser reduction in specificity to 79.11%, a NPV of 64.77%, and negative LR of 0.37.

Lastly, the Tammaro scoring system had a sensitivity of 79.57%, specificity of 60.76%, and NPV of 66.67%. The negative LR was 0.34.

Adding NG lavage data to the GBS with coffee grounds and red blood serving as a positive result with a value of 1 additional point, the sensitivity increased to 99.57% and the specificity remained unchanged at 22.78%. The NPV increased to 97.3% and the negative LR was 0.02.

The majority of patients in our study were admitted to the hospital for management of UGIB. 82 patients (20.87%) were discharged and managed as outpatients. Of these only 4 (1%) met our criteria for having a significant UGIB and 29 (7.4%) of these patients had a Blatchford score of 0.

4. Discussion

One of the most important steps in the management of acute upper GI bleeding occurs in the initial triage of these patients. The clinical presentation of UGIB can vary widely and determining which patients will require urgent evaluation can be difficult. Moreover, this decision is often made by ED providers without the aid of an experienced gastroenterologist. In an effort to avoid discharging patients home with the potential for worsening bleeding, the majority of patients presenting with UGIB are admitted to the hospital for an urgent evaluation, which often culminates in upper endoscopy [4]. On the other hand, if hospital admission is not needed because outpatient evaluation and follow-up are safe, then this cost and patient inconvenience can be avoided.

Several scoring systems have been developed as clinical decision tools prior to endoscopy which may facilitate appropriate triage in the ED. Of these, the best studied is the GBS system which has been validated in numerous studies [4–9, 19, 20]. However, these scorings systems have, for the most part, been evaluated in a non-US patient population. This raises the question of the generalizability of these studies to US practice as the underlying populations and common work-flow patterns could differ. While differences in population characteristics (e.g., age, gender, race/ethnicity, comorbidities) may not affect the sensitivity and specificity of the scoring system, positive and negative predictive values are dependent on prevalence which could vary by patient mix. In addition, we wondered if US providers would reject scoring systems that did not include NG lavage, a frequent triage procedure in the US, and whether the impact of using a score on triage practices (e.g., the proportion of cases admitted that could have been managed out of the hospital) would vary with admission thresholds in different settings.

Our retrospective study is one of the few to test several GIB prediction scoring systems in a US based population. More specifically, we examined the test characteristics on a large sample of patients presenting to the ED of a major academic medical center. It is also the first study to date to directly compare these four scoring algorithms in the same patient population.

Overall, the scoring system with the highest sensitivity was the GBS. In our patient population this scoring system was able to correctly identify patients with evidence of significant upper GI bleeding in nearly 99% of cases. For the purposes of our analysis, we focused on sensitivity and negative predictive values and were less concerned with correspondingly lower specificity.

Compared to the other scoring algorithms, the Clinical Rockall had a high sensitivity but remained inferior to the GBS in all evaluated capacities. The Tammaro score had modest sensitivity with slightly improved specificity compared to the GBS. The NPV of the Clinical Rockall and Tammaro scores were in our opinions inadequate to safely determine patients at low risk of having a significant UGIB who could be discharged without endoscopy. Of note, the original Rockall score included endoscopic data and was developed to guide discharge decisions *after* urgent endoscopy. Therefore, it is

TABLE 4: Test parameters for each scoring system.

Prediction scoring system	Sensitivity	95% CI	Specificity	95% CI	NPV	95% CI	Negative LR	95% CI
Blatchford (GBS)	**98.30**	96.64–99.95	22.78	16.24–29.33	90.00	80.70–99.30	0.07	0.0–0.15
GBS + NGL	**99.57**	98.74–100.00	22.78	16.24–29.33	97.30	92.07–100.00	0.02	−0.02–0.06
Clinical Rockall Score (≥1)	**92.77**	89.45–96.08	32.28	24.99–39.57	75.00	64.71–85.29	0.22	0.11–0.34
Adamopoulos (≥7)	**29.79**	23.94–35.63	92.41	88.27–96.54	46.95	41.40–52.49	0.76	0.69–0.83
Adamopoulos (≥4)	**71.06**	65.27–76.86	79.11	72.78–85.45	64.77	58.03–71.51	0.37	0.29–0.44
Tamarro	**79.57**	74.42–84.73	60.76	53.15–68.37	66.67	58.97–74.37	0.34	0.24–0.43

not too surprising that the Clinical Rockall score, which does not include any findings from endoscopy, does not perform as well as an initial triage tool prior to endoscopy.

In the largest prior study from the US both the GBS and Clinical Rockall score were evaluated retrospectively with a similar clinical endpoint of significant GI hemorrhage. This analysis revealed sensitivities of 99% and 100% for the GBS and clinical Rockwall, respectively. However, the specificities were only 6% and 4% respectively (using standard cutoff values) [20]. The investigators concluded that the scoring systems were of limited value and recommended instead clinical decision-making in consultation with GI specialists. We agree that careful clinical assessment is important; however, we disagree regarding the value of GBS to aid appropriate triage from the ED. The high sensitivity of the GBS scoring algorithm allows the test to be useful in determining patients appropriate for outpatient management.

A 2015 study suggested that the cutoff for the GBS could be increased to ≤1 to increase the specificity while maintaining a sensitivity of 99% [21]. This change in cutoff would allow more patients to be considered low risk for the purposes of triage. We performed a secondary analysis of the GBS in our data set with a ≤1 cutoff and this resulted in a sensitivity of 96.15%. While we were not able to replicate a sensitivity of 99% our results still suggest that this higher cutoff might be reasonable to consider.

Our study also evaluated the use of NG lavage as a triage tool. This test is still used widely in clinical practice in spite of published test characteristics with sensitivities of 42–84%, specificities of 54–91%, and NPV of 64–85% [15, 16] and data suggesting that use of NG lavage does not significantly alter mortality, hospital length of stay, transfusion requirements, or the need for surgery [22]. Our analysis revealed that incorporation of the NG lavage data into the GBS did improve the sensitivity as well as the NPV with no effect on the specificity. However, the sensitivity increased only marginally and was over 95% prior to addition of the NG lavage data. Therefore, any added benefit from NG lavage appears minimal. While there may be a role for an NG lavage in an effort to clear gastric contents prior to endoscopic evaluation, the value in the diagnostic evaluation of an acute UGIB appears negligible which is consistent with the prior studies.

Although the incidence of UGIB in the US has been decreasing, likely because of wide spread proton pump inhibitor (PPI) therapy, treatment of *Helicobacter pylori (H. pylori)* infection and decreased *H. pylori* incidence [23],

the advent of new anticoagulant and antiplatelet agents and increased use of newer cardiac devices and therapies may affect these trends. Regardless, the financial burden of UGIB management on the health care system remains high. Estimated costs for the inpatient management of upper GI bleeding range from $3,180 to $14,301 [24, 25]. Outpatient management of upper GI bleeding has fewer costs, even when endoscopy is required. Use of GBS to facilitate appropriate discharge could decrease costs without compromising patient safety.

Our study was a retrospective analysis and accordingly was subject to certain inherit biases. To avoid ascertainment bias the data were abstracted and verified by multiple researchers and the abstraction protocol was standardized. Moreover, the data points used were largely fixed values and less susceptible to individual interpretation. Patients were called after discharge if outcome data were not complete to avoid attrition bias. This was a single center study at a large academic center and hence may be less clearly representative of other patient populations. However, we do feel that the population was adequately representative of large US academic hospitals and as such the results are generalizable to that clinical setting. Our outcome was significant UGIB which does not have a standard definition clinically or in research. The findings of high-risk stigmata on endoscopy or documentation of intervention (i.e., transfusion, surgery) or death have been used in various combinations in other studies. However, the clinical use of transfusion was not standardized at our institution at the time of the study. While this could have potentially misclassified a patient's outcome, it should not have affected the *relative* performance of the scoring systems. Some of the scoring algorithms were not originally validated for the purposes of triaging significant upper GIB such as the Adamopoulos score which was originally aimed at targeting those in need of urgent endoscopy, or the Clinical Rockall score which aimed to predict risk of death following acute UGIB. For that reason we performed separate analyses using altered cutoff values, which favored increased sensitivity for these scores. Lastly, the analysis of NG lavage was based on clinical practice and may have selected for certain clinical presentations and characteristics of patients. However, our findings did not suggest that this procedure contributed substantially to the diagnosis of a significant UGIB and as such this influence was likely minimal. Moreover, the results obtained are consistent with the majority of recently published studies evaluating the utility of this exam.

In conclusion, of the four scoring systems compared, the GBS demonstrated the highest sensitivity and NPV for identifying a patient with a significant UGIB. Therefore, patients with a 0 score can be safely managed as an outpatient. Our results also suggest that performing an NG lavage adds little to the diagnosis of significant UGIB. In an era of increasing cost consciousness and efforts to reduce unnecessary spending, a simple tool that may facilitate more cost-effective management of UGIB should be considered.

Competing Interests

The authors of this manuscript certify that they have no financial or nonfinancial conflict of interests to disclose.

Authors' Contributions

Hassan K. Dakik participated in study concept and design, data acquisition, analysis and interpretation of data, drafting manuscript, and revision. F. Douglas Srygley participated in study concept and design and acquisition of data. Shih-Ting Chiu participated in analysis and interpretation of data. Shein-Chung Chow participated analysis and interpretation of data. Deborah A. Fisher participated study concept and design, acquisition of data, analysis and interpretation of data, drafting manuscript, and critical revision.

References

[1] Y. Zhao and W. Encinosa, *Hospitalizations for Gastrointestinal Bleeding 1998 and 2006*, HCUP Statistical Brief #65, Agency for Healthcare Research and Quality, Rockville, Md, USA, 1998 http://www.hcup-us.ahr.gov/reports/statbriefs/sb65.pdf.

[2] B. L. Cryer, C. M. Wilcox, H. J. Henk, G. Zlateva, L. Chen, and V. Zarotsky, "The economics of upper gastrointestinal bleeding in a US managed-care setting: a retrospective, claims-based analysis," *Journal of Medical Economics*, vol. 13, no. 1, pp. 70–77, 2010.

[3] A. N. Barkun, M. Bardou, E. J. Kuipers et al., "International consensus recommendations on the management of patients with nonvariceal upper gastrointestinal bleeding," *Annals of Internal Medicine*, vol. 152, no. 2, pp. 101–113, 2010.

[4] A. Stanley, D. Ashley, H. Dalton et al., "Outpatient management of patients with low-risk upper-gastrointestinal haemorrhage: multicentre validation and prospective evaluation," *The Lancet*, vol. 373, no. 9657, pp. 42–47, 2009.

[5] O. Blatchford, W. R. Murray, and M. Blatchford, "A risk score to predict need for treatment for upper-gastrointestinal haemorrhage," *Lancet*, vol. 356, no. 9238, pp. 1318–1321, 2000.

[6] I.-C. Chen, M.-S. Hung, T.-F. Chiu, J.-C. Chen, and C.-T. Hsiao, "Risk scoring systems to predict need for clinical intervention for patients with nonvariceal upper gastrointestinal tract bleeding," *American Journal of Emergency Medicine*, vol. 25, no. 7, pp. 774–779, 2007.

[7] T. Masaoka, H. Suzuki, S. Hori, N. Aikawa, and T. Hibi, "Blatchford scoring system is a useful scoring system for detecting patients with upper gastrointestinal bleeding who do not need endoscopic intervention," *Journal of Gastroenterology and Hepatology*, vol. 22, no. 9, pp. 1404–1408, 2007.

[8] R. Srirajaskanthan, R. Conn, C. Bulwer, and P. Irving, "The Glasgow Blatchford scoring system enables accurate risk stratification of patients with upper gastrointestinal haemorrhage," *International Journal of Clinical Practice*, vol. 64, no. 7, pp. 868–874, 2010.

[9] J. Romagnuolo, A. N. Barkun, R. Enns, D. Armstrong, and J. Gregor, "Simple clinical predictors may obviate urgent endoscopy in selected patients with nonvariceal upper gastrointestinal tract bleeding," *Archives of Internal Medicine*, vol. 167, no. 3, pp. 265–270, 2007.

[10] L. Tammaro, M. C. di Paolo, A. Zullo et al., "Endoscopic findings in patients with upper gastrointestinal bleeding clinically classified into three risk groups prior to endoscopy," *World Journal of Gastroenterology*, vol. 14, no. 32, pp. 5046–5050, 2008.

[11] A. B. Adamopoulos, N. M. Baibas, S. P. Efstathiou et al., "Differentiation between patients with acute upper gastrointestinal bleeding who need early urgent upper gastrointestinal endoscopy and those who do not. A Prospective Study," *European Journal of Gastroenterology and Hepatology*, vol. 15, no. 4, pp. 381–387, 2003.

[12] F. D. Srygley, C. J. Gerardo, T. Tran, and D. A. Fisher, "Does this patient have a severe upper gastrointestinal bleed?" *JAMA*, vol. 307, no. 10, pp. 1072–1079, 2012.

[13] A. M. Aljebreen, C. A. Fallone, and A. N. Barkun, "Nasogastric aspirate predicts high-risk endoscopic lesions in patients with acute upper-GI bleeding," *Gastrointestinal Endoscopy*, vol. 59, no. 2, pp. 172–178, 2004.

[14] D. J. Pallin and J. R. Saltzman, "Is nasogastric tube lavage in patients with acute upper GI bleeding indicated or antiquated?" *Gastrointestinal Endoscopy*, vol. 74, no. 5, pp. 981–984, 2011.

[15] M. D. Witting, L. Magder, A. E. Heins, A. Mattu, C. A. Granja, and M. Baumgarten, "Usefulness and validity of diagnostic nasogastric aspiration in patients without hematemesis," *Annals of Emergency Medicine*, vol. 43, no. 4, pp. 525–532, 2004.

[16] C. Roth, S. A. Rusincovitch, M. M. Horvath et al., "DEDUCE clinical text: an ontology-based module to support self-service clinical notes exploration and cohort development," *AMIA Summits on Translational Science Proceedings*, vol. 2013, article 227, 2013.

[17] T. A. Rockall, R. F. A. Logan, H. B. Devlin, and T. C. Northfield, "Risk assessment after acute upper gastrointestinal haemorrhage," *Gut*, vol. 38, no. 3, pp. 316–321, 1996.

[18] J. H. Forrest, N. D. C. Finlayson, and D. J. C. Shearman, "Endoscopy in gastrointestinal bleeding," *The Lancet*, vol. 304, no. 7877, pp. 394–397, 1974.

[19] S. H. Pang, J. Y. L. Ching, J. Y. W. Lau, J. J. Y. Sung, D. Y. Graham, and F. K. L. Chan, "Comparing the Blatchford and pre-endoscopic Rockall score in predicting the need for endoscopic therapy in patients with upper GI hemorrhage," *Gastrointestinal Endoscopy*, vol. 71, no. 7, pp. 1134–1140, 2010.

[20] S. Chandra, E. P. Hess, D. Agarwal et al., "External validation of the Glasgow-Blatchford bleeding score and the Rockall score in the US setting," *American Journal of Emergency Medicine*, vol. 30, no. 5, pp. 673–679, 2012.

[21] S. B. Laursen, H. R. Dalton, I. A. Murray et al., "Performance of new thresholds of the glasgow blatchford score in managing patients with upper gastrointestinal bleeding," *Clinical Gastroenterology and Hepatology*, vol. 13, no. 1, pp. 115.e2–121.e2, 2015.

[22] E. S. Huang, S. Karsan, F. Kanwal, I. Singh, M. Makhani, and B. M. Spiegel, "Impact of nasogastric lavage on outcomes in acute

GI bleeding," *Gastrointestinal Endoscopy*, vol. 74, no. 5, pp. 971–980, 2011.

[23] L. Laine, H. Yang, S.-C. Chang, and C. Datto, "Trends for incidence of hospitalization and death due to GI complications in the United States from 2001 to 2009," *American Journal of Gastroenterology*, vol. 107, no. 8, pp. 1190–1195, 2012.

[24] D. R. Parker, X. Luo, J. J. Jalbert, and A. R. Assaf, "Impact of upper and lower gastrointestinal blood loss on healthcare utilization and costs: a systematic review," *Journal of Medical Economics*, vol. 14, no. 3, pp. 279–287, 2011.

[25] C. T. Whelan, C. Chen, P. Kaboli, J. Siddique, M. Prochaska, and D. O. Meltzer, "Upper versus lower gastrointestinal bleeding: a direct comparison of clinical presentation, outcomes, and resource utilization," *Journal of Hospital Medicine*, vol. 5, no. 3, pp. 141–147, 2010.

16

Duodenal Rare Neuroendocrine Tumor: Clinicopathological Characteristics of Patients with Gangliocytic Paraganglioma

Yoichiro Okubo,[1] Tomoyuki Yokose,[1] Osamu Motohashi,[2] Yohei Miyagi,[3] Emi Yoshioka,[1] Masaki Suzuki,[1] Kota Washimi,[1] Kae Kawachi,[1] Madoka Nito,[4] Tetsuo Nemoto,[5] Kazutoshi Shibuya,[5] and Yoichi Kameda[1]

[1]Department of Pathology, Kanagawa Cancer Center, 2-3-2 Nakao, Asahi-Ku, Yokohama, Kanagawa 241-8515, Japan
[2]Department of Gastroenterology, Kanagawa Cancer Center, 2-3-2 Nakao, Asahi-Ku, Yokohama, Kanagawa 241-8515, Japan
[3]Molecular Pathology and Genetics Division, Kanagawa Cancer Center Research Institute, 2-3-2 Nakao, Asahi-Ku, Yokohama, Kanagawa 241-8515, Japan
[4]Department of Thoracic Surgery, Kanagawa Cancer Center, 2-3-2 Nakao, Asahi-Ku, Yokohama, Kanagawa 241-8515, Japan
[5]Department of Surgical Pathology, Toho University School of Medicine, 6-11-1 Omori-Nishi, Ota-Ku, Tokyo 143-8541, Japan

Correspondence should be addressed to Yoichiro Okubo; yoichiro0207@hotmail.com

Academic Editor: Niccola Funel

Gangliocytic paraganglioma (GP) has been regarded as a rare benign tumor that commonly arises from the second part of the duodenum. As GP does not exhibit either prominent mitotic activity or Ki-67 immunoreactivity, it is often misdiagnosed as neuroendocrine tumor (NET) G1. However, the prognosis might be better in patients with GP than in those with NET G1. Therefore, it is important to differentiate GP from NET G1. Moreover, our previous study indicated that GP accounts for a substantial, constant percentage of duodenal NETs. In the present article, we describe up-to-date data on the clinicopathological characteristics of GP and on the immunohistochemical findings that can help differentiate GP from NET G1, as largely revealed in our new and larger literature survey and recent multi-institutional retrospective study. Furthermore, we would like to refer to differential diagnosis and clinical management of this tumor and provide intriguing information about the risk factors for lymph node metastasis on GP.

1. Introduction

The incidence of neuroendocrine tumors (NETs) has been increasing worldwide [1]; however, the reasons for this increase are unclear [1]. The current World Health Organization classification proposed a grading system for NETs based on the proliferative activity of tumor cells (the number of mitoses or the Ki-67 labeling index) [2–4]. Specifically, NETs have been classified as G1, G2, and G3 (neuroendocrine carcinoma). Patients with NET G1 have a relatively good prognosis; however, it has been reported that the 5-year survival rate of patients with NET G1 was approximately 80–90% [5]. We would like to emphasize that clinicians and pathologist should be aware of the existence of gangliocytic paraganglioma (GP), which is often misdiagnosed as NET G1 [6]. GP has been regarded as an extremely rare NET [7].

Dahl et al. [8] first reported this tumor as ganglioneuroma in 1957, and Kepes and Zacharias [9] named this tumor "gangliocytic paraganglioma" in 1971. Previous studies [7, 10] have reported on the clinicopathological characteristics of GP. These studies stated that this rare tumor typically occurs in the second part of the duodenum, includes 3 characteristic components (epithelioid, spindle-shaped, and ganglion-like cells), and shows a good prognosis. On the other hand, few cases with lymph node and/or liver metastasis [11–13] and 1 fatal duodenal GP case after distant metastasis (pelvic lesion and liver mass) [11] have been reported. As most previous studies included a single patient or a small group of patients, we previously evaluated the details of this tumor in accordance with the Preferred Reporting Items for Systematic Reviews and Meta-Analyses (PRISMA) style [14] as much as possible and elucidated some aspects of the epidemiology and clinicopathological characteristics of GP. Thereafter, we perused studies on GP and obtained new knowledge through a multi-institutional retrospective study of GP [6]. We found that the prognosis might be better in patients with GP than in those with NET G1, and we believe that it is important to differentiate between GP and NET G1. In this review article, we describe up-to-date data of the clinicopathological characteristics of GP, based on a new and larger literature survey and the results of our recent retrospective study [6].

2. Benefits of Conducting a Literature Survey

Our previous multi-institutional retrospective study [6] shed some light on clinicopathological findings of GP. However, since GP is an extremely rare neuroendocrine tumor, a large study design is difficult and standard clinical management of this tumor has not been established. Accordingly, we would like to emphasize the benefits of literature survey. This research method can provide the researcher with up-to-date key to the deciphering of GP.

3. Literature Survey and Data Collection Method

In January 2016, we conducted a comprehensive literature survey using the PubMed (http://www.ncbi.nlm.nih.gov/pubmed/) and Igaku Chuo Zasshi (http://www.jamas.or.jp/; Japanese medical database) databases. Namely, we assessed English and Japanese language case reports of GP using these medical databases and search term was "gangliocytic paraganglioma." In the resent review, no advance search systems of PubMed database were used, whereas for the Igaku Chuo Zasshi search, the "shoreihoukoku" (Japanese word for case report) option was used. We then reviewed all abstracts of selected publications to identify GP cases.

In addition, since gangliocytic paraganglioma has been reported by other names (e.g., ganglioneuroma [8], nonchromaffin paraganglioma [15, 16], and paraganglioma [17, 18]) until named "gangliocytic paraganglioma" by Kepes and Zacharias in 1971 [9] and becoming widespread, some GP cases were not identified in the first databases search. We therefore checked the references of selected publications collected by first database search. With reference to our previous research [7], we added some publications as GP and these publications met the following criteria: (1) the characteristic three components could be confirmed in the manuscript or a figure and (2) the paper was cited in other publications as a GP report.

Subsequently, we extracted and sampled the raw data from the selected publications in relation to factors, such as age, sex, site of the tumor, tumor size, medical treatment method, outcome, lymph node metastasis, depth of tumor invasion, diagnostic rate using biopsy specimens before medical treatment, clinical symptoms, and immunohistochemical findings. In this literature survey, data collection was performed in accordance with the PRISMA style [14] as much as possible. In addition, we performed appropriate statistical analyses using the extracted data. The nonparametric Mann–Whitney U test or χ^2 test was used for statistical analysis. All

statistical analyses were performed using IBM SPSS Statistics version 20 (IBM Corp., Armonk, NY, USA). Differences were considered significant at $P < 0.05$ [19].

4. Overall Findings of Literature Survey of GP

We retrieved 21,581 English and 40 Japanese (total 21,621) publications by conducting a search of "gangliocytic paraganglioma" using the PubMed and Igaku Chuo Zasshi databases. Among these publications, 123 English and 30 Japanese publications were recognized and selected as case reports of GP. The remaining 21,468 publications were excluded from this survey. We then reviewed the references of all the selected publications of GP; however, no additional GP case reports were found. Consequently, 254 patients with GP were finally assessed (totally, 123 English and 30 Japanese publications reported 254 patients with GP).

The patient age at the time of diagnosis ranged from 15 to 84 years (n = 254; mean ± standard deviation (SD), 53.22 ± 12.13). The sex ratio was 152 : 100 (male : female; n = 252, 2 not reported). The tumor size at the time of diagnosis ranged from 5.5 to 100 mm (n = 194, 60 not reported; mean ± SD, 25.73 ± 1422 mm). The duodenum was found to be the most common site of the disease (90.2%, 229/254), followed by the respiratory system (2.4%, 6/254) [20–25], low-level spinal cord (2.0%, 5/254) [26–30], jejunum (1.2%, 3/254) [31–33], esophagus (0.8%, 2/254) [34, 35], and appendix (0.8%, 2/254) [36, 37]. There were individual cases involving the stomach [31], ileum [38], retromediastinum [39], pancreas [40], thymus [41], and mature teratoma [42], as well as a case of double focus in the duodenum and pancreas [43]. These data are summarized in Figure 1. As most of the cases of GP were associated with the duodenum, we additionally conducted detailed clinicopathological examinations and statistical analyses for duodenal GP.

5. Clinical Findings of Duodenal GP

A total of 230 patients with duodenal GP were identified from the PubMed and Igaku Chuo Zasshi databases (including the case of double focus in the duodenum and pancreas [43]). The patient's age at the time of diagnosis ranged from 15 to 84 years (n = 230; mean ± SD, 53.60 ± 11.79). The sex ratio was 136 : 92 (male : female; n = 228, 2 not reported). Gastrointestinal bleeding was the most common symptom of this tumor (40.9%, 94/230), followed by abdominal pain (40.0%, 92/230), anemia (17.0%, 39/230), incidental findings (9.6%, 22/230), nausea (6.1%, 14/230), weight loss (4.8%, 11/230), and jaundice (4.4%, 10/230). These findings are summarized in Figure 2.

The documented follow-up period ranged from 3 months [44] to 300 months [45], and recurrence of GP was reported in only 2 patients [11, 46]. Unfortunately, 1 of these patients died from GP [11]. Although 26 patients underwent an endoscopic procedure for treatment, only 1 patient required additional surgical intervention owing to the presence of a tumor residue following the initial procedure [47].

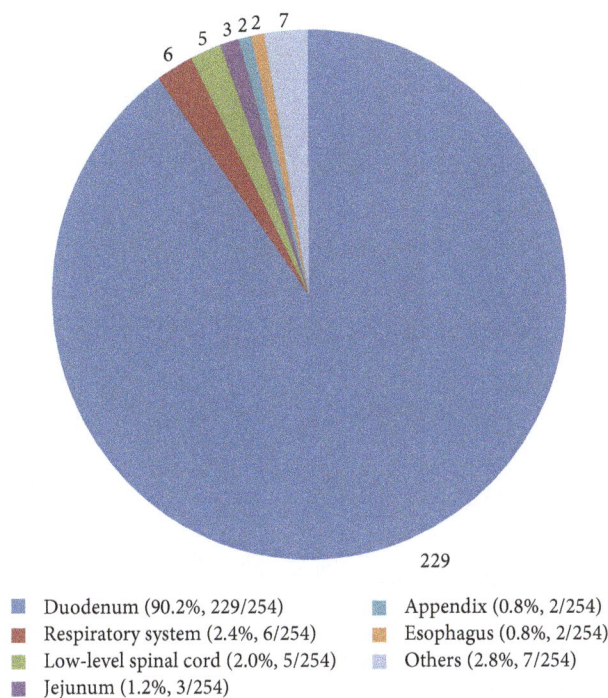

FIGURE 1: In the present literature survey, the duodenum was found to be the most common site of gangliocytic paraganglioma (90.2%, 229/254), followed by the respiratory system (2.4%, 6/254), low-level spinal cord (2.0%, 5/254), jejunum (1.2%, 3/254), esophagus (0.8%, 2/254), appendix (0.8%, 2/254), and others (2.8%, 7/254).

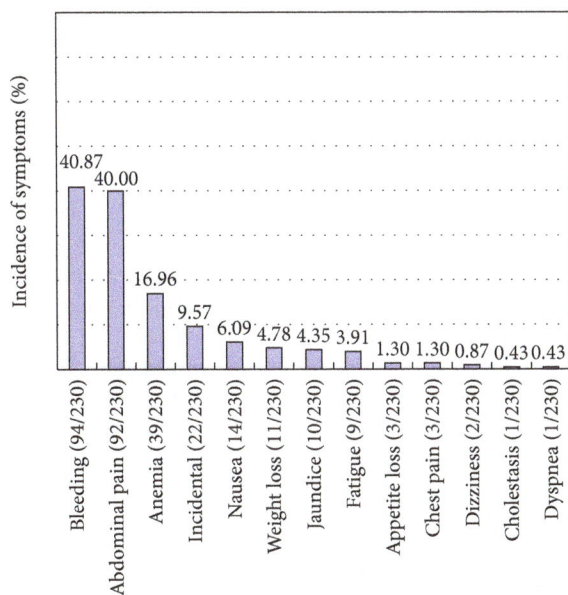

FIGURE 2: In the present literature survey, gastrointestinal bleeding was the most common symptom of gangliocytic paraganglioma (GP; 40.9%, 94/230), followed by abdominal pain (40.0%, 92/230), anemia (17.0%, 39/230), incidental findings (9.6%, 22/230), nausea (6.1%, 14/230), weight loss (4.8%, 11/230), and jaundice (4.4%, 10/230). It has been largely accepted that gastrointestinal bleeding and abdominal pain commonly occur in patients with GP; however, our survey revealed that obstructive jaundice is less common in patients with GP, although GP commonly occurs in the second part of the duodenum.

6. Histopathological Findings of Duodenal GP

In the selected cases, the tumor size at the time of diagnosis ranged from 5.5 to 100 mm ($n = 172$, 58 not reported; mean ± SD, 25.33 ± 13.41 mm). The depth of tumor invasion was described in 153 patients. Of the 153 patients, 81 had GP within the submucosa or sphincter of Oddi layer and 72 had GP exceeding the submucosa or sphincter of Oddi layer. Moreover, 25 patients showed lymph node metastasis [6, 10–13, 18, 46–60], 3 patients showed pancreatic metastasis and/or invasion [51, 55, 57], and 3 patients showed liver metastasis [11–13]. As mentioned previously, GP is an extremely rare NET, and the histopathological diagnosis of GP requires confirmation of the presence of epithelioid, spindle-shaped, and ganglion-like cells. However, the distribution of the 3 characteristic tumor cells varied from case to case, even among patients with GP [6, 61]. As histopathological findings vary widely (Figure 3), pathologists should recognize this fact when diagnosing GP. Furthermore, diagnosis using biopsy specimens obtained before surgical intervention or an endoscopic procedure has been regarded as extremely difficult in the literature. In fact, histopathological findings of biopsy specimens obtained before surgical intervention were described in 60 patients. However, among these 60 patients, 10 were successfully diagnosed with GP, 40 showed no evidence of tumor cells (specimens did not contain tumor cells), 9 were diagnosed or suspected with a different NET (6 carcinoid tumors, 2 paragangliomas, and 1 ganglioneuroma), and 1 showed atypical cells (details unknown). Therefore, in the literature, only 16.7% (10/60) of the patients with GP were accurately diagnosed using biopsy specimens.

7. Immunohistochemical Findings of Duodenal GP

In the present literature survey, we only assessed the cases in which the positive or negative result of the immuno-histochemical analysis was clearly mentioned. Thus, the denominators for the collected immunohistochemical data varied for each kind of immunohistochemical item. The representative findings for each of the 3 characteristic tumor cells are presented below.

In epithelioid cells, CD56 showed the highest positive rate (100%, 27/27), followed by synaptophysin (96.2%, 76/79), neuron-specific enolase (NSE; 95.7%, 90/94), progesterone receptor (93.3%, 14/15), pancreatic polypeptide (91.5%, 86/94), somatostatin (82.6%, 76/92), chromogranin A (74.8%, 98/131), cytokeratins (58.8%, 50/85), vimentin (38.0%, 3/8), and estrogen receptor (23.1%, 3/13).

In spindle-shaped cells, S-100 showed the highest positive rate (96.6%, 144/149), followed by NSE (85.0%, 68/80), neurofilament (69.1%, 47/68), vimentin (60.0%, 3/5), Bcl-2 (58.3%, 7/12), synaptophysin (54.4%, 31/57), CD56 (50.0%, 9/18), CD34 (33.3%, 1/3), calcitonin (20.0%, 4/20), and vasoactive intestinal peptide (13.3%, 4/30).

In ganglion-like cells, CD56 showed the highest positive rate (100%, 19/19), followed by synaptophysin (98.4%,

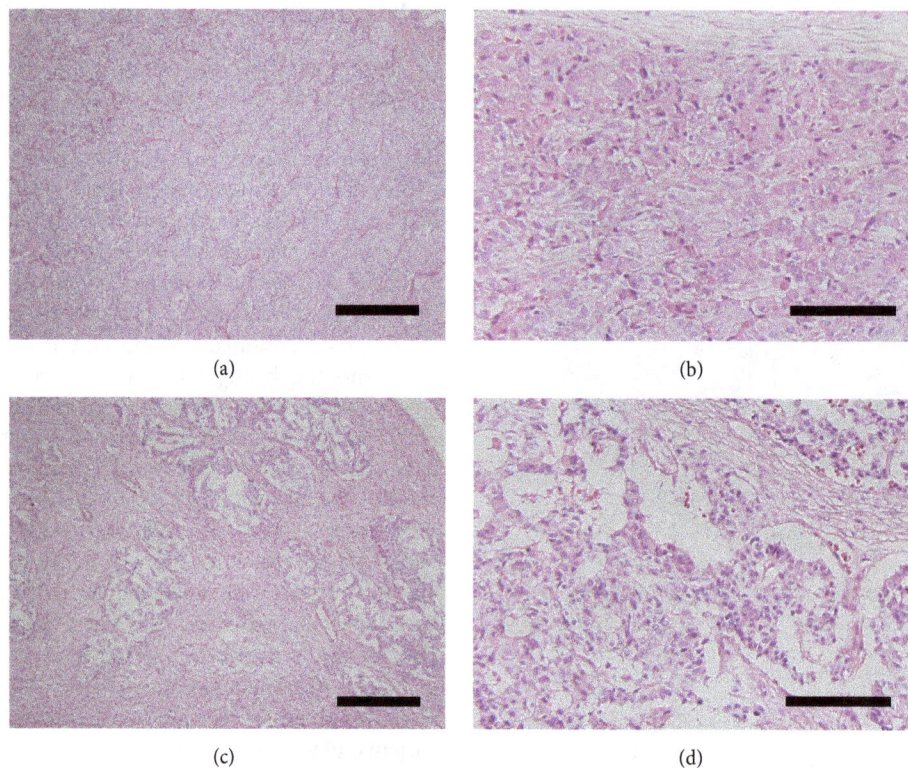

FIGURE 3: (a) Photomicrograph showing a low-power field of the gangliocytic paraganglioma (GP) site with a dense proliferation of epithelioid cells. Nested and compactly arranged epithelioid cells comprise the majority of the tumor (HE staining; magnification, ×100; the scale bar represents 300 μm). (b) Photomicrograph showing a high-power field of the GP site. The epithelioid cells have round to oval-shaped nuclei, inconspicuous nucleoli, and eosinophilic cytoplasm. Spindle-shaped cells surround the nests of epithelioid cells and are aligned in a single layer (HE staining; magnification, ×400; the scale bar represents 100 μm). (c) Photomicrograph showing a low-power field of the GP site with sporadic proliferation of epithelioid cells. A chaotic arrangement of epithelioid cells and a predominance of stromal cells are seen (HE staining; magnification, ×100; the scale bar represents 300 μm). (d) The epithelioid cells show a random arrangement, and spindle cells in the stroma are arranged in an irregular pattern (HE staining; magnification, ×400; the scale bar represents 100 μm).

61/62), NSE (87.0%, 80/92), somatostatin (51.3%, 41/80), Bcl-2 (36.4%, 4/11), pancreatic polypeptide (32.1%, 27/84), chromogranin A (28.9%, 28/97), neurofilament (27.3%, 18/66), vimentin (25.0%, 1/4), and S-100 (23.9%, 28/117). The immunohistochemical findings are summarized in Table 1.

8. Statistical Analysis of Clinicopathological Data

We assessed the significant risk factors associated with lymph node metastasis and depth of invasion (indicators of tumor growth) of duodenal GP. When we used evidence of lymph node metastasis as an indicator of progression, a significant difference was found only for the tumor size among the clinicopathological findings between patients with and those without lymph node metastasis (Mann–Whitney U test, $P = 0.009$). The tumor size was larger in patients with lymph node metastasis than in those without metastasis. In contrast, no significant differences were found in age and sex between patients with and those without lymph node metastasis (Mann–Whitney U test, $P = 0.105$, and χ^2 test, $P = 0.390$, resp.). These results are summarized in Table 2.

In addition, comparisons of clinicopathological findings between patients with GP within and those with GP exceeding the submucosa or sphincter of Oddi layer revealed significant differences in sex and the rate of lymph node metastasis (χ^2 test, $P = 0.032$ and $P = 0.019$, resp.). The number of female patients and the rate of lymph node metastasis were higher among patients with GP exceeding the submucosa or sphincter of Oddi layer than among those with GP within the submucosa or sphincter of Oddi layer. These results are summarized in Table 3.

No significant differences were noted in tumor size and patient age between male and female patients. In addition, Spearman's rank correlation coefficient was calculated to assess any potential relationship between tumor size and patient age; however, no significant relationship was noted. These results are consistent with those of our previous study [7].

Tumor size and depth of invasion were significant risk factors for lymph node metastasis. In addition, as approximately half of the patients with GP (47.1%, 72/153) had lesions exceeding the submucosa or sphincter of Oddi layer, detailed imaging examinations to determine depth of invasion are important. On the other hand, although the overall mean

TABLE 1: Immunohistochemical findings in each tumor component of gangliocytic paraganglioma.

Immunohistochemical marker	Epithelioid cells	Spindle-shaped cells	Ganglion-like cells
Bcl-2	16.7% (2/12)	58.33% (7/12)	36.36% (4/11)
Calcitonin	20.8% (5/24)	20.0% (4/20)	21.05% (4/19)
CD34	0% (0/2)	33.33% (1/3)	0% (0/1)
CD56	100% (27/27)	50% (9/18)	100% (19/19)
Chromogranin A	74.8% (98/131)	8.8% (9/102)	28.9% (28/97)
Cytokeratins	58.8% (50/85)	6.0% (4/67)	3.0% (2/66)
C-kit	0% (0/8)	0% (0/8)	16.7% (4/11)
Corticotropin	0% (0/0)	0% (0/3)	0% (0/2)
Estrogen receptor	23.1% (3/13)	0% (0/12)	0% (0/11)
Gastrin	4.5% (3/67)	0% (0/62)	0% (0/60)
Glucagon	6.1% (3/49)	0% (0/44)	2.3% (1/43)
Insulin	4.3% (2/47)	0% (0/42)	0% (0/41)
Neurofilament	21.7% (15/69)	69.1% (47/68)	27.3% (18/66)
Neuron-specific enolase	95.7% (90/94)	85.0% (68/80)	87.0% (80/92)
p53	0% (0/13)	0% (0/12)	0% (0/11)
Progesterone receptor	93.3% (14/15)	0% (0/12)	0% (0/12)
Pancreatic polypeptide	91.5% (86/94)	0% (0/83)	32.1% (27/84)
S-100	10.2% (13/128)	96.6% (144/149)	23.9% (28/117)
Serotonin	20.0% (12/60)	1.5% (1/66)	16.7% (9/54)
Somatostatin	82.6% (76/92)	8.7% (6/69)	51.3% (41/80)
Synaptophysin	96.2% (76/79)	54.4% (31/57)	98.4% (61/62)
Vimentin	37.5% (3/8)	60.0% (3/5)	25.0% (1/4)
Vasoactive intestinal peptide	12.1% (4/33)	13.3% (4/30)	10.3% (3/29)

The positive or negative rates in the extracted cases of duodenal gangliocytic paraganglioma are summarized. Listing in alphabetical number.

TABLE 2: Comparison of clinicopathological data between patients with and those without lymph node metastasis.

	Patients with lymph node metastasis	Patients without lymph node metastasis	Statistical analysis
Number of patients	25	205	
Age (years), range	16–74 (median, 50.0)	15–84 (median, 54.0)	No significant difference was found (Mann–Whitney U test, $P = 0.105$)
Tumor size (mm), range	10–90 (median, 30.0)	5.5–100 (median, 20.0)	Significant difference was found (Mann–Whitney U test, $P = 0.009$)
Sex (male : female)	13 : 12	125 : 78 (2 not reported)	No significant difference was found (χ^2 test, $P = 0.390$)

A significant difference was found for the tumor size between patients with and those without lymph node metastasis (Mann–Whitney U test, $P = 0.009$). This fact means that the size of tumor lesions was significantly larger in patients with lymph node metastasis than in those without lymph node metastasis.

tumor size of duodenal GP was 25.3 mm, the mean and median tumor size of duodenal GP associated with lymph node metastasis were 32.3 and 30.0 mm. Therefore, it might be necessary to perform imaging examinations for confirmation of the existence of lymph node metastasis if the tumor size is larger than 30 mm. Meanwhile, tumor size larger than 30 mm has another important clinical significance, because several recent reports indicate that endoscopic polypectomy is the treatment of choice, except in cases where the tumor is >30 mm [62–67]. We therefore conducted further statistical analysis between tumor size and rate of lymph node metastasis. In the present survey, 185 cases described both tumor size and presence or absence of lymph node metastasis. We carried out statistical examinations for confirmation of the existence of lymph node metastasis if the tumor size is larger than 30 mm. As a result, rate of lymph node metastasis in GP

TABLE 3: Comparison of clinicopathological data between patients with gangliocytic paraganglioma (GP) within and those with GP exceeding the submucosa or sphincter of Oddi layer.

	GP within the submucosa or sphincter of Oddi layer	GP exceeding the submucosa or sphincter of Oddi layer	Statistical analysis
Number of patients	81	72	
Age (years), range	16–84 (median, 50.0)	15–73 (median, 57.0)	Significant difference was found (Mann–Whitney U test, $P = 0.016$)
Tumor size (mm), range	5.5–65 (median, 21.0)	8–100 (median, 20.0)	No significant difference was found (Mann–Whitney U test, $P = 0.175$)
Sex (male to female)	55 : 26	36 : 36	Significant difference was found (χ^2 test, $P = 0.032$)
Rate of lymph node metastasis	7.4% (6/81)	20.8% (15/72)	Significant difference was found (χ^2 test, $P = 0.019$)

Significant differences were found for age, sex, and the rate of lymph node metastasis between patients with GP within the submucosa or sphincter of Oddi layer and those with GP exceeding the submucosa or sphincter of Oddi layer.

TABLE 4: Comparison of rate of lymph node metastasis in patients with gangliocytic paraganglioma focusing on tumor size (30 mm).

	Tumor size is within 30 mm	Tumor size is larger than 30 mm
Total number of patients	156	29
Number of patients with lymph node metastasis	16	9
Number of patients without lymph node metastasis	140	20
Rate of lymph node metastasis	10.3% (16/156)	31.0% (9/29)
Statistical analysis	Significant difference was found (χ^2 test, $P = 0.019$)	

Significant difference was found between them (χ^2 test, $P = 0.006$). This fact indicated that GP larger than 30 mm is significant risk factor of lymph node metastasis in gangliocytic paraganglioma.

within 30 mm (tumor size) was 16 of 156 cases (10.3%) and the rate in GP larger than 30 mm (tumor size) was 9 of 29 cases (31.0%), respectively. In addition, significant difference was found between them (χ^2 test, $P = 0.006$). This fact indicated that GP larger than 30 mm is also significant risk factor of lymph node metastasis. This fact indicated that GP larger than 30 mm is risk factor of not only clinical complications but also lymph node metastasis. These results are summarized in Table 4.

In the present review, sex was not significantly associated with tumor size and the rate of lymph node metastasis. However, female sex was associated with GP exceeding the submucosa or sphincter of Oddi layer. This finding indicates that female patients mainly show vertical tumor growth. Epithelioid cells (typically the main component of

GP) showed positive immunoreactivity for the progesterone receptor, and some investigators reported that progesterone regulates neural differentiation [68, 69], suggesting that the vertical growth of GP might be influenced by progesterone exposure. However, our survey might be affected by publication bias, because the findings were based on a cumulative case series. Therefore, further studies are required to confirm our findings. For example, analyses of gene expression using stored formalin-fixed paraffin-embedded tissue which is widely employed in routine works for surgical pathology may be necessary, as in other fields [70–72].

9. Differential Diagnosis of GP

The diagnosis of GP using specimens obtained during surgical removal or endoscopic resection is not always difficult, because the characteristic 3 components can be confirmed with ease. In contrast, the diagnosis using biopsy specimens has been regarded as extremely difficult. In fact, our present review found that the biopsy diagnostic rate before surgical intervention was only 16.7% (10/60) in the literature. The differential diagnoses include gastrointestinal stromal tumor, smooth muscle tumor, NET, ganglioneuroma, and paraganglioma. Gastrointestinal stromal tumor, smooth muscle tumor, and adenocarcinoma can easily be excluded with immunohistochemical staining for S100 protein, synaptophysin, and/or chromogranin A. Ganglioneuroma lacks the epithelioid component, while GP usually shows a prominent epithelioid component. Paraganglioma lacks ganglion-like cells, and it is very rare in the duodenum [73]. Although NET G1 is the most important differential diagnosis, GP has often been misdiagnosed as NET G1 owing to its low cell proliferative activity. In fact, positive immunoreactivity for neuroendocrine markers and neither mitosis nor prominent Ki-67 immunoreactivity in GP are similar to the findings in

NET G1. Nevertheless, as a benign course is more common in cases of GP than in cases of NET G1, it is important to clearly differentiate GP from NET G1. In our multi-institutional retrospective study, we found that the typical epithelioid cells of GP exhibited positive immunoreactivity for the progesterone receptor and pancreatic polypeptide, whereas tumor cells of NET G1 were negative for both markers [6]. Therefore, immunohistochemical analysis of the progesterone receptor and pancreatic polypeptide can assist in differentiating GP from NET G1, even with biopsy specimens.

10. Clinical Management of GP

Although GP has been considered an extremely benign neuroendocrine tumor, a previous report mentioned that a patient died from GP [11] and our literature survey found that gastrointestinal bleeding, which can cause severe anemia, was the most common symptom. Furthermore, 25 of 230 cases of GP showed lymph node metastasis and 1 patient has been reported as showing a recurrence due to a residue of a previous tumor at his initial surgical intervention [46]. These findings indicate that surgical or endoscopic intervention for GP is needed and observation with careful follow-up may be undesirable.

In the literature survey, we found that 26 patients underwent an endoscopic procedure for treatment, while only 1 patient required additional surgical intervention owing to the presence of a tumor residue following the initial procedure [47]. These findings indicate that endoscopic procedures can yield favorable results in patients with duodenal GP, if indicated.

Although 2 patients received irradiation after surgical interventions [11, 60], we believe that patients without residual tumors do not require adjuvant therapy because no recurrence or metastasis has been reported in such patients. However, it is still unclear whether a residual tumor can be controlled with irradiation or chemotherapy alone without surgical intervention. Further evaluation of the incidence of GP is warranted. GP has been regarded as an extremely rare NET; however, we previously found that 4 of 10 patients (40.0%) with duodenal NET G1 actually had GP [6]. This suggests that GP accounts for a substantial, constant percentage of duodenal NETs.

11. Conclusion

Our new and larger literature survey provided up-to-date clinicopathological information of GP. Since the first case report published by Dahl et al. [8] in 1957, 254 cases of GP have been reported. Our previous literature survey [7] published in 2011 found 192 cases of GP. Therefore, 62 new cases have been identified in the past 5 years, indicating that clinicians and/or pathologists are gradually recognizing the existence of GP and that GP accounts for a substantial percentage of duodenal NETs. As the prognosis differs between GP and NET G1, it is important to differentiate between them.

We emphasize the usefulness of immunohistochemical analysis of the progesterone receptor and pancreatic polypeptide for differentiating GP from NET G1, and we believe that this can help improve the clinical management of GP. We found that 1 patient died from GP [11] and that 25 and 3 patients with GP showed lymph node and liver metastases, respectively. To elucidate the risk factors for metastasis and tumor progression of GP, further investigations on GP are required.

Competing Interests

The authors declare that there are no competing interests regarding the publication of this paper.

Acknowledgments

This work was supported by a Grant-in-Aid for Scientific Research from the Ministry of Education, Culture, Sports, Science, and Technology of Japan (no. 26860774) and a research grant from the Kanagawa Cancer Center (no. 28-07). The authors also thank Sachie Osanai and Rie Kajihara for their excellent pathological and technical support and Keisuke Kazama, Tetsuta Satoyoshi, Atsushi Wada, and Takao Ishiwatari for their clinicopathological advice.

References

[1] J. Hallet, C. H. L. Law, M. Cukier, R. Saskin, N. Liu, and S. Singh, "Exploring the rising incidence of neuroendocrine tumors: a population-based analysis of epidemiology, metastatic presentation, and outcomes," Cancer, vol. 121, no. 4, pp. 589–597, 2015.

[2] K. Öberg and D. Castellano, "Current knowledge on diagnosis and staging of neuroendocrine tumors," Cancer and Metastasis Reviews, vol. 30, supplement 1, no. 1, pp. 3–7, 2011.

[3] K. E. Öberg, "Gastrointestinal neuroendocrine tumors," Annals of Oncology, vol. 21, no. 7, pp. vii72–vii80, 2010.

[4] Y. Okubo, O. Motohashi, N. Nakayama et al., "The clinicopathological significance of angiogenesis in hindgut neuroendocrine tumors obtained via an endoscopic procedure," Diagnostic Pathology, vol. 11, article 128, 2016.

[5] U.-F. Pape, H. Jann, J. Müller-Nordhorn et al., "Prognostic relevance of a novel TNM classification system for upper gastroenteropancreatic neuroendocrine tumors," Cancer, vol. 113, no. 2, pp. 256–265, 2008.

[6] Y. Okubo, T. Nemoto, M. Wakayama et al., "Gangliocytic paraganglioma: a multi-institutional retrospective study in Japan," BMC Cancer, vol. 15, no. 1, article no. 269, 2015.

[7] Y. Okubo, M. Wakayama, T. Nemoto et al., "Literature survey on epidemiology and pathology of gangliocytic paraganglioma," BMC Cancer, vol. 11, article 187, 2011.

[8] E. V. Dahl, J. M. Waugh, and D. C. Dahlin, "Gastrointestinal ganglioneuromas; brief review with report of a duodenal ganglioneuroma," The American Journal of Pathology, vol. 33, no. 5, pp. 953–965, 1957.

[9] J. J. Kepes and D. L. Zacharias, "Gangliocytic paragangliomas of the duodenum. A report of two cases with light and electron microscopic examination," Cancer, vol. 27, no. 1, pp. 61–67, 1971.

[10] Y. Okubo, T. Yokose, M. Tuchiya et al., "Duodenal gangliocytic paraganglioma showing lymph node metastasis: a rare case report," *Diagnostic Pathology*, vol. 5, no. 1, article 27, 2010.

[11] B. Li, Y. Li, X.-Y. Tian, B.-N. Luo, and Z. Li, "Malignant gangliocytic paraganglioma of the duodenum with distant metastases and a lethal course," *World Journal of Gastroenterology*, vol. 20, no. 41, pp. 15454–15461, 2014.

[12] S. M. Amin, N. Wewer Albrechtsen, J. Forster, and I. Damjanov, "Gangliocytic paraganglioma of duodenum metastatic to lymph nodes and liver and extending into the retropancreatic space," *Pathologica*, vol. 105, no. 3, pp. 90–93, 2013.

[13] C. Rowsell, N. Coburn, and R. Chetty, "Gangliocytic paraganglioma: a rare case with metastases of all 3 elements to liver and lymph nodes," *Annals of Diagnostic Pathology*, vol. 15, no. 6, pp. 467–471, 2011.

[14] D. Moher, A. Liberati, J. Tetzlaff, and D. G. Altman, "Preferred reporting items for systematic reviews and meta-analyses: the PRISMA statement," *International Journal of Surgery*, vol. 8, no. 5, pp. 336–341, 2010.

[15] I. Babaryka, "Polypoid nonchromaffin paraganglioma of the duodenum," *Virchows Archiv A Pathological Anatomy and Histology*, vol. 377, no. 2, pp. 181–187, 1978.

[16] S. Weitzner, "Benign nonchromaffin paraganglioma of the duodenum. Report of a case and review of the literature," *The American Journal of Gastroenterology*, vol. 53, no. 4, pp. 365–369, 1970.

[17] A. H. Qizilbash, "Benign paraganglioma of the duodenum. Case report with light and electron microscopic examination and brief review of literature," *Archives of Pathology and Laboratory Medicine*, vol. 96, no. 4, pp. 276–280, 1973.

[18] M. Buchler, P. Malfertheiner, K. Baczako, W. Krautzberger, and H. G. Beger, "A metastatic endocrine-neurogenic tumor of the ampulla of Vater with multiple endocrine immunoreaction—malignant paraganglioma?" *Digestion*, vol. 31, no. 1, pp. 54–59, 1985.

[19] T. Ishiwatari, Y. Okubo, N. Tochigi et al., "Remodeling of the pulmonary artery induced by metastatic gastric carcinoma: a histopathological analysis of 51 autopsy cases," *BMC Cancer*, vol. 14, no. 1, article no. 14, 2014.

[20] P. Sinkre, G. Lindberg, and J. Albores-Saavedra, "Nasopharyngeal gangliocytic paraganglioma," *Archives of Pathology and Laboratory Medicine*, vol. 125, no. 8, pp. 1098–1100, 2001.

[21] M. Hironaka, M. Fukayama, N. Takayashiki, K. Saito, Y. Sohara, and N. Funata, "Pulmonary gangliocytic paraganglioma: case report and comparative immunohistochemical study of related neuroendocrine neoplasms," *American Journal of Surgical Pathology*, vol. 25, no. 5, pp. 688–693, 2001.

[22] A.-R. Kee, C. H. Forrest, B. A. Brennan, J. M. Papadimitriou, and R. J. Glancy, "Gangliocytic paraganglioma of the bronchus: a case report with follow-up and ultrastructural assessment," *American Journal of Surgical Pathology*, vol. 27, no. 10, pp. 1380–1385, 2003.

[23] M. A. Paláu, M. J. Merino, and M. Quezado, "Corticotropin-producing pulmonary gangliocytic paraganglioma associated with Cushing's syndrome," *Human Pathology*, vol. 37, no. 5, pp. 623–626, 2006.

[24] H. Gucer and O. Mete, "Endobronchial gangliocytic paraganglioma: not all keratin-positive endobronchial neuroendocrine neoplasms are pulmonary carcinoids," *Endocrine pathology*, vol. 25, no. 3, pp. 356–358, 2014.

[25] D. Lin, Y. Hu, X. Xing et al., "Pulmonary gangliocytic paraganglioma: a case report and review of the literature," *International Journal of Clinical and Experimental Pathology*, vol. 7, no. 1, pp. 432–437, 2014.

[26] R. I. Lerman, E. S. Kaplan, and L. Daman, "Ganglioneuroma-paraganglioma of the intradural filum terminale. Case report," *Journal of Neurosurgery*, vol. 36, no. 5, pp. 652–658, 1972.

[27] J. F. Llena, H. S. Wisoff, and A. Hirano, "Gangliocytic paraganglioma in cauda equina region, with biochemical and neuropathological studies. Case report," *Journal of Neurosurgery*, vol. 56, no. 2, pp. 280–282, 1982.

[28] M. Djindjian, P. Ayache, P. Brugieres, D. Malapert, M. Baudrimont, and J. Poirier, "Giant gangliocytic paraganglioma of the filum terminale. Case report," *Journal of Neurosurgery*, vol. 73, no. 3, pp. 459–461, 1990.

[29] M. Vural, A. Arslantas, S. Isiksoy, B. Adapinar, M. Atasoy, and F. Soylemezoglu, "Gangliocytic paraganglioma of the cauda equina with significant calcification: first description in pediatric age," *Zentralblatt fur Neurochirurgie*, vol. 69, no. 1, pp. 47–50, 2008.

[30] M. Sable, A. Nalwa, V. Suri et al., "Gangliocytic paraganglioma of filum terminale: report of a rare case," *Neurology India*, vol. 62, no. 5, pp. 543–545, 2014.

[31] A. P. Burke and E. B. Helwig, "Gangliocytic paraganglioma," *American Journal of Clinical Pathology*, vol. 92, no. 1, pp. 1–9, 1989.

[32] R. J. Reed, P. J. Caroca Jr., and J. C. Harkin, "Gangliocytic paraganglioma," *American Journal of Surgical Pathology*, vol. 1, no. 3, pp. 207–216, 1977.

[33] W. Aung, H. J. Gallagher, W. P. Joyce, D. Bouchier Hayes, and M. Leader, "Gastrointestinal haemorrhage from a jejunal gangliocytic paraganglioma," *Journal of Clinical Pathology*, vol. 48, no. 1, pp. 84–85, 1995.

[34] D. M. Weinrach, K. L. Wang, M. G. Blum, A. V. Yeldandi, and W. B. Laskin, "Multifocal presentation of gangliocytic paraganglioma in the mediastinum and esophagus," *Human Pathology*, vol. 35, no. 10, pp. 1288–1291, 2004.

[35] K. Harries, T. Nunn, V. Shah, D. Richards, and J. M. Manson, "First reported case of esophageal paraganglioma. A review of the literature of gastrointestinal tract paraganglioma including gangliocytic paraganglioma," *Diseases of the Esophagus*, vol. 17, no. 2, pp. 191–195, 2004.

[36] S. Van Eeden, G. J. A. Offerhaus, H. L. Peterse, K. P. Dingemans, and H. L. G. Blaauwgeers, "Gangliocytic paraganglioma of the appendix," *Histopathology*, vol. 36, no. 1, pp. 47–49, 2000.

[37] M. Q. Abdelbaqi, M. Tahmasbi, and M. Ghayouri, "Gangliocytic paraganglioma of the appendix with features suggestive of malignancy, a rare case report and review of the literature," *International Journal of Clinical and Experimental Pathology*, vol. 6, no. 9, pp. 1948–1952, 2013.

[38] D. Sirohi, P. Sengupta, H. Kumar, and P. P. Rao, "Gangliocytic paraganglioma: a rare presentation as intestinal intussusception," *Indian Journal of Pathology and Microbiology*, vol. 53, no. 4, pp. 775–777, 2010.

[39] V. T. De Montpréville, S. Mussot, N. Gharbi, P. Dartevelle, and E. Dulmet, "Paraganglioma with ganglioneuromatous component located in the posterior mediastinum," *Annals of Diagnostic Pathology*, vol. 9, no. 2, pp. 110–114, 2005.

[40] S. Tomic and T. Warner, "Pancreatic somatostatin-secreting gangliocytic paraganglioma with lymph node metastases," *The American Journal of Gastroenterology*, vol. 91, no. 3, pp. 607–608, 1996.

[41] J. W. Yang, J. Han, H. W. Lee, S. Y. Cho, and H. K. Kim, "A rare case of thymic gangliocytic paraganglioma," *Journal of Pathology and Translational Medicine*, vol. 50, no. 2, pp. 165–167, 2016.

[42] A. Mahdavi, B. Silberberg, V. K. Malviya, A. H. Braunstein, and J. Shapiro, "Gangliocytic paraganglioma arising from mature cystic teratoma of the ovary," *Gynecologic Oncology*, vol. 90, no. 2, pp. 482–485, 2003.

[43] K. Kawaguchi, T. Takizawa, M. Koike, I. Tabata, and N. Goseki, "Multiple paraganglioneuromas," *Virchows Archiv A Pathological Anatomy and Histopathology*, vol. 406, no. 3, pp. 373–380, 1985.

[44] A. G. Hernandez, E. D. Lanuza, A. C. Matias et al., "Large gangliocytic paraganglioma of the duodenum: a rare entity," *World Journal of Gastrointestinal Surgery*, vol. 7, no. 8, pp. 170–173, 2015.

[45] B. W. Scheithauer, F. E. Nora, J. LeChago et al., "Duodenal gangliocytic paraganglioma: clinicopathologic and immunocytochemical study of 11 cases," *American Journal of Clinical Pathology*, vol. 86, no. 5, pp. 559–565, 1986.

[46] D. B. Dookhan, M. Miettinen, G. Finkel, and Z. Gibas, "Recurrent duodenal gangliocytic paraganglioma with lymph node metastases," *Histopathology*, vol. 22, no. 4, pp. 399–401, 1993.

[47] A. Witkiewicz, A. Galler, C. J. Yeo, and S. D. Gross, "Gangliocytic paraganglioma: case report and review of the literature," *Journal of Gastrointestinal Surgery*, vol. 11, no. 10, pp. 1351–1354, 2007.

[48] M. Fiscaletti, A. Fornelli, N. Zanini et al., "Segmental groove pancreatitis and duodenal gangliocytic paraganglioma with lymph node metastasis: a newly described association," *Pancreas*, vol. 40, no. 7, pp. 1145–1147, 2011.

[49] S. Hashimoto, S. Kawasaki, K. Matsuzawa, H. Harada, and M. Makuuchi, "Gangliocytic paraganglioma of the papilla of vater with regional lymph node metastasis," *American Journal of Gastroenterology*, vol. 87, no. 9, pp. 1216–1218, 1992.

[50] S. Ogata, T. Horio, Y. Sugiura, S. Aiko, and S. Aida, "Duodenal gangliocytic paraganglioma with regional lymph node metastasis and a glandular component," *Pathology International*, vol. 61, no. 2, pp. 104–107, 2011.

[51] B. Wang, Y. Zou, H. Zhang et al., "Duodenal gangliocytic paraganglioma: report of two cases and review of literature," *International Journal of Clinical and Experimental Pathology*, vol. 8, no. 9, pp. 9752–9759, 2015.

[52] H. Shi, J. Han, N. Liu et al., "A gangliocytic patially glandular paraganglioma with lymph node metastasis," *Diagnostic Pathology*, vol. 9, article 63, 2014.

[53] K. Inai, T. Kobuke, S. Yonehara, and S. Tokuoka, "Duodenal gangliocytic paraganglioma with lymph node metastasis in a 17-year-old boy," *Cancer*, vol. 63, no. 12, pp. 2540–2545, 1989.

[54] J. E. Dowden, K. F. Staveley-O'Carroll, E. T. Kimchi, E. R. Camp, K. A. Morgan, and D. B. Adams, "Ampullary gangliocytic paraganglioma with lymph node metastasis," *American Surgeon*, vol. 81, no. 11, pp. E359–E360, 2015.

[55] P. Bucher, Z. Mathe, L. Bühler et al., "Paraganglioma of the ampulla of vater: a potentially malignant neoplasm," *Scandinavian Journal of Gastroenterology*, vol. 39, no. 3, pp. 291–295, 2004.

[56] V. Sundararajan, T. M. Robinson-Smith, and A. M. Lowy, "Duodenal gangliocytic paraganglioma with lymph node metastasis: a case report and review of the literature," *Archives of pathology & laboratory medicine*, vol. 127, no. 3, pp. e139–e141, 2003.

[57] C. M. Mann, S. R. Bramhall, J. A. Buckels, and P. Taniere, "An unusual case of duodenal obstruction-gangliocytic paraganglioma," *Journal of Hepato-Biliary-Pancreatic Surgery*, vol. 16, no. 4, pp. 562–565, 2009.

[58] M. Barret, G. Rahmi, J.-P. Duong Van Huyen, B. Landi, C. Cellier, and A. Berger, "Duodenal gangliocytic paraganglioma with lymph node metastasis and an 8-year follow-up: a case report," *European Journal of Gastroenterology and Hepatology*, vol. 24, no. 1, pp. 90–94, 2012.

[59] S. M. Dustin, K. A. Atkins, V. M. Shami, R. B. Adams, and E. B. Stelow, "The cytologic diagnosis of gangliocytic paraganglioma: a case report," *Diagnostic Cytopathology*, vol. 41, no. 7, pp. 650–653, 2013.

[60] A. Wong, A. R. Miller, J. Metter, and C. R. Thomas Jr., "Locally advanced duodenal gangliocytic paraganglioma treated with adjuvant radiation therapy: case report and review of the literature," *World Journal of Surgical Oncology*, vol. 3, no. 1, article 15, 2005.

[61] N. Funel, "The role of miR-21 and miR-211 on MMP9 regulation in pancreatic ductal adenocarcinoma: cooperation in invasiveness behaviors?" *Epigenomics*, vol. 7, no. 3, pp. 333–335, 2015.

[62] D. Libânio, M. N. Costa, P. Pimentel-Nunes, and M. Dinis-Ribeiro, "Sa1001 risk factors for bleeding after gastric endoscopic submucosal dissection—a systematic review and meta-analysis," *Gastrointestinal Endoscopy*, vol. 83, no. 5, pp. AB198–AB199, 2016.

[63] A. Manuel Vázquez, A. Carabias Hernández, T. Carrascosa Mirón et al., "What to do with an intraductal papillary mucinous pancreatic neoplasm? our experience," *Cirugía Española*, vol. 94, no. 8, pp. 467–472, 2016.

[64] B. Yilmaz, E. C. Roach, S. Koklu, O. Aydin, O. Unlu, and Y. A. Kilic, "Air leak syndrome after endoscopic retrograde cholangiopancreatography: a rare and fatal complication," *World Journal of Gastroenterology*, vol. 21, no. 15, pp. 4770–4772, 2015.

[65] K. Higa, Y. Yamaguchi, K. Aoki, M. Toki, K. Nakamura, and S. Takahashi, "Endoscopic treatment for hemorrhagic peptic ulcer in patients aged 70 years or more," *Journal of Japanese Society of Gastroenterology*, vol. 108, no. 3, pp. 418–428, 2011.

[66] J. M. Church, "Experience in the endoscopic management of large colonic polyps," *ANZ Journal of Surgery*, vol. 73, no. 12, pp. 988–995, 2003.

[67] N. Funel, M. Del Chiaro, D. L. Cahen, and J. Laukkarinen, "Pancreatic cancer," *Gastroenterology Research and Practice*, vol. 2015, Article ID 809036, 2 pages, 2015.

[68] A. Bukovsky, M. R. Caudle, and M. Svetlikova, "Steroid-mediated differentiation of neural/neuronal cells from epithelial ovarian precursors in vitro," *Cell Cycle*, vol. 7, no. 22, pp. 3577–3583, 2008.

[69] L. Liu, J. Wang, L. Zhao et al., "Progesterone increases rat neural progenitor cell cycle gene expression and proliferation via extracellularly regulated kinase and progesterone receptor membrane components 1 and 2," *Endocrinology*, vol. 150, no. 7, pp. 3186–3196, 2009.

[70] K. Aki, Y. Okubo, H. Nanjo et al., "Genomic analysis of single nucleotide polymorphisms Asp299Gly and Thr399Ile in Japanese patients with invasive aspergillosis," *Japanese Journal of Infectious Diseases*, vol. 68, no. 4, pp. 330–332, 2015.

[71] Y. Okubo, N. Tochigi, M. Wakayama et al., "How histopathology can contribute to an understanding of defense mechanisms against cryptococci," *Mediators of Inflammation*, vol. 2013, Article ID 465319, 11 pages, 2013.

[72] Y. Okubo, T. Ishiwatari, H. Izumi et al., "Pathophysiological implication of reversed CT halo sign in invasive pulmonary mucormycosis: a rare case report," *Diagnostic Pathology*, vol. 8, no. 1, article 82, 2013.

[73] H. K. Park and H. S. Han, "Duodenal gangliocytic paraganglioma with lymph node metastasis," *Archives of Pathology and Laboratory Medicine*, vol. 140, no. 1, pp. 94–98, 2016.

17

From Pathogenesis, Clinical Manifestation, and Diagnosis to Treatment: An Overview on Autoimmune Pancreatitis

Ou Cai and Shiyun Tan

Department of Gastroenterology, Renmin Hospital of Wuhan University, Wuhan, Hubei, China

Correspondence should be addressed to Shiyun Tan; tanshiyun@medmail.com.cn

Academic Editor: Shahram Golbabapour

Autoimmune pancreatitis (AIP) is a special type of chronic pancreatitis which is autoimmune mediated. The international consensus diagnostic criteria (ICDC) 2011 proposed two types of AIP: type I is associated with histological pattern of lymphoplasmacytic sclerosing pancreatitis (LPSP), characterized by serum IgG4 elevation, whereas type 2 is named idiopathic duct-centric pancreatitis (IDCP), with granulocytic epithelial lesion (GEL) and immunoglobulin G4 (IgG4) negative. The pathogenic mechanism is unclear now; based on genetic factors, disease specific or related antigens, innate and adaptive immunity may be involved. The most common clinical manifestations of AIP are obstructive jaundice and upper abdominal pain. The diagnosis can be made by a combination of parenchymal and ductal imaging, serum IgG4 concentrations, pancreatic histology, extrapancreatic disease, and glucocorticoid responsiveness according to ICDC 2011. Because of the clinical and imaging similarities with pancreatic cancer, general work-up should be done carefully to exclude pancreatic malignant tumor before empirical trial of glucocorticoid treatment. Glucocorticoid is the most common drug for AIP to induce remission, while there still exists controversy on steroid maintenance and treatment for relapse. Further studies should be done to identify more specific serum biomarkers for AIP, the pathogenic mechanisms, and the treatment for relapse.

1. Introduction

Autoimmune pancreatitis (AIP) is a special form of chronic pancreatitis that is autoimmune mediated [1]. Autoimmunity is defined as acquired immune reactivity against self-antigens. Autoimmune diseases (AIDs) occur when autoimmune responses lead to tissue damage. AIDs are often classified into two patterns; some are organ specific, for example, diabetes mellitus, in which the pancreas is the target organ, whereas others are systemic, for example, systemic lupus erythematosus (SLE), in which many tissues and organs of the body are damaged. Some common AIDs include diabetes mellitus type 1, Grave's disease, multiple sclerosis, psoriasis, rheumatoid arthritis, and SLE. AIP belongs to and shares some characteristics with AID in pathophysiology, clinical manifestations, and treatment and of course has its uniqueness. The prevalence rate of AIP in Japan was 4.6 per 100,000 individuals in 2011 and the annual incidence rate was 1.4 per 100,000 individuals [2]. In 1961, Sarles et al. [3]

first reported a case about nonalcoholic chronic pancreatitis accompanied by hypergammaglobulinemia and predicted its association with an autoimmune process. In 1995, Yoshida et al. [4] first proposed the clinical entity of autoimmune pancreatitis. From then on, more and more scholars have paid attention to this rare type of chronic pancreatitis and substantial progress has been made in the recognition of AIP. The international consensus diagnostic criteria (ICDC) 2011 [5] proposed two forms of AIP: type I is associated with histological pattern of lymphoplasmacytic sclerosing pancreatitis (LPSP), accompanied with the serum immunoglobulin G4 (IgG4) elevation, whereas type 2 is characterized by idiopathic duct-centric pancreatitis (IDCP), with granulocytic epithelial lesion (GEL) and IgG4 negative [5, 6]. The diagnosis of AIP depends on serum IgG4 concentration, pancreatic histology, pancreatic parenchymal and duct imaging, other organ involvement, and steroid reaction and is most often confused with pancreatic cancer, especially the focal AIP exhibiting mass formation [5, 7, 8]. Therefore, some patients with focal AIP have undergone surgical resection due to the suspicion of malignancy, despite recent improvements in radiological imaging modalities [9–13]. Kobayashi et al. [8] reported 11 (72.2%) AIP patients had undergone surgery due to a preoperative diagnosis of mass formation pancreatitis with possible cancer revealed to be focal AIP. Hence, we sought to prepare an updated review about AIP to get a comprehensive knowledge about it.

2. Classification

The international consensus diagnostic criteria (ICDC) 2011 [5] had classified AIP into two types. Type 1 called lymphoplasmacytic sclerosing pancreatitis (LPSP), or without granulocyte epithelial lesions (GELs), has some characteristic features in histopathology: dense infiltration of plasma cells and lymphocytes; peculiar storiform fibrosis; obliterative phlebitis [15]; elevated IgG4-positive plasma cells (generally >50 cells per high-power field [HPF] [16]). It generally is believed to be the pancreatic manifestation of an IgG4 related systematic disease and is often accompanied with some extrapancreatic lesions, such as sclerosing cholangitis, sclerosing sialadenitis, and retroperitoneal fibrosis [5, 15, 17]. This type of AIP usually presents with obstructive jaundice in elderly male subjects and responds well to steroid therapy [2, 5, 18].

Type 2 called idiopathic duct-centric pancreatitis (IDCP) has the unique characteristic feature of intraluminal and intraepithelial neutrophils in medium-sized and small ducts as well as in acini in histopathology, which is not seen in LPSP [5]. Also, they share some features in histopathology, such as periductal lymphoplasmacytic infiltration and storiform fibrosis. IDCP often has no or few IgG4-positive cells (<10 cells/HPF) and it seems to be a pancreatic-specific disorder, because it is IgG4 negative and is not associated with other organ involvement (OOI) [5]. Patients in IDCP are often a decade younger and do no show gender preference. IDCP lacks a serological marker and for its diagnosis pancreatic histology is a must [5]. The comparisons between the two types of AIP are in Table 1.

3. Pathogenesis

Recent studies have suggested several possible pathogenic factors in the development of AIP, though its pathogenic mechanism remains unclear. Based on genetic factors, disease specific or related antigens, innate and adaptive immunity may be involved [19].

3.1. Genetic Factors. Kawa et al. [20] first revealed that the susceptibility of AIP in Japanese patients may be associated with class II antigen haplotype of the major histocompatibility complex (HLA-DRB1*0405-DQB1*0401). Later, Umemura et al. found that serum IgG4 concentrations in Japanese patients with AIP were significantly positively correlated with the number of susceptible Fc receptor-like 3 (FCRL3) genes alleles [21] expressed on B cells in 2006 and cytotoxic T lymphocyte antigen 4 (CTLA-4) [22] expressed

TABLE 1: Comparisons of the two types of AIP.

Characteristics	Type 1	Type 2
Other nomenclatures [5]	LPSP AIP without GEL IgG4 related	IDCP AIP with GEL IgG4 unrelated
Ethnic [5]	Asia > United States, Europe	Europe > United States > Asian
Age [2, 5, 18]	60 years or older	A decade younger
Sex [5]	Usually male	Equal
Symptom [5]	Obstructive jaundice often Abdominal pain rare Pancreas swelling common	Obstructive jaundice often Abdominal pain common Pancreas swelling common
Serology [2, 5]	High serum IgG4, auto-Ab+	Normal serum IgG4, auto-Ab−
Histopathology [5]	Lymphocyte and plasmacyte infiltration and fibrosis Infiltration of IgG4 plasma cells	Granulocyte epithelial lesion often with destruction and obliteration of the pancreatic duct
Extrapancreatic lesion [5, 15, 17]	Sclerosing cholangitis Sclerosing sialadenitis Retroperitoneal fibrosis, etc.	Unrelated with OOI
Ulcerative colitis [2, 5]	Rare	Often
Histology needed for diagnosis [5]	No	Yes
Respond to steroid [2, 5]	Responsive	Responsive
Relapse rate [5]	High	Low

on CD4$^+$ and CD8$^+$ T cells in 2008. In 2011, Ota et al. evaluated the association of AIP with single nucleotide polymorphisms (SNPs) and provided the evidence of KCNA3 [23] association with AIP. Chang et al. revealed the association of cystic fibrosis transmembrane conductance regulator (CFTR) gene variants [24] with AIP. Although the functions of the CFTR variants and their roles in the pathogenesis of AIP were not elucidated that clear, CFTR variants may play roles as disease modifiers in AIP (seen in Table 2). Undeniably, FCRL3 is found to be associated with various autoimmune diseases, such as rheumatoid arthritis, autoimmune thyroid disease, and SLE in Japanese populations [25, 26].

3.2. Immunogenic Factors. AIP is an autoimmune-mediated disease and abnormal immune response may play an important role in its pathophysiology. More than one autoantibody is seen in AIP patients and some other antigens like lactoferrin (LF), carbonic anhydrase (CA) II [27, 28], pancreatic secretory trypsin inhibitor (PSTI) [29], amylase alpha 2A [30], and type IV collagen [31] may also be involved in the

TABLE 2: Genetic factors in the pathogenesis of AIP.

Gene related	Cells involved	Sites related	Possible function in AIP	Referencing
HLA-DRB1*0405-DQB1*0401	T cells	HLA-DRB1*0405-DQB1*0401 haplotype	Inducing an autoimmune response; genetic marker for non-HLA gene associated disease susceptibility	Kawa et al. [20]
FCRL3	B cells	FCRL3-110 alleles	Susceptibility with AIP	Umemura et al. [21]
CTLA4	T cells	+6230G/G +49A/A	Being related with AIP resistance; marker of risk of relapse in AIP	Umemura et al. [22]
KCNA3	T cells	SNP (rs2840381, rs1058184, rs2640480, rs1319782)	T cell proliferation and activation	Ota et al. [23]
CFTR	—	Variants (1556V, 5T, S42F, etc.)	Predictors of a slow and reduced response to steroid treatment in AIP	Chang et al. [24]

TABLE 3: Symptoms of AIP in different studies.

Year	Number of patients	Ethnic	Male : female	Jaundice	Abdominal pain	Weight loss	No symptoms
2008 [41]	25	Chinese	22 : 3	18 (72%)	11 (44%)	10 (40%)	3 (12%)
2011 [42]	731	8 countries	—	Type 1 AIP 75% Type 2 AIP 47%	Type 1 AIP 41% Type 2 AIP 68%	—	—
2015 [43]	705	Chinese	4.47 : 1	63.4%	62.3%	45.1%	2.9%
2016 [44]	52	Spain	—	27 (51.9%)	34 (65.4%)	—	—

pathogenesis of AIP. While combining amylase alpha 2A with IgG4 in diagnosing AIP, the specificity can be 99%, higher than the specificity of 96% while using IgG4 only in a clinical study [32].

As for innate immune response, Watanabe et al. reported that activation of toll-like receptors (TLRs) and nucleotide-binding oligomerization domain- (NOD-) like receptors (NLRs) in monocytes and basophils of patients with IgG4 related disease (IgG4-RD) induced IgG4 production by B cells via B cell activating factor (BAFF) [33, 34]. What is more, Fukui et al. reported that abundant infiltration of TLR-7 positive M2 macrophages was observed in the pancreatic tissues in type 1 AIP patients [35].

As for adaptive immune response, B cells and T cells are unavoidable topics. A recent study showed that increased CD19+CD24highCD38high regulatory B cells (Bregs) might suppress the disease activity of type 1 AIP, while the decreased CD19+CD24highCD27+ Bregs may be involved in the development of type 1 AIP [36]. Circulatory naïve regulatory T cells (Tregs) are significantly decreased in peripheral blood, while memory T cells are significantly increased in type 1 AIP patients [37]. In addition, prominent infiltration of Tregs with upregulation of IL-10 is observed in the liver of type 1 AIP patients [38]. Li et al. found significant CD8+ T lymphocyte infiltration in the pancreas and extrapancreatic lesions in a case of AIP misdiagnosed as pancreatic cancer, indicating that CD8+ T lymphocyte might have some effect on the cause of AIP [39].

4. Clinical Manifestation

The clinical manifestations of AIP are complex and lack of specificity; therefore, it is extremely difficult to diagnose AIP from symptoms only. Type 1 AIP is typically diagnosed later in life (the mean age at diagnosis is older than 60 years) [2, 18]. Obstructive painless jaundice and upper abdominal pain are the most common complaints. Other rare symptoms include body weight loss, general fatigue, and even no symptoms [40]. A series of studies have been focused on the symptoms and treatments of AIP in different countries and have got different results [41–44] (shown in Table 3). A retrospective study from China showed that the jaundice accounted for 72% and abdominal pain was 44% [41]. Another multicenter study in Spain indicated that abdominal pain accounted for 65.7% and obstructive jaundice was 51.9% in AIP patients [44]. Ueki et al. [45] reveal that type 2 AIP can have the symptoms of acute, constant abdominal pain like in acute pancreatitis, different from the character of chronic pancreatitis.

Besides, AIP can cause extrapancreatic lesions including sclerosing cholangitis, retroperitoneal fibrosis, lachrymal and salivary gland lesions, pulmonary lesions including hilar lymphadenopathy, and tubulointerstitial nephritis, hypophysitis, chronic thyroiditis, and prostatitis [5, 15, 17, 40, 46–50] and biliary tract is the most commonly involved extrapancreatic site [43, 46], which probably explains why there is painless jaundice in AIP patients.

AIP has certain comorbidities. Finkelberg et al. [51] reported that, in AIP patients, approximately 50% have

TABLE 4: Comparisons of diagnostic criteria in different countries.

Diagnostic criteria	Japanese criteria(2006) [55]	SIHORts (2006) [57]	Korean criteria (2007) [56]	Asian criteria (2008) [58]
A: imaging	Diffuse or segmental narrowing of the MPD; diffuse or localized enlargement of the pancreas	Typical imaging features: diffusely enlarged gland with delayed (rim) enhancement; diffusely irregular and attenuated MPD Atypical imaging features: focal pancreatic mass, focal pancreatic duct stricture	Diffuse enlargement of pancreas and diffuse or segmental irregular narrowing of MPD	Typical imaging features: diffusely enlarged gland with delayed (rim) enhancement; diffusely irregular and attenuated MPD Atypical imaging features: focal pancreatic mass, focal pancreatic duct stricture
B: serology	High serum γ globulin, IgG, IgG4, or the presence of autoantibodies	Elevated serum IgG4 level	Elevated levels of IgG and/or IgG4 or detected autoantibodies	High level of serum IgG or IgG4 or detected autoantibodies
C: histology	Infiltration of lymphocytes and plasma cells	Lymphoplasmacytic infiltrate with storiform fibrosis showing abundant (>10 cells/HPF) IgG4-positive cells	Fibrosis and lymphoplasmacytic infiltration	Lymphoplasmacytic infiltration with fibrosis, with abundant IgG4-positive cell infiltration
D: other organ involvement	Not included	Biliary stricture, parotid/lacrimal gland involvement, mediastinal lymphadenopathy, retroperitoneal fibrosis	Included	Not included
E: steroid effect	Not included	Included	Included	Included
Definite diagnosis	Criterion A + B Criterion A + C	Criterion A + B Criterion A + C Criterion A + D Criterion A + E	Criterion A + B Criterion A + C Criterion A + D Criterion A + E	Criterion A + B Criterion A + C Histology shows the presence of lymphoplasmacytic sclerosing pancreatitis in the resected pancreas

diabetes. More and more attention is focused on the relationship between AIP and inflammatory bowel disease, and the prevalence of IBD in patients with AIP seems to be increased compared to the general population, with 6 to 27% of AIP patients having concomitant IBD [45, 52, 53], especially in type 2 AIP.

5. Diagnosis

5.1. Diagnosis Criteria for AIP. In 2002, the Japan Pancreas Society (JPS) [54] first proposed the diagnostic criteria for AIP and made the image abnormal findings such as irregular narrowing of the main pancreatic duct (MPD) (>one-third of the entire pancreas) and parenchymal swelling as necessity, accompanied with either of the following two: (1) serology showing hypergammaglobulinemia (>2 g/dL, autoantibodies) and serum IgG elevation (>1800 mg/dL) and (2) characteristic pathological findings including lymphoplasmacytic infiltration with fibrosis. The JPS criterion was revised in 2006 [55], and it first proposed the IgG4 elevation as the

serology finding, which is important for the diagnosis of AIP even until now. Because of the limitations in JPS, 2006 [55], Korean Kim criteria [56] occurred, including four parts of imaging, laboratory examinations, histology, and steroid effect. Subsequently, HISORt [14, 57] (based on the four parts in Korean criteria, other organ involvement was added), Asian [58] (histology only can be used to diagnose AIP when it meets the demand), and Manheim criteria [59] have been proposed around the world. In 2011, Shimosegawa et al. [5] first proposed the ICDC for AIP, which is the most accepted major diagnostic criterion. Later, JPS 2011 [60, 61] was proposed in response to the ICDC's inclusion of response to steroid treatment. Table 4 shows the comparisons of diagnostic criteria in different countries.

There are several diagnostic criteria for AIP in different countries, but ICDC is the first universally accepted criterion of AIP because it considers ethnic and region differences and classifies AIP into two subtypes. The diagnosis of AIP includes five dimensions: serology, histology, imaging, other organ involvement, and steroid effect.

5.2. Serology Changes in AIP. Since being proposed by JPS 2006, serum IgG4 elevation is widely used in the diagnosis of AIP. However, IgG4 has its limitations. Studies have shown that 4–10% of both healthy controls and controls with other diseases have high serum IgG4 concentrations [62–64]. In addition, about 20% of patients with AIP have normal serum IgG4 concentrations at presentation [63, 65]. A systematic review with meta-analysis about IgG and IgG4 shows that the pooled sensitivity of serum IgG4 was 0.74 and the pooled specificity was 0.94 [66]. An ideal serological marker should be both sensitive and specific, while IgG4 is neither sufficiently sensitive nor specific. Besides, elevated IgG4 is seen only in type 1 AIP whereas type 2 AIP often has normal IgG4 level. Considering these two factors, searching for new serological marker is essential and valuable. Song et al. [67] proposed combining measurement of serum IgG and IgG4 instead of IgG4 alone to increase the sensitivity in diagnosing AIP. Recently, Hao et al. [68] explored that hybrid kappa (κ)/lambda (λ) antibody, which composes a substantial portion of IgG4 in normal human serum and is formed by two IgG4 heavy chains plus one κ and one λ light chain, is a new serological marker for diagnosing AIP. The sensitivity and specificity of hybrid κ/λ antibody were 80.3% and 91%, respectively. While combining serum IgG4 and the hybrid κ/λ antibody, the diagnostic sensitivity could be increased from 78.7% to 90.2% compared with serum IgG4 alone without sacrificing specificity significantly.

5.3. Imaging Features of AIP in Different Examinations. Ultrasound (US) is widely used for its noninvasiveness, low price, and easy operation. US can present the diffuse enlargement and hypoechoic pancreas, but it cannot show the irregular narrowing or stenosis of the pancreatic duct. Quantitative perfusion analysis in pancreatic contrast enhanced ultrasound (DCE-US) can show the vascular lesions of pancreas and play a significant role in differentiating AIP from pancreatic cancer [69].

Computed tomography (CT) is the most important tool to diagnose AIP and distinguish it from pancreatic cancer. The typical image finding is diffuse morphological pancreatic parenchymal enlargement and the atypical findings include focal enlargement of the pancreas, no enlargement or normal pancreas, and mixed patterns [57, 70–73]. AIP demonstrates a diminished pattern of enhancement in the arterial phase and a relatively increased or prolonged enhancement in the delayed or venous phase [72, 74]. And a capsule-like low density rim is a distinctive finding on CT in AIP [72]. However, if there is low density mass on contrast enhanced CT, pancreatic cancer should be considered.

Magnetic resonance imaging (MRI) has advantages over CT on the capsule-like imaging of the pancreatic duct and surrounding lesions, which is the result of the fibrosis of the pancreas. The typical MRI findings include hypointense signal on T1 weighted images and relatively T2 hyperintense signal [75]. Diffusion weighted imaging (DWI) has been increasingly utilized as a MRI sequence for evaluating pancreas [76–78]. Kim et al. [79] found that while perfusion fraction (f) is 0.933, it is most useful for differentiating

AIP and normal pancreas and its sensitivity is 85.7% and specificity is 100%. And perfusion fraction (f) and perfusion-related diffusion coefficient (D_{fast}) are more useful than pure molecule diffusion coefficient (D_{slow}) in differentiating pancreatic diseases from normal pancreas.

Magnetic Resonance Cholangiopancreatography (MRCP) is widely used for its advantage of high quality image and noninvasiveness, but for its less sensitivity in the focal form of AIP and pancreatic cancer, it cannot replace ERCP completely. MRCP could show the diffused narrow or segmental stenosis of main pancreatic ducts, the pancreatic segment of common bile duct stricture, proximal bile duct dilation, and gallbladder enlargement [80].Endoscopic retrograde cholangiopancreatography (ERCP) is an invasive method but it is feasible in treatment and diagnosis of AIP and the incidence of ERCP-related adverse events is low in patients with type 1 AIP [81]. Ductal imaging, ERCP, may show a long, narrow ductal stricture, or multiple, noncontinuous strictures without marked upstream dilation, and side branches arising from the stricture [82, 83]. The multicenter study carried out by Sugumar et al. [84] has highlighted that the ability of ERCP to diagnose AIP based on ERCP feature alone is limited, but taken together with clinical symptoms, serology, and/or histology it can be useful.

Endoscopic Ultrasound (EUS) can be utilized to evaluate the pancreatic parenchyma, bile duct, and pancreatic duct, as well as in evaluating the bile duct stricture. The EUS guided fine needle aspiration (EUS-FNA) is not included in ICDC as a method for histopathologic diagnosis of AIP because of the difficulty in obtaining adequate specimens for histological analysis. Although EUS-FNA has its limitations for 20.5% unsuccessful adequate tissue sampling, 23 of the 53 undetermined patients could be diagnosed as definitive type 1 AIP without the aid of pancreatic imaging, serology, other organ involvement, and response to steroids [84], which is unique. The nationwide epidemiology survey of AIP in Japan in 2011 found that the use of EUS-FNA increased to 63.8% from 48.4% and the utility of EUS-FNA for establishing of AIP will be further validated in the future [2, 85–87].

Positron Emission Computed Tomography (PET) can get the total image of every part of the body and it is especially sensitive in finding tumors. PET is more sensitive than conventional imaging to detect organ involvement and uptake of fluorodeoxyglucose in organs other than the pancreas often suggests AIP when the clinical characteristic, histology, and serum detection incline the diagnosis of IgG4 related disease [88, 89].

Every imaging method has its cons and pros (shown in Table 5). What should be emphasized is that methods are not isolated; we can combine two or more methods when needed. Uchida et al. [90] stated that in their institution they initially use CT scans to evaluate the enlarged pancreas followed by evaluation of the main pancreatic duct by ERP. For pancreatic head lesions with obstructive jaundice or biliary enzyme abnormality due to biliary stricture, they first perform diagnostic and therapeutic ERCP. For pancreatic head lesions without obstructive jaundice, they perform

TABLE 5: Cons and pros of different kinds of imaging.

Imaging	Imaging findings	Advantage	Disadvantage	When to select
US	Diffuse enlargement, hypoechoic pancreas	Low price, noninvasive, and easy to operate	Lack of specificity	Physical examination
CT	Diffuse morphological pancreatic parenchymal enlargement, focal enlargement of the pancreas [72]	Being noninvasive, being easy to operate, high quality image for pancreatic parenchymal enlargement, differentiating AIP from pancreatic cancer	Less sensitivity in the pancreatic and bile duct lesion than MRCP and MRI	Evaluate the pancreatic parenchyma and differentiate AIP from pancreatic cancer
MRI	Hypointense signal on T1 weighted images and relatively T2 hyperintense signal [75]	Being noninvasive, being easy to operate, showing the pancreatic fibrosis	Less sensitivity in pancreatic parenchymal than CT	Evaluate the pancreatic parenchyma
MRCP	Diffused narrow or segmental stenosis of main pancreatic ducts, the pancreatic segment of common bile duct stricture, proximal bile duct dilation, and gallbladder enlargement [80]	Being noninvasive, being easy to operate, presenting the pancreatic duct and bile duct and their relationship	Less sensitivity in the focal lesion of pancreatic parenchymal than CT	Evaluate the bile duct, pancreatic duct, and bile duct stricture
ERCP	Diffuse, irregular narrowing of the MPD [82, 83]	Diagnosis and treatment simultaneously, especially in the case of jaundice	Invasive	Evaluating the bile duct, pancreatic duct, and bile duct stricture, treatment for jaundice
EUS-FNA	—	Get the tissue with much less wound than surgery	Invasive May not get adequate tissue	Get the pancreatic tissue sample
PET	Uptake of fluorodeoxyglucose in organs other than the pancreas [88, 89]	Other organ involvement is easily detected	Expensive	Assess the other organ involvement, exclude malignant tumor

EUS-FNA followed by diagnostic and therapeutic ERCP. For pancreatic body or tail lesions, they first perform EUS-FNA.

6. Differential Diagnosis and the Strategy for Distinguishing AIP from Pancreatic Cancer

As a new and relatively rare pancreatic lesion, AIP is easy to be neglected and misdiagnosed as pancreatic cancer for its clinical and imaging features. As is proposed in ICDC, IgG4 elevation is a high-specific serum marker for AIP [49, 50]. However, Ngwa et al. [91] reported that 10.1% of 548 patients with pancreatic cancer have elevated serum IgG4, which may be confusing when serum IgG4 is used to differentiate pancreatic cancer and AIP. Serum CA19-9 was stated to be useful for distinguishing AIP from pancreatic cancer [92], while CA19-9 can also be elevated in other pancreatic diseases or in other pathological states [93]. Thus, so far, a simple serological marker for the differential diagnosis of AIP from pancreatic cancer is still lacking. What is worse, the differentiation by imaging also presents some problems, especially pancreatic cancer and the focal AIP exhibiting mass formation [7, 8]. Thus, a thorough work-up is essential before either surgery or steroid treatment is planned.

Here we present the American diagnostic strategy to differentiate AIP from pancreatic cancer. In patients with obstructive jaundice and/or pancreatic mass CT findings typical for AIP, the presence of any collateral evidence for AIP (elevated IgG4 or autoantibodies or other organ involvement)

is sufficient to make the diagnosis. On the other hand, those with any of the features highly suggestive of pancreatic cancer should generally be managed as cancer unless there is clear evidence of other organ involvement suggestive of AIP. Patients without typical findings of AIP, including those with indeterminate CT findings, should undergo work-up for cancer. If negative, additional collateral evidence for AIP (serum IgG4) should be sought. Diagnosis of AIP is confirmed by pancreatic core biopsy, steroid trial and surgical resection [14] (Figure 1).

7. Treatment for AIP

Glucocorticoids are the routine drug for AIP and rapid response to steroid treatment is one of the primary characteristics of AIP. A poor response to steroid therapy might suggest misdiagnosis, especially in the case of pancreatic cancer. Hart et al. [18] conducted a multicenter, international analysis (1064 patients), showing that 99% of type 1 AIP and 92% of type 2 AIP got clinical remission after steroid treatment. Before induction of remission by an initial steroid therapy, management of blood glucose and biliary drainage is recommended in patients with diabetes mellitus and obstructive jaundice. Generally, patients are given initial oral prednisolone dose of 0.6 mg/Kg/day for induction of remission, which is administered for 2 to 4 weeks. The dose is then tapered by 5 mg every 1 to 2 weeks to a maintenance dose (2.5–5 mg/day) that should be continued for three years as

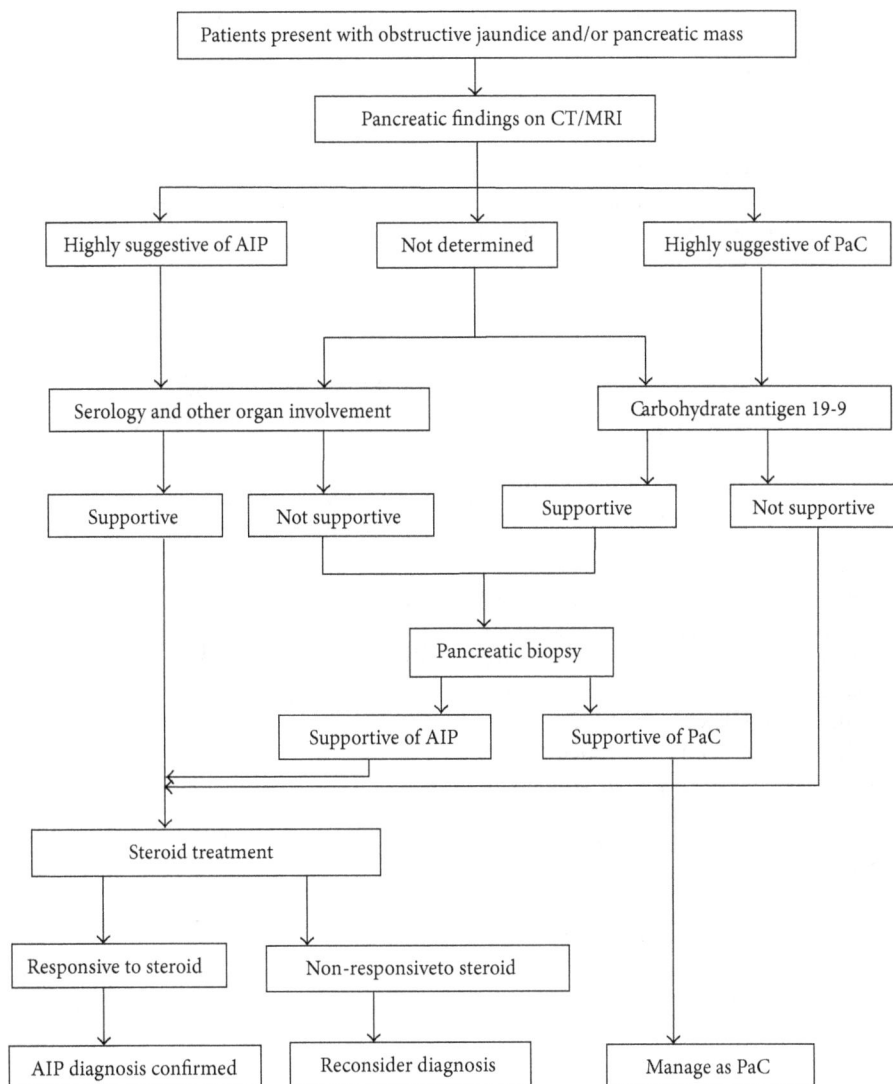

FIGURE 1: Strategy for distinguishing AIP from pancreatic cancer [14]. CT: computed tomography; MRI: magnetic resonance imaging; PaC: pancreatic cancer; OOI/O: other organ involvement; S: serology; CA19-9: carbohydrate antigen 19-9.

maintenance therapy in Japan [94] and the regimen is utilized in most Asian countries. In a multicenter study in Japan, Kamisawa et al. [95] reported that relapse occurred significantly less during maintenance steroid therapy than after the discontinuation of therapy (23% versus 34%, $P < 0.05$), while in European and American countries, maintenance therapy is not commonly used. Ghazale et al. [96] conducted a study and the initial steroid regimen was as follows: prednisolone 40 mg/day orally for 4 weeks, then tapering by 5 mg/week until 11 weeks, and then having a maintenance dose from 12 weeks (Table 6). As a result, 16 (53%) of 30 patients associated with sclerosing cholangitis relapsed during a median follow-up of 29.5 months. Moreover, long time maintenance steroid therapy may cause steroid-related side effects and not all patients can tolerate them. Therefore, whether a maintenance therapy is needed or not needs international discussion.

In a multicenter study in Japan, the cumulative rate of relapse after starting steroid therapy was 56% at 1 year, 76%

at two years, and 92% after 3 years [95]. Hart et al. [18] found the relapse was related to IgG4 related sclerosing cholangitis, no business with serum IgG4 level or pancreatic parenchyma involvement (diffuse or focal pancreatic parenchyma enlargement), while Shimizu et al. [97] confirmed that the rate of decrease in serum IgG4 level was significantly higher in nonrelapse group than in the relapse group after steroid treatment and it might be a predictor of a relapse of AIP. The treatment for relapse is restarting steroids. Whether or not to use alternative immunosuppressant, such as azathioprine, methotrexate, and mycophenolate mofetil [5, 18], depends on the patient's reaction to re-steroid therapy and his tolerance to steroid. Unfortunately, in some cases, the patients cannot tolerate both steroid and immunosuppressant and require drug discontinuation. Rituximab, a monoclonal CD20 antibody, has been shown to be useful in treating AIP patients [98, 99]. The effectiveness of rituximab shed light on the role of B cells in the pathogenesis of AIP because of the B cell depletion. As

TABLE 6: Management strategy of AIP based on immunology therapy.

Time	0–12 weeks	12 weeks–6 months	6 months–3 years
Japan and Asian countries [94]			
Objective	Induction of remission	Maintenance therapy	
Drug	Prednisolone	Prednisolone	
Dose	0.6 mg/Kg/day for 2–4 weeks, tapered by 5 mg every 1-2 weeks to a maintenance dose	2.5–5.0 mg/day	
American and European countries [19]			
Objective	Induction of remission	Maintenance therapy	Observation
Drug	Prednisolone	Prednisolone	Immunomodulator/rituximab (when relapsing)
Dose	30–40 mg/day for 2–4 weeks, tapered by 5 mg every 1-2 weeks to a maintenance dose	5.0–7.5 mg/day	Undetermined

rituximab is the only drug for induction of remission other than glucocorticoids, it would be extremely useful in patients who are unable to tolerate high-dose corticosteroids, require high doses of prednisolone to maintain remission, or have failed to respond to immunomodulator therapy. Currently approved for treating B cell lymphoma and rheumatoid arthritis, rituximab's approval for treating AIP will come true.

The prognosis of AIP is good in general and the long-term complication is rare. Pancreatic duct stones and canceration are the main sequelae [18]. Kanno et al. [2] conducted the nationwide epidemiological survey in Japan in 2011 and found that during the course of observation (1623.3 days), malignant tumors were detected in 109 of 923 patients (11.2%). Shiokawa et al. [100] reported that AIP patients had a high risk of having various cancers, while Hart et al. [101] reported that cancer risk of AIP patients was similar to that of control subjects. Whether AIP is the risk factor for developing cancer needs further investigation.

8. Conclusion

In conclusion, AIP is a special type of chronic pancreatitis, whose pathogenic mechanism, maybe a combination of genetic factors and immunity abnormality, needs more work to be clarified. The diagnosis of AIP depends on serology, imaging, histology, other organ involvement, and reaction to steroids, while high sensitive serum biomarkers for AIP subtypes lack. AIP reacts well to steroids, but controversy exists on the steroid maintenance and treatment for relapse. For AIP shares similarity with pancreatic cancer in clinical and imaging characteristics, general work-up is necessary to differentiate them. Future research may be focused on the pathogenesis, the novel serum biomarker, and the relapse treatment for AIP.

Competing Interests

The authors declare that they have no competing interests.

References

[1] T. Kamisawa, T. Tabata, S. Hara et al., "Recent advances in autoimmune pancreatitis," *Frontiers in Physiology*, vol. 3, article no. 374, 2012.

[2] A. Kanno, A. Masamune, K. Okazaki et al., "Nationwide epidemiological survey of autoimmune pancreatitis in Japan in 2011," *Pancreas*, vol. 44, no. 4, pp. 535–539, 2015.

[3] H. Sarles, J.-C. Sarles, R. Muratore, and C. Guien, "Chronic inflammatory sclerosis of the pancreas—an autonomous pancreatic disease?" *The American Journal of Digestive Diseases*, vol. 6, no. 7, pp. 688–698, 1961.

[4] K. Yoshida, F. Toki, T. Takeuchi, S.-I. Watanabe, K. Shiratori, and N. Hayashi, "Chronic pancreatitis caused by an autoimmune abnormality—proposal of the concept of autoimmune pancreatitis," *Digestive Diseases and Sciences*, vol. 40, no. 7, pp. 1561–1568, 1995.

[5] T. Shimosegawa, S. T. Chari, L. Frulloni et al., "International consensus diagnostic criteria for autoimmune pancreatitis: guidelines of the international association of pancreatology," *Pancreas*, vol. 40, no. 3, pp. 352–358, 2011.

[6] S. Fritz, F. Bergmann, L. Grenacher et al., "Diagnosis and treatment of autoimmune pancreatitis types 1 and 2," *British Journal of Surgery*, vol. 101, no. 10, pp. 1257–1265, 2014.

[7] S. Hoshimoto, K. Aiura, M. Tanaka, M. Shito, T. Kakefuda, and H. Sugiura, "Mass-forming type 1 autoimmune pancreatitis mimicking pancreatic cancer," *Journal of Digestive Diseases*, vol. 17, no. 3, pp. 202–209, 2016.

[8] G. Kobayashi, N. Fujita, Y. Noda, K. Ito, and J. Horaguchi, "Autoimmune pancreatitis: with special reference to a localized variant," *Journal of Medical Ultrasonics*, vol. 35, no. 2, pp. 41–50, 2008.

[9] S. Ben Abid, R. Hefaiedh, S. Zghab, N. Miloudi, L. Gharbi, and M. T. Khalfallah, "Pseudotumoral autoimmune pancreatitis mimicking a pancreatic cancer: a very difficult disease to diagnose," *Clinics and Practice*, vol. 2, no. 4, 2012.

[10] K. Dede, F. Salamon, A. Taller, and A. Bursics, "Autoimmune pancreatitis mimicking pancreatic tumor," *Magyar Sebészet*, vol. 67, no. 1, pp. 18–23, 2014.

[11] R. S. C. Lo, R. K. Singh, A. S. Austin, and J. G. Freeman, "Autoimmune pancreatitis presenting as a pancreatic mass

mimicking malignancy," *Singapore Medical Journal*, vol. 52, no. 4, pp. e79–e81, 2011.

[12] I. Matsumoto, M. Shinzeki, H. Toyama et al., "A focal mass-forming autoimmune pancreatitis mimicking pancreatic cancer with obstruction of the main pancreatic duct," *Journal of Gastrointestinal Surgery*, vol. 15, no. 12, pp. 2296–2298, 2011.

[13] G.-F. Sun, C.-J. Zuo, C.-W. Shao, J.-H. Wang, and J. Zhang, "Focal autoimmune pancreatitis: radiological characteristics help to distinguish from pancreatic cancer," *World Journal of Gastroenterology*, vol. 19, no. 23, pp. 3634–3641, 2013.

[14] S. T. Chari, N. Takahashi, M. J. Levy et al., "A diagnostic strategy to distinguish autoimmune pancreatitis from pancreatic cancer," *Clinical Gastroenterology and Hepatology*, vol. 7, no. 10, pp. 1097–1103, 2009.

[15] T. Kamisawa, Y. Zen, S. Pillai, and J. H. Stone, "IgG4-related disease," *The Lancet*, vol. 385, no. 9976, pp. 1460–1471, 2015.

[16] V. Deshpande, Y. Zen, J. K. Chan et al., "Consensus statement on the pathology of IgG4-related disease," *Modern Pathology*, vol. 25, no. 9, pp. 1181–1192, 2012.

[17] S. Kawa, K. Okazaki, T. Kamisawa et al., "Amendment of the Japanese consensus guidelines for autoimmune pancreatitis, 2013 II. Extrapancreatic lesions, differential diagnosis," *Journal of Gastroenterology*, vol. 49, pp. 765–784, 2014.

[18] P. A. Hart, T. Kamisawa, W. R. Brugge et al., "Long-term outcomes of autoimmune pancreatitis: a multicentre, international analysis," *Gut*, vol. 62, no. 12, pp. 1771–1776, 2013.

[19] K. Okazaki and K. Uchida, "Autoimmune pancreatitis: the past, present, and future," *Pancreas*, vol. 44, no. 7, pp. 1006–1016, 2015.

[20] S. Kawa, M. Ota, K. Yoshizawa et al., "HLA DRB1*0405-DQB1*0401 haplotype is associated with autoimmune pancreatitis in the Japanese population," *Gastroenterology*, vol. 122, no. 5, pp. 1264–1269, 2002.

[21] T. Umemura, M. Ota, H. Hamano, Y. Katsuyama, K. Kiyosawa, and S. Kawa, "Genetic association of Fc receptor-like 3 polymorphisms with autoimmune pancreatitis in Japanese patients," *Gut*, vol. 55, no. 9, pp. 1367–1368, 2006.

[22] T. Umemura, M. Ota, H. Hamano et al., "Association of autoimmune pancreatitis with cytotoxic T-lymphocyte antigen 4 gene polymorphisms in Japanese patients," *The American Journal of Gastroenterology*, vol. 103, no. 3, pp. 588–594, 2008.

[23] M. Ota, T. Ito, T. Umemura et al., "Polymorphism in the KCNA3 gene is associated with susceptibility to autoimmune pancreatitis in the Japanese population," *Disease Markers*, vol. 31, no. 4, pp. 223–229, 2011.

[24] M.-C. Chang, I.-S. Jan, P.-C. Liang et al., "Cystic fibrosis transmembrane conductance regulator gene variants are associated with autoimmune pancreatitis and slow response to steroid treatment," *Journal of Cystic Fibrosis*, vol. 14, no. 5, article 1230, pp. 661–667, 2015.

[25] Y. Kochi, R. Yamada, A. Suzuki et al., "A functional variant in FCRL3, encoding Fc receptor-like 3, is associated with rheumatoid arthritis and several autoimmunities," *Nature Genetics*, vol. 37, pp. 478–485, 2005.

[26] K. Ikari, S. Momohara, T. Nakamura et al., "Supportive evidence for a genetic association of the FCRL3 promoter polymorphism with rheumatoid arthritis," *Annals of the Rheumatic Diseases*, vol. 65, no. 5, pp. 671–673, 2006.

[27] H. Nishi, A. Tojo, M. L. Onozato et al., "Anti-carbonic anhydrase II antibody in autoimmune pancreatitis and tubulointerstitial nephritis," *Nephrology Dialysis Transplantation*, vol. 22, no. 4, pp. 1273–1275, 2007.

[28] K. Okazaki, K. Uchida, M. Ohana et al., "Autoimmune-related pancreatitis is associated with autoantibodies and a Th1/Th2-type cellular immune response," *Gastroenterology*, vol. 118, no. 3, pp. 573–581, 2000.

[29] M. Asada, A. Nishio, K. Uchida et al., "Identification of a novel autoantibody against pancreatic secretory trypsin inhibitor in patients with autoimmune pancreatitis," *Pancreas*, vol. 33, no. 1, pp. 20–26, 2006.

[30] T. Endo, S. Takizawa, S. Tanaka et al., "Amylase α-2A autoantibodies novel marker of autoimmune pancreatitis and fulminant type 1 diabetes," *Diabetes*, vol. 58, no. 3, pp. 732–737, 2009.

[31] Q.-C. Liu, F. Dong, J.-F. Pan et al., "Antibodies to type IV collagen induce type 1 autoimmune pancreatitis," *Inflammation*, vol. 39, no. 2, pp. 592–600, 2016.

[32] M. S. Castañón, V. Zuliani, A. Amodio et al., "Role of amylase-α2A autoantibodies in the diagnosis of autoimmune pancreatitis," *Pancreas*, vol. 44, no. 7, pp. 1078–1082, 2015.

[33] T. Watanabe, K. Yamashita, S. Fujikawa et al., "Involvement of activation of toll-like receptors and nucleotide-binding oligomerization domain-like receptors in enhanced IgG4 responses in autoimmune pancreatitis," *Arthritis and Rheumatism*, vol. 64, no. 3, pp. 914–924, 2012.

[34] T. Watanabe, K. Yamashita, T. Sakurai et al., "Toll-like receptor activation in basophils contributes to the development of IgG4-related disease," *Journal of Gastroenterology*, vol. 48, no. 2, pp. 247–253, 2013.

[35] Y. Fukui, K. Uchida, Y. Sakaguchi et al., "Possible involvement of Toll-like receptor 7 in the development of type 1 autoimmune pancreatitis," *Journal of Gastroenterology*, vol. 50, no. 4, pp. 435–444, 2015.

[36] K. Sumimoto, K. Uchida, T. Kusuda et al., "The role of CD19$^+$CD24^{high} CD38^{high} and CD19$^+$CD24^{high}CD27$^+$ regulatory B cells in patients with type 1 autoimmune pancreatitis," *Pancreatology*, vol. 14, no. 3, pp. 193–200, 2014.

[37] H. Miyoshi, K. Uchida, T. Taniguchi et al., "Circulating naïve and CD4$^+$CD25high regulatory T cells in patients with autoimmune pancreatitis," *Pancreas*, vol. 36, no. 2, pp. 133–140, 2008.

[38] T. Kusuda, K. Uchida, H. Miyoshi et al., "Involvement of inducible costimulator- and interleukin 10-positive regulatory T cells in the development of IgG4-related autoimmune pancreatitis," *Pancreas*, vol. 40, no. 7, pp. 1120–1130, 2011.

[39] S.-Y. Li, X.-Y. Huang, Y.-T. Chen, Y. Liu, and S. Zhao, "Autoimmune pancreatitis characterized by predominant CD8$^+$ T lymphocyte infiltration," *World Journal of Gastroenterology*, vol. 17, no. 41, pp. 4635–4639, 2011.

[40] K. Okazaki, S. Kawa, T. Kamisawa et al., "Amendment of the Japanese consensus guidelines for autoimmune pancreatitis, 2013 I. Concept and diagnosis of autoimmune pancreatitis," *Journal of Gastroenterology*, vol. 49, pp. 567–588, 2014.

[41] Y. Song, Q.-D. Liu, N.-X. Zhou, W.-Z. Zhang, and D.-J. Wang, "Diagnosis and management of autoimmune pancreatitis: experience from China," *World Journal of Gastroenterology*, vol. 14, no. 4, pp. 601–606, 2008.

[42] T. Kamisawa, S. T. Chari, S. A. Giday et al., "Clinical profile of autoimmune pancreatitis and its histological subtypes: an international multicenter survey," *Pancreas*, vol. 40, no. 6, pp. 809–814, 2011.

[43] Q. Meng, L. Xin, W. Liu et al., "Diagnosis and treatment of autoimmune pancreatitis in China: a systematic review," *PLoS ONE*, vol. 10, no. 6, Article ID e0130466, 2015.

[44] A. López-Serrano, J. Crespo, I. Pascual et al., "Diagnosis, treatment and long-term outcomes of autoimmune pancreatitis in Spain based on the International Consensus Diagnostic Criteria: a multi-centre study," *Pancreatology*, vol. 16, no. 3, pp. 382–390, 2016.

[45] T. Ueki, K. Kawamoto, Y. Otsuka et al., "Prevalence and clinicopathological features of autoimmune pancreatitis in Japanese patients with inflammatory bowel disease," *Pancreas*, vol. 44, no. 3, pp. 434–440, 2015.

[46] T. Milosavljevic, M. Kostic-Milosavljevic, I. Jovanovic, and M. Krstic, "Extraintestinal manifestations of autoimmune pancreatitis," *Digestive Diseases*, vol. 30, no. 2, pp. 220–223, 2012.

[47] H. Umehara, K. Okazaki, Y. Masaki et al., "A novel clinical entity, IgG4-related disease (IgG4RD): general concept and details," *Modern Rheumatology*, vol. 22, no. 1, pp. 1–14, 2012.

[48] M. Dahlgren, A. Khosroshahi, G. P. Nielsen, V. Deshpande, and J. H. Stone, "Riedel's thyroiditis and multifocal fibrosclerosis are part of the IgG4-related systemic disease spectrum," *Arthritis Care and Research*, vol. 62, no. 9, pp. 1312–1318, 2010.

[49] W. Cheuk, H. K. L. Yuen, S. Y. Y. Chu, E. K. W. Chiu, L. K. Lam, and J. K. C. Chan, "Lymphadenopathy of IgG4-related sclerosing disease," *American Journal of Surgical Pathology*, vol. 32, no. 5, pp. 671–681, 2008.

[50] J. H. Stone, A. Khosroshahi, V. Deshpande et al., "Recommendations for the nomenclature of IgG4-related disease and its individual organ system manifestations," *Arthritis and Rheumatism*, vol. 64, no. 10, pp. 3061–3067, 2012.

[51] D. L. Finkelberg, D. Sahani, V. Deshpande, and W. R. Brugge, "Autoimmune pancreatitis," *New England Journal of Medicine*, vol. 355, no. 25, pp. 2670–2676, 2006.

[52] D. Yadav and A. B. Lowenfels, "The epidemiology of pancreatitis and pancreatic cancer," *Gastroenterology*, vol. 144, no. 6, pp. 1252–1261, 2013.

[53] G. Maconi, R. Dominici, M. Molteni et al., "Prevalence of pancreatic insufficiency in inflammatory bowel diseases. Assessment by fecal elastase-1," *Digestive Diseases and Sciences*, vol. 53, no. 1, pp. 262–270, 2008.

[54] Members of the Criteria Committee for Autoimmune Pancreatitis of the Japan Pancreas Society, "Diagnostic criteria for autoimmune pancreatitis by the Japan Pancreas Society," *Journal of Japan Pancreas Society*, vol. 17, pp. 585–587, 2002 (Japanese).

[55] K. Okazaki, S. Kawa, T. Kamisawa et al., "Clinical diagnostic criteria of autoimmune pancreatitis: revised proposal," *Journal of Gastroenterology*, vol. 41, no. 7, pp. 626–631, 2006.

[56] S. Kwon, M.-H. Kim, and E. K. Choi, "The diagnostic criteria for autoimmune chronic pancreatitis: it is time to make a consensus," *Pancreas*, vol. 34, no. 3, pp. 279–286, 2007.

[57] S. T. Chari, T. C. Smyrk, M. J. Levy et al., "Diagnosis of autoimmune pancreatitis: the Mayo clinic experience," *Clinical Gastroenterology and Hepatology*, vol. 4, no. 8, pp. 1010–1016, 2006.

[58] M. Otsuki, J. B. Chung, K. Okazaki et al., "Asian diagnostic criteria for autoimmune pancreatitis: consensus of the Japan-Korea symposium on autoimmune pancreatitis," *Journal of Gastroenterology*, vol. 43, no. 6, pp. 403–408, 2008.

[59] A. Schneider and J. M. Löhr, "Autoimmune pancreatitis," *Internist*, vol. 50, no. 3, pp. 318–330, 2009.

[60] The Japan Pancreas Society the Ministry of Health and Welfare Investigation Research Team for Intractable Pancreatic Disease, "Clinical diagnostic criteria for autoimmune pancreatitis 2011 (proposal)," *Suizo*, vol. 27, no. 1, pp. 17–25, 2012 (Japanese).

[61] T. Shimosegawa, The working Group Members of the Japan Pancreas Society Research Committee for Intractable Pancreatic Disease by the Ministry of Labor, Health, and Welfare of Japan, "The amendment of the clinical diagnostic criteria in Japan (JPS2011) in response to the proposal of the international consensus of diagnostic criteria (ICDC) for autoimmune pancreatitis," *Pancreas*, vol. 41, no. 8, pp. 1341–1342, 2012.

[62] A. Ghazale, S. T. Chari, T. C. Smyrk et al., "Value of serum IgG4 in the diagnosis of autoimmune pancreatitis and in distinguishing it from pancreatic cancer," *American Journal of Gastroenterology*, vol. 102, no. 8, pp. 1646–1653, 2007.

[63] T. Tabata, T. Kamisawa, K. Takuma et al., "Serum IgG4 concentrations and IgG4-related sclerosing disease," *Clinica Chimica Acta*, vol. 408, no. 1-2, pp. 25–28, 2009.

[64] R. Sadler, R. W. Chapman, D. Simpson et al., "The diagnostic significance of serum IgG4 levels in patients with autoimmune pancreatitis: A UK Study," *European Journal of Gastroenterology and Hepatology*, vol. 23, no. 2, pp. 139–145, 2011.

[65] R. P. Sah and S. T. Chari, "Serologic issues in IgG4-related systemic disease and autoimmune pancreatitis," *Current Opinion in Rheumatology*, vol. 23, no. 1, pp. 108–113, 2011.

[66] M.-J. Lian, S. Liu, G.-Y. Wu, and S.-Y. Liu, "Serum IgG4 and IgG for the diagnosis of autoimmune pancreatitis: a systematic review with meta-analysis," *Clinics and Research in Hepatology and Gastroenterology*, vol. 40, no. 1, pp. 99–109, 2016.

[67] T. J. Song, M.-H. Kim, S.-H. Moon et al., "The combined measurement of total serum igg and IgG4 may increase diagnostic sensitivity for autoimmune pancreatitis without sacrificing specificity, compared with IgG4 alone," *American Journal of Gastroenterology*, vol. 105, no. 7, pp. 1655–1660, 2010.

[68] M. Hao, W. Li, L. Yi et al., "Hybrid kappa\lambda antibody is a new serological marker to diagnose autoimmune pancreatitis and differentiate it from pancreatic cancer," *Scientific Reports*, vol. 6, Article ID 27415, 2016.

[69] F. Vitali, L. Pfeifer, C. Janson et al., "Quantitative perfusion analysis in pancreatic contrast enhanced ultrasound (DCE-US): a promising tool for the differentiation between autoimmune pancreatitis and pancreatic cancer," *Zeitschrift für Gastroenterologie*, vol. 53, no. 10, pp. 1175–1181, 2015.

[70] K. D. Bodily, N. Takahashi, J. G. Fletcher et al., "Autoimmune pancreatitis: pancreatic and extrapancreatic imaging findings," *American Journal of Roentgenology*, vol. 192, no. 2, pp. 431–437, 2009.

[71] D. V. Sahani, S. P. Kalva, J. Farrell et al., "Autoimmune pancreatitis: imaging features," *Radiology*, vol. 233, no. 2, pp. 345–352, 2004.

[72] N. Takahashi, J. G. Fletcher, J. L. Fidler, D. M. Hough, A. Kawashima, and S. T. Chari, "Dual-phase CT of autoimmune pancreatitis: A Multireader Study," *American Journal of Roentgenology*, vol. 190, no. 2, pp. 280–286, 2008.

[73] R. Rotzinger, H. Blaker, M. Bahra, T. Denecke, and C. Grieser, "CT and MRI findings of autoimmune polymorph bifocal pancreatitis mimicking pancreatic adenocarcinoma: a case report and review of the literature," *Journal of Investigative Medicine High Impact Case Reports*, vol. 3, no. 1, 2015.

[74] E. Buscarini, L. Frulloni, S. De Lisi, M. Falconi, P. Testoni, and A. Zambelli, "Autoimmune pancreatitis: a challenging diagnostic puzzle for clinicians," *Digestive and Liver Disease*, vol. 42, no. 2, pp. 92–98, 2010.

[75] H. Irie, H. Honda, S. Baba et al., "Autoimmune pancreatitis: CT and MR characteristics," *American Journal of Roentgenology*, vol. 170, no. 5, pp. 1323–1327, 1998.

[76] N. Kartalis, T. L. Lindholm, P. Aspelin, J. Permert, and N. Albiin, "Diffusion-weighted magnetic resonance imaging of pancreas tumours," *European Radiology*, vol. 19, no. 8, pp. 1981–1990, 2009.

[77] N. Inan, A. Arslan, G. Akansel, Y. Anik, and A. Demirci, "Diffusion-weighted imaging in the differential diagnosis of cystic lesions of the pancreas," *American Journal of Roentgenology*, vol. 191, no. 4, pp. 1115–1121, 2008.

[78] Y. Fukukura, K. Takumi, K. Kamimura et al., "Pancreatic adenocarcinoma: variability of diffusion-weighted MR imaging findings," *Radiology*, vol. 263, pp. 732–740, 2012.

[79] B. Kim, S. S. Lee, Y. S. Sung et al., "Intravoxel incoherent motion diffusion-weighted imaging of the pancreas: characterization of benign and malignant pancreatic pathologies," *Journal of Magnetic Resonance Imaging*, vol. 45, no. 1, pp. 260–269, 2016.

[80] G. Carbognin, V. Girardi, C. Biasiutti et al., "Autoimmune pancreatitis: imaging findings on contrast-enhanced MR, MRCP and dynamic secretin-enhanced MRCP," *Radiologia Medica*, vol. 114, no. 8, pp. 1214–1231, 2009.

[81] I. Naitoh, T. Nakazawa, F. Okumura et al., "Endoscopic retrograde cholangiopancreatography-related adverse events in patients with type 1 autoimmune pancreatitis," *Pancreatology*, vol. 16, no. 1, pp. 78–82, 2016.

[82] T. Nakazawa, H. Ohara, H. Sano et al., "Cholangiography can discriminate sclerosing cholangitis with autoimmune pancreatitis from primary sclerosing cholangitis," *Gastrointestinal Endoscopy*, vol. 60, no. 6, pp. 937–944, 2004.

[83] S.-H. Moon and M.-H. Kim, "The role of endoscopy in the diagnosis of autoimmune pancreatitis," *Gastrointestinal Endoscopy*, vol. 76, no. 3, pp. 645–656, 2012.

[84] A. Sugumar, M. J. Levy, T. Kamisawa et al., "Endoscopic retrograde pancreatography criteria to diagnose autoimmune pancreatitis: an international multicentre study," *Gut*, vol. 60, pp. 666–670, 2011.

[85] A. Kanno, A. Masamune, F. Fujishima et al., "Diagnosis of autoimmune pancreatitis by EUS-guided FNA using a 22-gauge needle: A Prospective Multicenter Study," *Gastrointestinal Endoscopy*, vol. 84, no. 5, pp. 797.e1–804.e1, 2015.

[86] A. Kanno, K. Ishida, S. Hamada et al., "Diagnosis of autoimmune pancreatitis by EUS-FNA by using a 22-gauge needle based on the International Consensus Diagnostic Criteria," *Gastrointestinal Endoscopy*, vol. 76, no. 3, pp. 594–602, 2012.

[87] T. Ishikawa, A. Itoh, H. Kawashima et al., "Endoscopic ultrasound-guided fine needle aspiration in the differentiation of type 1 and type 2 autoimmune pancreatitis," *World Journal of Gastroenterology*, vol. 18, no. 29, pp. 3883–3888, 2012.

[88] M. Ebbo, A. Grados, E. Guedj et al., "Usefulness of 2-[^{18}F]-fluoro-2-deoxy-d-glucose–positron emission tomography/computed tomography for staging and evaluation of treatment response in IgG4-related disease: A Retrospective Multicenter Study," *Arthritis Care and Research*, vol. 66, no. 1, pp. 86–96, 2014.

[89] Y. Y. Ozaki, K. Oguchi, H. Hamano et al., "Differentiation of autoimmune pancreatitis from suspected pancreatic cancer by fluorine-18 fluorodeoxyglucose positron emission tomography," *Journal of Gastroenterology*, vol. 43, no. 2, pp. 144–151, 2008.

[90] K. Uchida, H. Miyoshi, T. Ikeura, M. Shimatani, M. Takaoka, and K. Okazaki, "Clinical and pathophysiological issues associated with type 1 autoimmune pancreatitis," *Clinical Journal of Gastroenterology*, vol. 9, no. 1, pp. 7–12, 2016.

[91] T. Ngwa, R. Law, P. Hart, T. C. Smyrk, and S. T. Chari, "Serum IgG4 elevation in pancreatic cancer: diagnostic and prognostic significance and association with autoimmune pancreatitis," *Pancreas*, vol. 44, no. 4, pp. 557–560, 2015.

[92] M. J. van Heerde, J. Buijs, B. E. Hansen et al., "Serum level of ca 19-9 increases ability of IgG4 test to distinguish patients with autoimmune pancreatitis from those with pancreatic carcinoma," *Digestive Diseases and Sciences*, vol. 59, no. 6, pp. 1322–1329, 2014.

[93] M.-C. Chang, Y.-T. Chang, T.-C. Su et al., "Adiponectin as a potential differential marker to distinguish pancreatic cancer and chronic pancreatitis," *Pancreas*, vol. 35, no. 1, pp. 16–21, 2007.

[94] T. Kamisawa, K. Okazaki, S. Kawa et al., "Amendment of the Japanese Consensus Guidelines for Autoimmune Pancreatitis, 2013 III. Treatment and prognosis of autoimmune pancreatitis," *Journal of Gastroenterology*, vol. 49, no. 6, pp. 961–970, 2014.

[95] T. Kamisawa, T. Shimosegawa, K. Okazaki et al., "Standard steroid treatment for autoimmune pancreatitis," *Gut*, vol. 58, no. 11, pp. 1504–1507, 2009.

[96] A. Ghazale, S. T. Chari, L. Zhang et al., "Immunoglobulin G4-associated cholangitis: clinical profile and response to therapy," *Gastroenterology*, vol. 134, no. 3, pp. 706–715, 2008.

[97] K. Shimizu, J. Tahara, Y. Takayama et al., "Assessment of the rate of decrease in serum IgG4 level of autoimmune pancreatitis patients in response to initial steroid therapy as a predictor of subsequent relapse," *Pancreas*, vol. 45, no. 9, pp. 1341–1346, 2016.

[98] P. A. Hart, M. D. Topazian, T. E. Witzig et al., "Treatment of relapsing autoimmune pancreatitis with immunomodulators and rituximab: the mayo clinic experience," *Gut*, vol. 62, no. 11, pp. 1607–1615, 2013.

[99] M. Topazian, T. E. Witzig, T. C. Smyrk et al., "Rituximab therapy for refractory biliary strictures in immunoglobulin G4-associated cholangitis," *Clinical Gastroenterology and Hepatology*, vol. 6, no. 3, pp. 364–366, 2008.

[100] M. Shiokawa, Y. Kodama, K. Yoshimura et al., "Risk of cancer in patients with autoimmune pancreatitis," *American Journal of Gastroenterology*, vol. 108, no. 4, pp. 610–617, 2013.

[101] P. A. Hart, R. J. Law, R. A. Dierkhising, T. C. Smyrk, N. Takahashi, and S. T. Chari, "Risk of cancer in autoimmune pancreatitis: a case-control study and review of the literature," *Pancreas*, vol. 43, no. 3, pp. 417–421, 2014.

18

Nutrition and IBD: Malnutrition and/or Sarcopenia?
A Practical Guide

F. Scaldaferri,[1] M. Pizzoferrato,[1] L. R. Lopetuso,[1] T. Musca,[1] F. Ingravalle,[1]
L. L. Sicignano,[1] M. Mentella,[2] G. Miggiano,[2] M. C. Mele,[2] E. Gaetani,[1] C. Graziani,[1]
V. Petito,[1] G. Cammarota,[1] E. Marzetti,[3] A. Martone,[3] F. Landi,[3] and A. Gasbarrini[1]

[1]*Gastroenterology Division, Catholic University of Sacred Heart, Rome, Italy*
[2]*Nutrition Team, Catholic University of Sacred Heart, Rome, Italy*
[3]*Gerontology Division, Catholic University of Sacred Heart, Rome, Italy*

Correspondence should be addressed to F. Scaldaferri; francoscaldaferri@gmail.com

Academic Editor: Alfred Gangl

Malnutrition is a major complication of inflammatory bowel disease (IBD). This mini review is focusing on main determinants of malnutrition in IBD, the most important components of malnutrition, including lean mass loss and sarcopenia, as an emerging problem. Each one of these components needs to be well considered in a correct nutritional evaluation of an IBD patient in order to build a correct multidisciplinary approach. The review is then focusing on possible instrumental and clinical armamentarium for the nutritional evaluation.

1. Introduction

Malnutrition is a major complication of inflammatory bowel disease (IBD) and it is primarily responsible for chronic weight loss. Existing data suggest that malnutrition affects a large portion of patients with inflammatory bowel disease (IBD), estimated in 65–75% of patients with Crohn's disease (CD) and in 18–62% of patients with ulcerative colitis (UC). Based on BMI analysis, malnutrition prevalence seems to be higher in CD compared to UC, although several authors reported similar prevalence of malnutrition in both conditions [1–4]. In pediatric patients, malnutrition is main cause of growth retardation and it could anticipate gastrointestinal symptoms. Prevalence of malnutrition in pediatric patients seems to be higher in CD patients than in UC patients [5, 6].

Impairment of nutritional status has a multifactorial etiology. Main reasons include suboptimal energy intake, malabsorption, enteric nutrient loss, increased basal energy expenditure, and medications. In clinical settings, IBD patients are commonly found to be underweight, with several nutritional deficiencies, alterations of anthropometric parameters, in body composition of fat, and muscle mass and with low bone mineral density [2, 3, 7].

2. Main Determinants of Malnutrition in IBD

The *decrease of oral food intake* is one of the most important reasons for malnutrition in patient with IBD. Two main mechanisms are reported. The first is connected to the disease itself: patients avoid eating due to symptoms such as nausea, abdominal pain, vomiting, and diarrhea during disease inflammatory activity. The second is connected to fasting due to hospitalization or prolonged restrictive diets [8, 9]. Moreover, energy intake is also linked to disease localization in CD patients, with a reduction of energy intake only in ileal and ileocolonic disease [10].

Existing data correlate malabsorption *to inflammatory cytokines* released from immune cells within gut mucosa of CD and UC patients during active and remission phases. Malabsorption mechanisms are related to epithelial alterations such as impaired epithelial transport and loss of epithelial integrity. Other important mechanisms seem to be bacterial overgrowth and increased intestinal mobility [11,12]. Malabsorption seems to play a major role in patients with BMI less than 18.5 kg/m^2 [4, 13].

Gastrointestinal nutrient loss is strictly connected to malabsorption and is caused by both epithelial alteration and disease activity, which mainly lead to loss in nutrient and in active phases of disease by inflammatory diarrhea. In particular, alterations of ionic transports cause dispersion of electrolytes and water in intestinal lumen. Inflammation can also lead to the ulceration of the bowel surfaces, which in turn determine chronic blood loss and proteins loss within the intestinal lumen. A correct management of IBD patients can prevent anemia and hypoalbuminemia [9, 11, 14].

Another important mechanism is *the biliary salt diarrhea*, usually associated with a terminal ileal disease, with an impaired absorption of fat-soluble vitamin and lipids. Fat malabsorption can lead to steatorrhea [15].

Several studies investigated the increased *energy expenditure* in IBD. There are two key points: the first is the comparison of energy requirement among CD and UC patients and controls and the second is the difference between carbohydrate metabolism and lipid metabolism.

The energy requirement in IBD patient can be valued with the Harris-Benedict formula for basal energy expenditure (BEE) or with indirect calorimetric measurements of resting energy expenditure (REE). BEE represents the energy expenditure required for the maintenance of vital functions at rest and during the fasting; REE, instead, represents the energy expenditure during nonfasting time, including BEE and the thermic effect of food. No significant differences were found in energy requirement among IBD patients and controls using BEE or REE [16]. However, there is a significant difference in basal energy expenditure between IBD patients with a regular body weight and IBD patients with reduced body weight. For instance, patients with body weight less than 90% of the ideal body weight have higher energy expenditure than patients with body weight more than 90% of the ideal value, estimated in up to 24% of energy expenditure per kilogram over the control patients [7, 16].

Other important evidences suggest major differences in carbohydrate oxidation and lipid oxidation in IBD. In particular, CD patients show higher lipid oxidation and lower carbohydrate oxidation rate in basal condition compared to UC patients and controls. UC patients show a little increase in lipid metabolism and similar carbohydrate utilization compared to controls [2, 10]. In children with IBD, the energy intake and metabolism rate are variable according to age and weight of each patient [5, 6].

Medications could have an impact on micronutrient absorption and utilization.

Glucocorticoids can interfere with calcium, phosphorus, and zinc absorption and utilization. They are also related to an impaired metabolism of vitamins C and D. Long-term glucocorticoid exposure is associated with bone alteration and osteoporosis.

Sulfasalazine is a folic acid antagonist and long-term therapies are related to anemia and hyperhomocysteinemia.

Cholestyramine can interfere with absorption of fat-soluble vitamins, iron, and B_{12} vitamin. Main side effect is steatorrhea due to impairment absorption of fats.

Moreover, the use of long-term parenteral nutrition can lead to micronutrient deficiencies, including vitamins A, D, and E, zinc, copper, and selenium [1, 15].

Main determinants of malnutrition in inflammatory bowel disease are summarized in Figure 1.

3. Clinical Aspects of Malnutrition in Patients with IBD

Micronutrient and vitamin deficiencies are common in IBD patients and preventions of those deficiencies are important to avoid clinical complications. Types of deficit depend on many factors as disease localization and extension, disease activity, alimentation, nutritional support, and medication used for IBD (Table 1).

The most common micronutrient deficiencies in IBD are iron, calcium, selenium, zinc, and magnesium depletion. Vitamin deficiencies include all vitamins and in particular B_{12}, folic acid (water soluble), and vitamins A, D, and K (fat-soluble) [1, 15].

Selenium, zinc, and magnesium depletions are caused by inadequate dietary intake and chronic loss for diarrhea. The exact prevalence in IBD is still unclear. Symptoms associated with deficiencies include bone health impairment, fatigue, poor wound healing, and cartilage degeneration [1, 15].

Several studies documented vitamin A deficiency in up to 90% of IBD patients as a result of inadequate intake, low BMI and low fat mass and ileal location of disease or bowel resection, ileal resection, disease duration, and higher CRP level. Vitamin A deficiency associates with poor wound healing, night blindness, and xerophthalmia [1, 15].

Vitamin K deficiency is also reported in IBD patients, with unknown prevalence. Main determinants of vitamin K deficiency are disease activity, use of antibiotics, and malabsorption, as the most important source of vitamin K is intestinal production by gut microbiota. Vitamin K deficiency contributes to alteration of coagulation factors and may contribute also to abnormal bone metabolism [1, 15].

Anemia is another clinical aspect of malnutrition in IBD; its prevalence covers up to 70% of pediatric patients and up to 50% of adult patients [17]. Anemia is usually associated with other important symptoms like fatigue, sleeping disorders, restless legs syndrome, attention deficit, discontentment, agitation, or female infertility. Diagnostic criteria are not different from anemia in other types of patients. Main causes of anemia include iron deficiency, B_{12} vitamin and folic acid deficiencies, bleeding from mucosal lesions, surgery, systemic inflammation, and medications. Iron deficiency is the most frequent cause of anemia in IBD patients, like in healthy people, with prevalence estimated in 36–90% [17]. It was demonstrated that iron deficiency has multifactorial etiology, including inadequate intake, blood loss from damaged intestinal wall, impairment absorption (disease localization in duodenum or proximal tract of jejunum), and impairment utilization (due to the systemic inflammatory status) [18, 19]. Furthermore, iron absorption and metabolism are regulated by Hepcidin and soluble transferrin receptors, the first being an important hormone depressing iron absorption and iron release from body stores in iron-overload and in inflammatory status; the second, conversely, increases during iron deficiency status and increases intestinal absorption and

TABLE 1: Micronutrient deficiencies in IBD.

Micronutrient	Physiopathology	Main symptoms of deficiency	Diagnosis
Iron	Chronic blood loss Impaired iron metabolism Inadequate intake	Anemia, fatigue, sleeping disorders, restless legs syndrome, attention deficit, discontentment, agitation, and female infertility	Transferrin sat <16% and serum ferritin <30 ng/mL
Calcium	Inadequate dietary intake Decreased intestinal/renal absorption	Decreased bone density, hyperparathyroidism, hypertension, and muscle spasm	Bone density scan Serum calcium < 8.5 mg/dl
Selenium	Not fully understood	Cardiomyopathy and cartilage degeneration	Serum selenium <70 μg/L
Zinc	Chronic diarrhea Malabsorption	Poor wound healing	Serum zinc <75 μg/mL
Magnesium	Chronic diarrhea Inadequate dietary intake	Fatigue	Serum magnesium <1.41 mEq/L
Vitamin B9	Inadequate dietary intake Malabsorption Medications (MTX)	Megaloblastic anemia, modestly increased risk of colonic dysplasia, and hyperhomocysteinemia	Serum folate < 2.5 ng/mL
Vitamin B_{12}	History of ileal/ileocolonic resection	Megaloblastic anemia and peripheral neuropathy	Serum B_{12} < 200 pg/mL
Vitamin D	Inadequate dietary intake Malabsorption	Abnormal bone metabolism	Serum 25OHD (<15 ng/mL deficiency, <20 ng/mL insufficiency, and >30 ng/mL optimum)
Vitamin A	Inadequate dietary intake Malabsorption	Poor wound healing, night blindness, and xeropthalmia	Serum retinol <30 μg/dL
Vitamin K	Inadequate dietary intake Malabsorption Use of antibiotics	Abnormal bone metabolism	Serum phylloquinone <1.1 ng/mL PT/INR

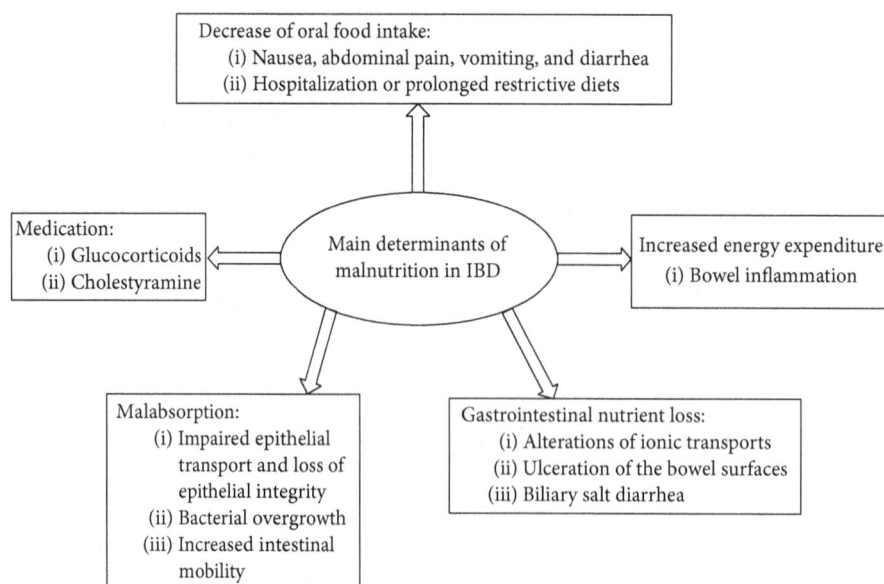

FIGURE 1: Main determinants of malnutrition in IBD.

release from stores. In active IBD, Hepcidin takes control of iron metabolism with development of anemia due to relative or absolute iron deficiency [20].

Main causes of non-iron deficiency anemia in IBD are anemia of chronic disease (ACD) and deficiencies of vitamin B_{12} and folic acid (vitamin B_9). ACD is perhaps the most frequent cause of anemia in hospitalized patients [17]. B_{12} deficiency is common in IBD patients, with estimated prevalence of 22% in CD patients and up to 3% in UC patients [1, 21]. B_{12} can be absorbed only in terminal ileal tract due to a complicated mechanism of absorption and all CD patients with ileal resection greater than 60 cm will develop

Nutrition and IBD: Malnutrition and/or Sarcopenia? A Practical Guide

159

B_{12} deficiency. It is associated with megaloblastic anemia and peripheral neuropathy. Low level of vitamin B_{12} can lead to hyperhomocysteinemia, which is an independent risk factor for venous thrombosis [22, 23].

Folic acid deficiency is more common in IBD patients and it is reported in 28.8% of the CD patients and 8.8% of ulcerative colitis (UC) patients [22]. Risk factors for deficiency include low dietary intake, active disease, malabsorption, and interaction with medicines as sulfasalazine or methotrexate treatment [22–24].

Low levels of calcium and vitamin D are common in patients with IBD, especially in those with duodenal and jejunal disease [1, 15]. Calcium deficiency is linked to vitamin D deficiency, because its absorption is governed by vitamin D levels, which can activate the calcium transporters. Vitamin D deficiency is related to inadequate daily intake, inflammation status, diarrhea, and glucocorticoid therapies. The prevalence among IBD patients is up to 70% in CD patients and up to 40% in UC patients. Vitamin D levels are also correlated to disease activity and existing data suggest that vitamin D could be a risk factor for IBD. Vitamin D is implicated in preserving mucosal integrity and mucosal healing capacity and its deficiency may compromise mucosal barrier, increasing risk for mucosal damage and for IBD. In particular, high levels of active vitamin D seem to reduce the risk of developing CD, while not changing significantly the risk for UC [1, 15, 25, 26].

Another significant aspect of malnutrition in IBD is linked to *alteration of body composition*, especially in alteration between fat mass (FM) and fat-free mass (FFM). FM consists of adipose tissues (both visceral and subcutaneous); instead FFM is the body portion which excludes adipose tissue and consists of water, proteins, and mineral and other components [3]. Although there are few small and heterogeneous studies that analyze the role of body composition alteration in IBD patients, it was demonstrated that one-third of CD patients had a significant reduction of body mass index, but only 5% were underweight by BMI criteria. Using second-line methods, it was demonstrated that 28% of CD patients had reduced FFM and 31% of these patients had a significant reduction in FM. Similar data were found in UC patients, in which significant BMI reduction was reported in 20% and a depletion of FFM and FM in 13%, while no one of UC patients was underweight by BMI criteria. These data suggest that BMI variations are not strictly connected to alteration in body compositions; in particular, there is no connection between FFM and FM depletion and BMI [27]. Conflicting data exist about the exact role of disease activity in body composition; several studies fail in finding connection between disease phase and alteration of BMI, FM, and FFM; others have shown a significant difference in these parameters; in particular, there is an important reduction of BMI and FM in active phase in CD patients, while in remission phase there is also FFM depletion. UC patients have a significant FM reduction in active phase compared to remission phase, but differences between active and remission phases were not significant for BMI and FFM [3]. Moreover, it was reported that FM depletion which occurred in active phase was partially recovered during remission phase instead of FFM which remained depleted also in remission phase.

4. The Deficit of Lean Mass in IBD and Sarcopenia: Emerging Aspects

Sarcopenia is a syndrome characterized by progressive and generalized loss of skeletal muscle mass and strength with risk of poor quality of life and physical disability. Principal mechanisms involved in genesis of sarcopenia are malnutrition, immobility, low protein synthesis, and increased proteolysis [28, 29]. Diagnosis of sarcopenia comprehends the demonstrations of both muscle mass and muscle strength. The gold standard to asses muscle mass is DXA, computed tomography (CT), or magnetic resonance imaging (MRI), but they have a limited use in clinical practice due to high costs. BIA can be a valid alternative to DXA due to lower cost instead of anthropometric measures. Muscle strength can be assessed with a grip strength test, which is of low cost and is an easy-to-handle technique, using a standard dynamometer [28]. Recent evidences suggest that prevalence of sarcopenia is up to 12% in CD patients evaluated with the appendicular skeletal muscle index (ASMI) asserted with whole-body DXA. Moreover, a multivariate analysis found that grip strength test was a positive predictor of low ASMI compared to BMI [30].

Consequences of sarcopenia are bone demineralization and pathological fractures, cardiovascular disease and higher probability of hospitalization, and reduction of mobility [29]. Furthermore, several studies associated sarcopenia with osteopenia: osteopenia has been evaluated as reduction of bone mineral density (BMD) with DXA and *t*-score analysis. Osteopenia was evident in 30% of CD patients in Bryant et al.'s study and in 36% of UC patients. Low lean mass, sarcopenia, and low BMI are all independent positive predictors for osteopenia and osteoporosis [30].

A correlation between IBD and obesity has also been described. The prevalence of obesity is quite different across different studies and likely this depends on obesity prevalence in general population. Up to 32.7% of IBD patients are obese, and in particular up to 30.3% of CD patients and up to 35.2% of UC patients [27, 31]. Obesity is associated with more anal and perianal complication [32]. Moreover, overweight patients had a better clinical course than normal weight patients. Obesity did not increase healthcare hospitalization and surgery operations. Clearly, more studies are needed to individuate the optimal therapy for IBD obese patients [33].

Two other teams investigated the influence of obesity on anti-TNF-alfa treatment with contrast results. Flores et al. found that IBD patients with BMI > 25 kg/m^2 are less likely to need anti-TNF therapy than normal or underweight patients and are less likely to need surgery or hospitalization. Overall, they define obesity as a marker of less severe disease [31]. Instead, Harper et al. reported that high BMI in IBD patients is associated with a greater need for Infliximab escalation dose and with higher loss of response, need for steroid therapy, and number of hospitalization days compared to normal BMI patients [34]. The reasons appear to be unclear and further investigations are needed.

Sarcopenia and obesity in IBD patients can lead to sarcopenic obesity. Sarcopenic obesity is defined in literature as a clinical condition in which criteria for sarcopenia met criteria for obesity; this syndrome is not simply the sum of the two conditions. Obesity and sarcopenia are both responsible of physical impairment and metabolic disorders and may act with each other. Sarcopenic obesity is related to a fast functional decline of patient's status, with a high risk of disability, mobility, and mortality; for these reasons diagnosis is important. Screen test can be simply grip strength test and BMI or otherwise body composition study with DXA [29].

5. Pathophysiology of Malnutrition and Sarcopenia in Inflammatory Bowel Disease

In healthy subjects, nutritional status and body composition are maintained by complex interactions between muscle, bone, and adipose tissue. This perfect balance permits the normal growth of body and the regulation of energy metabolism; moreover, it is crucial for the environmental adaptation of organism. Each factor of this balance is able to "communicate" with the others through a complex cell-signaling network, influencing the activation and the development of each other (Figure 2). Many pathological conditions can alter this balance, causing deregulation of energy metabolism and body composition, with hyperexpression and reduction of particular tissues. Inflammatory chronic diseases, infections, liver cirrhosis, and heart and kidney failure are the most diffuse diseases that are able to influence the nutritional status and the body composition through the deregulation of metabolism of muscle, bone, and adipose tissues.

In particular, inflammatory bowel diseases and other conditions characterized by chronic inflammation can alter the homeostasis of muscles, bones, and fat and are involved in the pathogenesis of malnutrition and dysregulated body composition (Figure 2). Therefore, it is crucial to analyze the role of inflammation for each factor involved in maintaining energy balance [35–37].

Skeletal muscle is the most diffuse tissue in human body and it is involved in many physiological functions like the uptake and the metabolism of glucose. Muscles are regulated by physiological stimuli and pathological conditions that influence size and mass through the control of protein turnover. In chronic inflammation, a shift of protein turnover poised toward protein degradation with subsequent reduction of myofibrillar proteins can be observed, resulting in loss of muscle mass and impaired muscular contraction. In inflammatory chronic diseases, muscle protein degradation seems to depend on a coordinated network of signaling pathways regulated by hormones and cytokines, which reduce synthesis and increase protein degradation. Current evidences indicate that several cellular pathways, involved in cellular growth, are deregulated during chronic inflammatory disorders, in particular the ubiquitin proteasome and the autophagy pathways. The most important pathway involved in muscle growth is the insulin/GH/IGF1 system. Normally, circulating GH binds to transmembrane GH receptors, activating the synthesis of IGF1 in liver and other tissues as bone and muscles. In bones, IGF1 stimulates the proliferation of chondrocytes and osteoblasts in the epiphysis of long bones, resulting in linear growth, while in muscular cells IGF1 enhances protein synthesis via P13K/AKT phosphorylation with activation of mTOR system and reduction of activation of ubiquitin ligands [38]. In IBD, as in chronic inflammatory conditions, a significant reduction in plasma and muscle IGF1 can be seen in response to the elevated concentrations of TNF-alpha and IL-6, cytokines that cause GH resistance in liver and muscles, inducing downregulation of mTOR pathway with activation of ubiquitin ligands and expression of enzymes involved in protein degradation, in particular atrogin-1, MuRF1, and MUSA1 [39–41]. On the contrary, during chronic inflammation, a significant activation of myostatin, a member of TGF-beta family, can be observed. Myostatin is able to induce degradation of sarcomeric proteins through the synthesis of atrogin-1 and MuRF1 via the upregulation of the transcription factors Smad2/3 and the suppression of Akt signaling [42, 43]. Moreover, in chronic inflammatory conditions, acute phase proteins and cytokines as TNF-alpha, IFN-gamma, and IL-6 exert a direct role in muscle wasting, in particular by activating the transcription factor NF-kB and the ubiquitin proteasome system and interfering with the myogenic program. For example, TNF-alpha can impair proliferation and differentiation of muscular steam cells, acting on NF-kB experimental model [44].

Viewed only as passive energy reservoir in past, it is now clear that adipose tissue is an important and active endocrine organ, involved in the modulation of energy metabolism and in the bone growth [45]. Adipose tissue has also a significant immunological role, in particular modulating the immune response via recruitment and activation of immune cells and differentiation of lymphocyte [46]. Dysregulation of adipose tissue is frequent in chronic conditions like diabetes, hypertension, and heart diseases, conditions which are all generally characterized by hyperexpression of fat tissue and low grade of inflammation.

In IBD, more in Crohn's disease, a significant increase in visceral adiposity can be observed, in particular in mesenteric fat. Moreover, the presence of an enlarged mesenteric adipose tissue that envelopes more than a half of the intestinal circumference in corresponding inflammatory lesions is reported. This type of adipose tissue, known as "creeping" fat, does not depend on BMI and it is an important indicator of disease activity, correlating with transmural inflammation and its complications (strictures and fistulas) [47, 48]. Mesenteric fat seems to be involved in the pathogenesis of Crohn's disease: adipocytes in mesenteric fat can produce inflammatory cytokines such as TNF-alpha, IFN-gamma, IL-6, and IL-1 and other adipokines as leptin and resistin. These molecules demonstrate a strong proinflammatory effect, activating immune response and deregulating intestinal homeostasis [36]. Moreover, it is now clear that adipocyte mass correlates with the degree of expression of these cytokines and disease activity [49].

In addition, adipose tissue can express several inflammatory adipokines as leptin. This adipokine is overexpressed in mesenteric fat in patients with active Crohn's disease compared with controls and it has significant proinflammatory

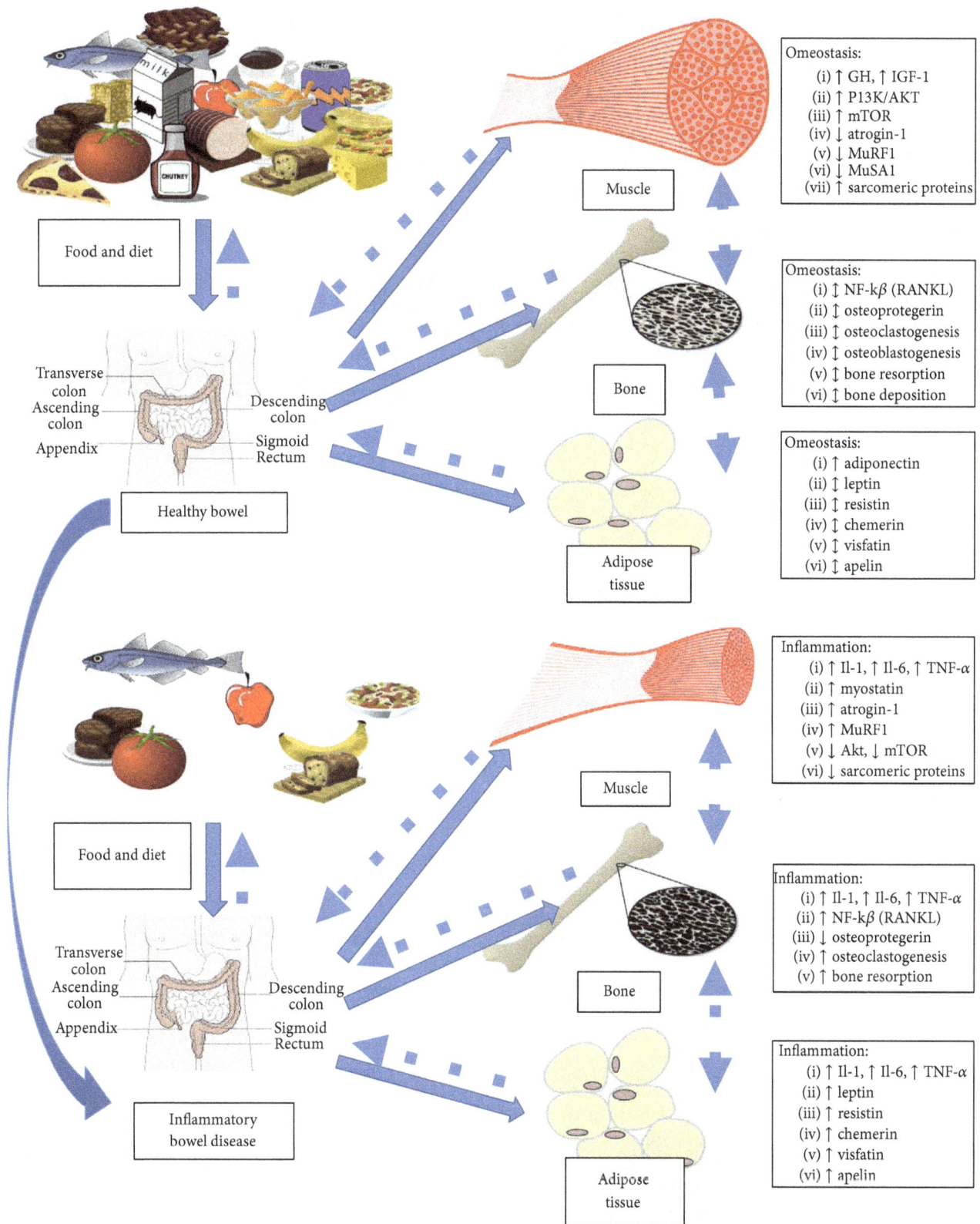

Figure 2: Pathophysiology of malnutrition and sarcopenia in inflammatory bowel disease. Interplay between nutrition, inflammation, muscle, bone, and adipose tissue in healthy subject and IBD.

activity [50]. Leptin indeed has structural and functional similarities with IL-6; it can stimulate the proliferation of blood mononuclear cells, increase the proliferation and the survival of CD4 T cells, stimulate the development of Th1 response, and promote dendritic cell differentiation via the activation of intracellular JAK-STAT pathways [51, 52]. Another adipokine hyperexpressed in mesenteric fat in Crohn's disease is resistin. Resistin is inducted by bacterial lipopolysaccharides and enhances the secretion of TNF-alpha and IL-12 in humans and the activation of mononuclear cells [53–55]. Other adipokines hyperexpressed in IBD seem to be visfatin and apelin which have significant proinflammatory activity, while the exact role of adiponectin is not clear yet [56, 57].

Skeletal homeostasis is a complex system, influenced by a delicate balance between bone formation and reabsorption, a process called bone remodeling. This delicate process is coordinated by a number of factors, severely impaired in patients with IBD. Although the pathogenic mechanism of bone loss in IBD has a multifactorial etiology, it is now clear that chronic inflammation plays a crucial role through inflammatory mediators like TNF-alpha, IL-6, and IL-1. In particular, these cytokines dysregulate the receptor activator of nuclear factor κB ligand (RANKL) osteoprotegerin (OPG) system: normally RANKL is a strong activator of osteoclastogenesis, while OPG is linked with osteoblastogenesis; thus the interaction of RANK on the surface of osteoclasts with its ligand RANKL induces osteoclastogenesis and conversely the interaction with the osteoblast derived soluble decoy receptor; osteoprotegerin (OPG) blocks RANK interaction inhibiting osteoclasts formation [58, 59]. In experimental models, proinflammatory cytokines induce RANKL and promote bone reabsorption with consecutive bone loss; moreover, activated T cells can directly trigger osteoclastogenesis through RANKL leading to bone [60].

Furthermore, it is now clear that bone metabolism is directly influenced by adipose tissue. Adipokines, indeed, seem to interfere in bone metabolism by altering the sensitive balance between osteoblasts and osteoclasts: in particular, resistin seems to increase the number of differentiated osteoclasts and stimulate the NF-kB promoter activity; when administered in vivo [61], adiponectin has a negative correlation with bone mass in vivo [62].

6. Nutritional Assessment of Inflammatory Bowel Disease

The assessment of nutritional status in IBD is the first step to identify malnutrition and/or sarcopenia status in order to set adequate and customized therapeutic regimens.

A correct nutritional assessment provides quantitative and qualitative evaluations, so that effectiveness of nutritional support could be measured and evaluated over time.

An accurate assessment of nutritional status could account for differential methods and diagnostic indicators, as a unique laboratory or instrumental marker is not available.

Main steps in a full evaluation require assessment of the energy balance, assessing anthropometric data, considering biochemical and clinical evaluation, and use of instrumental data.

The assessment of the energy balance is needed to establish the proper nutritional intervention and can be calculated on the basis of caloric intake and energy expenditure of patients with IBD. The caloric intake can be estimated by collecting food chart on eating habits (quantity and quality). Although the best estimation on energy expenditure can be measured by indirect calorimetry or predictive formulas, in current clinical practice, the formula of Harris-Benedict (rated basal metabolism or BEE) in combination with the possible factors of stress (TEE Kcal/day = BEE × stress factor) could be considered [63].

The evaluation of body composition needs to consider weight, height, BMI (body mass index), and body circumferences.

The body circumferences are indicators of the transverse dimensions of the body segments and of the muscle-fat areas of limbs; these parameters could be useful in patients with IBD to estimate nutritional status. Arm's and calf circumferences are the most useful indicators for the evaluation of energy reserves and muscle mass, also included in the evaluation test for screening malnutrition, known as MNA test.

BMI values <18.5 kg/m^2 are considered indicators of malnutrition [64], whereas values >25 kg/m^2 indicate overweight; patients with a BMI over >30 kg/m^2 are considered obese, while persons with a value inferior to 14-15 kg/m^2 of BMI are at risk for increased mortality due to malnutrition.

A full characterization of the body composition could be reached by the determination of lean body mass and adipose tissue, using specialized machineries, including dual-energy X-ray absorptiometry (DEXA), Bioimpedentiometry (BIA), TOBEC (Total Body Electrical Conductivity), ultrasound, CT (computed tomography), infrared interactance, and NMR (Nuclear Magnetic Resonance).

Among these, BIA and DEXA are considered the gold standard for measuring body composition [65].

DEXA is based on the principle of X-ray attenuation administered at two different energy levels; according to the intensity of the radiation registered after the passage through the tissues, the bone tissue can be differentiated from the soft parts, such as adipose tissue and muscle. The DEXA gives information on bone mineralization.

The BIA is an indirect technique for measuring body composition based on two physical principles: resistance (Rz) and reactance.

The resistance is the ability of all biological structures to "resist" (to counteract) the passage of electricity and it is inversely proportional to the water content: lean tissues are good conductors (containing water and electrolytes), while fatty tissues and bones are poor conductors (containing little water).

The reactance (Xc) is the opposing force to electricity measured at cell membranes levels; fat mass has low reactance, while lean body mass has high reactance.

The combined analysis of the two data allows us to calculate a new parameter, called "phase angle." In healthy subjects, normal values are considered between 6° and 8°; increased catabolic conditions like sarcopenia associated with decrease in these values below 6, while phase angle increases for muscle hypertrophy. Approximately, values of the phase angle under 4,5° indicate a possible expansion of the extracellular space and loss of cell membranes in forms of protein-energy malnutrition.

Among other methods, TOBEC (Total Body Electrical Conductivity) needs further explanation. It is based on the difference of electrical conductivity between lean and fat tissues. The electricity generates a weak magnetic field in a cylindrical chamber whose strength is related to the body composition. In about 10 seconds, TOBEC estimated lean body mass. It accounts for good accuracy, safety, and reliability; however, it cannot be used in case of major changes in weight or distributions of water or electrolytes [66].

The use of ultrasound on lean mass evaluation is limited, as it is strongly dependent on the operator [67].

Infrared interactance, based on the principle of absorption and reflection of spectroscopic light, has good potential but its application is limited [66].

CT is a technique that uses ionizing radiation to examine sections or layers body; despite its high accuracy, cost and radiation exposure do not justify its use in clinical practice.

The NMR (Nuclear Magnetic Resonance) is based on the principle of magnetic fields. NMR can be used for evaluation of the amount of total fat mass and analysis of the regional distribution of adipose tissue. The high cost of the instrumentation and the low practicality do not justify its use in the common practice.

Tables and nutritional questionnaires have been proposed to standardize the nutritional evaluation, assessing several items by numerical scores. Thanks to that, a degree of "the nutritional risk" associated with malnutrition is provided in order to influence the choice of the nutritional intervention.

The main screening tests for malnutrition are the following [68]:

(a) Instant Nutritional Assessment (INA)

(b) Malnutrition Universal Screening Tool (MUST)

(c) Nutritional Risk Screening (NRS)

(d) Mini Nutritional Assessment (MNA)

(e) Subjective Global Assessment (SGA)

INA, also called LAW (acronym coming from the first letters of each studied parameter), is based on three parameters: the count of lymphocytes in the blood, serum albumin, and the weight change per unit of time.

MUST, developed in the UK by the Malnutrition Advisory Group, is designed to identify patients at risk of malnutrition, which could benefit from nutritional intervention; it was first developed for community medicine but it had good success on hospitals evaluations because of its simplicity, reliability, and validity [69]. The nutritional risk is assessed with the identification of weight and height to calculate BMI, assessment of unintentional weight loss in the last 3–6 months, and the presence of any acute medical condition, in which there was an insufficient food intake calculated for a

period equal to or greater than 5 days. The total score ranges from 0 to 2, indicating the presence of a mild, moderate, or severe risk of malnutrition (low risk = 0, moderate risk = 1, and severe risk = 2) [70].

NRS is commonly used for hospitalized patients [71]. It starts by same parameters of MUST, adding the degree of severity of diseases and age.

NRS 2002 is divided into two parts: an initial screening consisting in 4 questions (BMI below 20.5, weight loss in the last three months, reduced food intake in the last week, and the presence of severe acute disease) and a second part consisting in the evaluation of degree of malnutrition associated with the severity of the disease and age. The second part of the questionnaire is completed if at least one of the four initial questions is positive; a score higher than 3 identifies patients at higher nutritional risk. These last patients require stronger therapeutic intervention.

MNA is a screening test for malnutrition mainly used in elderly people. It includes the assessments of general evaluation (lifestyle, physical activity, and medication), food chart analysis (number of meals, dysphagia, and autonomy), subjective symptoms (patient's perception of the health and nutrition), and detection of anthropometric parameters (reduction weight, BMI, circumference, and skinfolds). A total score below 17 is indicative of malnutrition, while a score between 17 and 23.5 is indicative of risk of malnutrition and a score greater than 24 indicates a good nutritional state [72]. MNA requires approximately 10 minutes, and that is one of the main reasons of success, as it is used in a large number of studies.

SGA is based on a standardized questionnaire that includes medical history (variations before treatment calorie, weight loss, gastrointestinal symptoms, and functional capacity) and goals (signs of malnutrition with the presence of edema and/or changing the dial fat and muscle) [73].

7. Conclusions

Nutritional aspects in inflammatory bowel disease are particularly relevant as they could potently contribute to disease morbidity and mobility. It can be argued that a poor nutritional status, selective malnutrition or sarcopenia, can be associated with poor clinical outcomes, response to therapy, and quality of life. For this reason, a multidisciplinary assessment of IBD is to be sustained, making closer gastroenterological assessment and nutritional assessment in a broader and harmonically defined picture, where instruments, clinical mind, and evaluation come closer.

Competing Interests

The authors declare that they have no competing interests.

Authors' Contributions

F. Scaldaferri and M. Pizzoferrato share equal contribution.

Acknowledgments

This work has been supported by Linea D.3.2-2013 grant (Catholic University of Sacred Heart) and Crohn's and Colitis Foundation of America (Research Fellowship Award, CON125252, to L. R. Lopetuso).

References

[1] R. Weisshof and I. Chermesh, "Micronutrient deficiencies in inflammatory bowel disease," *Current Opinion in Clinical Nutrition and Metabolic Care*, vol. 18, no. 6, pp. 576–581, 2015.

[2] E. Capristo, G. Mingrone, G. Addolorato, A. V. Greco, and G. Gasbarrini, "Metabolic features of inflammatory bowel disease in a remission phase of the disease activity," *Journal of Internal Medicine*, vol. 243, no. 5, pp. 339–347, 1998.

[3] R. Rocha, G. O. Santana, N. Almeida, and A. C. Lyra, "Analysis of fat and muscle mass in patients with inflammatory bowel disease during remission and active phase," *The British Journal of Nutrition*, vol. 101, no. 5, pp. 676–679, 2009.

[4] L. Valentini, L. Schaper, C. Buning et al., "Malnutrition and impaired muscle strength in patients with Crohn's disease and ulcerative colitis in remission," *Nutrition*, vol. 24, no. 7-8, pp. 694–702, 2008.

[5] R. J. Hill, G. J. Cleghorn, G. D. Withers et al., "Resting energy expenditure in children with inflammatory bowel disease," *Journal of Pediatric Gastroenterology and Nutrition*, vol. 45, no. 3, pp. 342–346, 2007.

[6] A. E. Wiskin, S. A. Wootton, T. M. Hunt et al., "Body composition in childhood inflammatory bowel disease," *Clinical Nutrition*, vol. 30, no. 1, pp. 112–115, 2011.

[7] L. R. Barot, J. L. Rombeau, I. D. Feurer, and J. L. Mullen, "Caloric requirements in patients with inflammatory bowel disease," *Annals of Surgery*, vol. 195, no. 2, pp. 214–218, 1982.

[8] X. Hébuterne, J. Filippi, R. Al-Jaouni, and S. Schneider, "Nutritional consequences and nutrition therapy in Crohn's disease," *Gastroentérologie Clinique et Biologique*, vol. 33, supplement 3, pp. S235–S244, 2009.

[9] A. J. Lucendo and L. C. De Rezende, "Importance of nutrition in inflammatory bowel disease," *World Journal of Gastroenterology*, vol. 15, no. 17, pp. 2081–2088, 2009.

[10] E. Capristo, G. Addolorato, G. Mingrone, A. V. Greco, and G. Gasbarrini, "Effect of disease localization on the anthropometric and metabolic features of Crohn's disease," *The American Journal of Gastroenterology*, vol. 93, no. 12, pp. 2411–2419, 1998.

[11] F. K. Ghishan and P. R. Kiela, "Epithelial transport in inflammatory bowel diseases," *Inflammatory Bowel Diseases*, vol. 20, no. 6, pp. 1099–1109, 2014.

[12] A. P. S. Urbano, L. Y. Sassaki, M. S. Dorna, M. A. B. L. Carvalhaes, L. A. Martini, and A. L. A. Ferreira, "Nutritional intake according to injury extent in ulcerative colitis patients," *Journal of Human Nutrition and Dietetics*, vol. 26, no. 5, pp. 445–451, 2013.

[13] N. Vaisman, I. Dotan, A. Halack, and E. Niv, "Malabsorption is a major contributor to underweight in Crohn's disease patients in remission," *Nutrition*, vol. 22, no. 9, pp. 855–859, 2006.

[14] G. Juckett and R. Trivedi, "Evaluation of chronic diarrhea," *American Family Physician*, vol. 84, no. 10, pp. 1119–1126, 2011.

[15] C. Hwang, V. Ross, and U. Mahadevan, "Micronutrient deficiencies in inflammatory bowel disease: from A to zinc," *Inflammatory Bowel Diseases*, vol. 18, no. 10, pp. 1961–1981, 2012.

[16] L. R. Barot, J. L. Rombeau, J. J. Steinberg, L. O. Crosby, I. D. Feurer, and J. L. Mullen, "Energy expenditure in patients with inflammatory bowel disease," *Archives of Surgery*, vol. 116, no. 4, pp. 460–462, 1981.

[17] A. U. Dignass, C. Gasche, D. Bettenworth et al., "European consensus on the diagnosis and management of iron deficiency and anaemia in inflammatory bowel diseases," *Journal of Crohn's & colitis*, vol. 9, no. 3, pp. 211–222, 2015.

[18] R. A. Alves, S. J. Miszputen, and M. S. Figueiredo, "Anemia in inflammatory bowel disease: prevalence, differential diagnosis and association with clinical and laboratory variables," *Sao Paulo Medical Journal*, vol. 132, no. 3, pp. 140–146, 2014.

[19] G. Weiss and C. Gasche, "Pathogenesis and treatment of anemia in inflammatory bowel disease," *Haematologica*, vol. 95, no. 2, pp. 175–178, 2010.

[20] G. Rogler and S. Vavricka, "Anemia in inflammatory bowel disease: an under-estimated problem?" *Frontiers in Medicine*, vol. 1, 2015.

[21] F. Bermejo, A. Algaba, I. Guerra et al., "Should we monitor vitamin B12 and folate levels in Crohn's disease patients?" *Scandinavian Journal of Gastroenterology*, vol. 48, no. 11, pp. 1272–1277, 2013.

[22] M. Yakut, Y. Üstün, G. Kabaçam, and I. Soykan, "Serum vitamin B12 and folate status in patients with inflammatory bowel diseases," *European Journal of Internal Medicine*, vol. 21, no. 4, pp. 320–323, 2010.

[23] Y. Erzin, H. Uzun, A. F. Celik, S. Aydin, A. Dirican, and H. Uzunismail, "Hyperhomocysteinemia in inflammatory bowel disease patients without past intestinal resections: correlations with cobalamin, pyridoxine, folate concentrations, acute phase reactants, disease activity, and prior thromboembolic complications," *Journal of Clinical Gastroenterology*, vol. 42, no. 5, pp. 481–486, 2008.

[24] K. Vagianos and C. N. Bernstein, "Homocysteinemia and B vitamin status among adult patients with inflammatory bowel disease: a one-year prospective follow-up study," *Inflammatory Bowel Diseases*, vol. 18, no. 4, pp. 718–724, 2012.

[25] J. Kong, Z. Zhang, M. W. Musch et al., "Novel role of the vitamin D receptor in maintaining the integrity of the intestinal mucosal barrier," *American Journal of Physiology—Gastrointestinal and Liver Physiology*, vol. 294, no. 1, pp. G208–G216, 2008.

[26] A. N. Ananthakrishnan, H. Khalili, L. M. Higuchi et al., "Higher predicted vitamin D status is associated with reduced risk of crohn's disease," *Gastroenterology*, vol. 142, no. 3, pp. 482–489, 2012.

[27] R. V. Bryant, M. J. Trott, F. D. Bartholomeusz, and J. M. Andrews, "Systematic review: body composition in adults with inflammatory bowel disease," *Alimentary Pharmacology & Therapeutics*, vol. 38, no. 3, pp. 213–225, 2013.

[28] A. J. Cruz-Jentoft, J. P. Baeyens, J. M. Bauer et al., "Sarcopenia: European consensus on definition and diagnosis," *Age and Ageing*, vol. 39, no. 4, Article ID afq034, pp. 412–423, 2010.

[29] V. Santilli, A. Bernetti, M. Mangone, and M. Paoloni, "Clinical definition of sarcopenia," *Clinical Cases in Mineral and Bone Metabolism*, vol. 11, no. 3, pp. 177–180, 2014.

[30] R. V. Bryant, S. Ooi, C. G. Schultz et al., "Low muscle mass and sarcopenia: common and predictive of osteopenia in inflammatory bowel disease," *Alimentary Pharmacology & Therapeutics*, vol. 41, no. 9, pp. 895–906, 2015.

[31] A. Flores, E. Burstein, D. J. Cipher, and L. A. Feagins, "Obesity in inflammatory bowel disease: a marker of less severe disease,"

Digestive Diseases and Sciences, vol. 60, no. 8, pp. 2436–2445, 2015.

[32] A. Blain, S. Cattan, L. Beaugerie, F. Carbonnel, J. P. Gendre, and J. Cosnes, "Crohn's disease clinical course and severity in obese patients," *Clinical Nutrition*, vol. 21, pp. 51–57, 2002.

[33] J. L. Seminerio, I. E. Koutroubakis, C. Ramos-Rivers et al., "Impact of obesity on the management and clinical course of patients with inflammatory bowel disease," *Inflammatory Bowel Diseases*, vol. 21, no. 12, pp. 2857–2863, 2015.

[34] J. W. Harper, M. N. Sinanan, and T. L. Zisman, "Increased body mass index is associated with earlier time to loss of response to infliximab in patients with inflammatory bowel disease," *Inflammatory Bowel Diseases*, vol. 19, no. 10, pp. 2118–2124, 2013.

[35] D. Costamagna, P. Costelli, M. Sampaolesi, and F. Penna, "Role of inflammation in muscle homeostasis and myogenesis," *Mediators of Inflammation*, vol. 2015, Article ID 805172, 14 pages, 2015.

[36] P. Gonçalves, F. Magro, and F. Martel, "Metabolic inflammation in inflammatory bowel disease: crosstalk between adipose tissue and bowel," *Inflammatory Bowel Diseases*, vol. 21, no. 2, pp. 453–467, 2015.

[37] S. Terzoudis, C. Zavos, and I. E. Koutroubakis, "The bone and fat connection in inflammatory bowel diseases," *Inflammatory Bowel Diseases*, vol. 20, no. 11, pp. 2207–2217, 2014.

[38] R. C. Olney, "Regulation of bone mass by growth hormone," *Medical and Pediatric Oncology*, vol. 41, no. 3, pp. 228–234, 2003.

[39] L. M. Difedele, J. He, E. L. Bonkowski et al., "Tumor necrosis factor α blockade restores growth hormone signaling in murine colitis," *Gastroenterology*, vol. 128, no. 5, pp. 1278–1291, 2005.

[40] C. Mammucari, S. Schiaffino, and M. Sandri, "Downstream of Akt: FoxO3 and mTOR in the regulation of autophagy in skeletal muscle," *Autophagy*, vol. 4, no. 4, pp. 524–526, 2008.

[41] L. A. Denson, M. A. Held, R. K. Menon, S. J. Frank, A. F. Parlow, and D. L. Arnold, "Interleukin-6 inhibits hepatic growth hormone signaling via upregulation of Cis and Socs-3," *American Journal of Physiology—Gastrointestinal and Liver Physiology*, vol. 284, no. 4, pp. G646–G654, 2003.

[42] A. U. Trendelenburg, A. Meyer, D. Rohner, J. Boyle, S. Hatakeyama, and D. J. Glass, "Myostatin reduces Akt/TORC1/p70S6K signaling, inhibiting myoblast differentiation and myotube size," *American Journal of Physiology—Cell Physiology*, vol. 296, no. 6, pp. C1258–C1270, 2009.

[43] R. S. Ahima and H.-K. Park, "Connecting myokines and metabolism," *Endocrinology and Metabolism*, vol. 30, no. 3, pp. 235–245, 2015.

[44] N. Bakkar, J. Wang, K. J. Ladner et al., "IKK/NF-κB regulates skeletal myogenesis via a signaling switch to inhibit differentiation and promote mitochondrial biogenesis," *The Journal of Cell Biology*, vol. 180, no. 4, pp. 787–802, 2008.

[45] E. A. Greco, A. Lenzi, and S. Migliaccio, "The obesity of bone," *Therapeutic Advances in Endocrinology and Metabolism*, vol. 6, no. 6, pp. 273–286, 2015.

[46] R. W. Grant and V. D. Dixit, "Adipose tissue as an immunological organ," *Obesity*, vol. 23, no. 3, pp. 512–518, 2015.

[47] I. Olivier, V. Théodorou, P. Valet et al., "Is Crohn's creeping fat an adipose tissue?" *Inflammatory Bowel Diseases*, vol. 17, no. 3, pp. 747–757, 2011.

[48] N. R. Borley, N. J. Mortensen, D. P. Jewell, and B. F. Warren, "The relationship between inflammatory and serosal connective tissue changes in ileal Crohn's disease: evidence for a possible causative link," *Journal of Pathology*, vol. 190, no. 2, pp. 196–202, 2000.

[49] A. Gambero, M. Maróstica, M. J. A. Saad, and J. Pedrazzoli Jr., "Mesenteric adipose tissue alterations resulting from experimental reactivated colitis," *Inflammatory Bowel Diseases*, vol. 13, no. 11, pp. 1357–1364, 2007.

[50] G. Paul, A. Schäffler, M. Neumeier et al., "Profiling adipocytokine secretion from creeping fat in Crohn's disease," *Inflammatory Bowel Diseases*, vol. 12, no. 6, pp. 471–477, 2006.

[51] G. Frühbeck, "Intracellular signalling pathways activated by leptin," *The Biochemical Journal*, vol. 393, no. 1, pp. 7–20, 2006.

[52] K. Karmiris, I. E. Koutroubakis, and E. A. Kouroumalis, "Leptin, adiponectin, resistin, and ghrelin—implications for inflammatory bowel disease," *Molecular Nutrition & Food Research*, vol. 52, no. 8, pp. 855–866, 2008.

[53] X.-D. Peng, H. Xie, Q. Zhao, X.-P. Wu, Z.-Q. Sun, and E.-Y. Liao, "Relationships between serum adiponectin, leptin, resistin, visfatin levels and bone mineral density, and bone biochemical markers in Chinese men," *Clinica Chimica Acta*, vol. 387, no. 1-2, pp. 31–35, 2008.

[54] N. Silswal, A. K. Singh, B. Aruna, S. Mukhopadhyay, S. Ghosh, and N. Z. Ehtesham, "Human resistin stimulates the proinflammatory cytokines TNF-α and IL-12 in macrophages by NF-κB-dependent pathway," *Biochemical and Biophysical Research Communications*, vol. 334, no. 4, pp. 1092–1101, 2005.

[55] A. Konrad, M. Lehrke, V. Schachinger et al., "Resistin is an inflammatory marker of inflammatory bowel disease in humans," *European Journal of Gastroenterology & Hepatology*, vol. 19, no. 12, pp. 1070–1074, 2007.

[56] A. Fukuhara, M. Matsuda, M. Nishizawa et al., "Visfatin: a protein secreted by visceral fat that Mimics the effects of insulin," *Science*, vol. 307, no. 5708, pp. 426–430, 2005.

[57] S. Han, G. Wang, S. Qiu et al., "Increased colonic apelin production in rodents with experimental colitis and in humans with IBD," *Regulatory Peptides*, vol. 142, no. 3, pp. 131–137, 2007.

[58] J. E. Aubin and E. Bonnelye, "Osteoprotegerin and its ligand: a new paradigm for regulation of osteoclastogenesis and bone resorption," *Medscape Women's Health*, vol. 5, article 5, 2000.

[59] J. E. Aubin and E. Bonnelye, "Osteoprotegerin and its ligand: a new paradigm for regulation of osteoclastogenesis and bone resorption," *Osteoporosis International*, vol. 11, no. 11, pp. 905–913, 2000.

[60] Y.-Y. Kong, W. J. Boyle, and J. M. Penninger, "Osteoprotegerin ligand: a common link between osteoclastogenesis, lymph node formation and lymphocyte development," *Immunology and Cell Biology*, vol. 77, no. 2, pp. 188–193, 1999.

[61] L. Thommesen, A. K. Stunes, M. Monjo et al., "Expression and regulation of resistin in osteoblasts and osteoclasts indicate a role in bone metabolism," *Journal of Cellular Biochemistry*, vol. 99, no. 3, pp. 824–834, 2006.

[62] Y. Shinoda, M. Yamaguchi, N. Ogata et al., "Regulation of bone formation by adiponectin through autocrine/paracrine and endocrine pathways," *Journal of Cellular Biochemistry*, vol. 99, no. 1, pp. 196–208, 2006.

[63] J. M. Miles, "Energy expenditure in hospitalized patients: implications for nutritional support," *Mayo Clinic Proceedings*, vol. 81, no. 6, pp. 809–816, 2006.

[64] D. D. Mijač, G. L. J. Janković, J. Jorga, and M. N. Krstić, "Nutritional status in patients with active inflammatory bowel disease: prevalence of malnutrition and methods for routine nutritional assessment," *European Journal of Internal Medicine*, vol. 21, no. 4, pp. 315–319, 2010.

[65] D. Royall, G. R. Greenberg, J. P. Allard, J. P. Baker, J. E. Harrison, and K. N. Jeejeebhoy, "Critical assessment of body-composition measurements in malnourished subjects with Crohn's disease: the role of bioelectric impedance analysis," *The American Journal of Clinical Nutrition*, vol. 59, no. 2, pp. 325–330, 1994.

[66] H. C. Lukaski, "Methods for the assessment of human body composition: traditional and new," *American Journal of Clinical Nutrition*, vol. 46, no. 4, pp. 537–556, 1987.

[67] D. R. Wagner, "Ultrasound as a tool to assess body fat," *Journal of Obesity*, vol. 2013, Article ID 280713, 9 pages, 2013.

[68] J. Kondrup, S. P. Allison, M. Elia, B. Vellas, and M. Plauth, "ESPEN guidelines for nutrition screening 2002," *Clinical Nutrition*, vol. 22, no. 4, pp. 415–421, 2003.

[69] A. Sandhu, M. Mosli, B. Yan et al., "Self-screening for malnutrition risk in outpatient inflammatory bowel disease patients using the Malnutrition Universal Screening Tool (MUST)," *Journal of Parenteral and Enteral Nutrition*, vol. 40, no. 4, pp. 507–510, 2016.

[70] C. A. Schneider, E. Ferrannini, R. Defronzo, G. Schernthaner, J. Yates, and E. Erdmann, "Effect of pioglitazone on cardiovascular outcome in diabetes and chronic kidney disease," *Journal of the American Society of Nephrology*, vol. 19, no. 1, pp. 182–187, 2008.

[71] J. Kondrup, H. H. Ramussen, O. Hamberg et al., "Nutritional risk screening (NRS 2002): a new method based on an analysis of controlled clinical trials," *Clinical Nutrition*, vol. 22, no. 3, pp. 321–336, 2003.

[72] A. M. Beck, L. Ovesen, and M. Osler, "The 'Mini Nutritional Assessment' (MNA) and the 'Determine Your Nutritional Health' Checklist (NSI Checklist) as predictors of morbidity and mortality in an elderly Danish population," *British Journal of Nutrition*, vol. 81, no. 1, pp. 31–36, 1999.

[73] A. S. Detsky, J. R. McLaughlin, J. P. Baker et al., "What is subjective global assessment of nutritional status?" *Journal of Parenteral and Enteral Nutrition*, vol. 11, no. 1, pp. 8–13, 1987.

19

Association of Fucosyltransferase 2 Gene Polymorphisms with Inflammatory Bowel Disease in Patients from Southeast China

Hao Wu,[1,2] Liang Sun,[2] Dao-po Lin,[2] Xiao-xiao Shao,[2] Sheng-long Xia,[2] and Ming Lv[1]

[1]Qilu Hospital, Shandong University, Ji'nan, Shandong 250012, China
[2]Department of Gastroenterology, The Second Affiliated Hospital, Wenzhou Medical University, Wenzhou, China

Correspondence should be addressed to Ming Lv; lvming@sdu.edu.cn

Academic Editor: Paolo Gionchetti

Aims. Fucosyltransferase 2 (*FUT2*) gene potentially affects the constituent of intestinal microbiota, which play a crucial role in the pathogenesis of inflammatory bowel disease (IBD). This study investigated the association of *FUT2* gene polymorphisms with IBD in southeast China. *Methods.* We collected 671 IBD patients and 502 healthy controls. *FUT2* gene polymorphisms (C357T, A385T, and G428A) were determined by SNaPshot. Frequencies of the *FUT2* genotypes, alleles, and haplotype between groups were compared by χ^2 test. *Results.* The allele and genotype frequencies of *FUT2* did not differ between ulcerative colitis patients and controls (all $P > 0.05$). However, mutant allele and genotype of *FUT2* (A385T) were significantly increased in Crohn's disease (CD) patients ($P = 0.024$, OR = 1.271, and 95% CI = 1.031–1.565; $P < 0.001$, OR = 1.927, and 95% CI = 1.353–2.747, resp.). The same conclusion was drawn from *FUT2* (G428A) ($P = 0.023$, OR = 3.324, and 95% CI = 1.108–9.968; $P = 0.044$, OR = 1.116–10.137, and 95% CI = 1.116–10.137, resp.). The haplotype TT formed with "C357T and A385T" was more prevalent in CD patients than in controls ($P = 0.020$, OR = 1.277, and 95% CI = 1.036–1.573). Besides, frequencies of mutant allele and genotype of *FUT2* (A385T) were significantly lower in patients with ileocolonic CD than in those with colonic CD ($P = 0.001$ and 0.002, resp.) and ileal CD ($P = 0.007$ and 0.004, resp.). *Conclusions.* FUT2 gene polymorphisms and haplotypes were associated with the susceptibility to CD but not UC.

1. Introduction

Inflammatory bowel disease (IBD), including ulcerative colitis (UC) and Crohn's disease (CD), has a rising global incidence rate in recent years [1, 2]. Although the pathogenesis of IBD is not yet fully clarified, it has been suggested to involve factors such as the environment, heredity, infection, and immunity. Gene polymorphisms in *NOD2, ATG16L1,* and *IRGM* have been commonly accepted as host factors in the predisposition of CD in western countries. However, these gene polymorphisms were not related to the predisposition of CD in Chinese population [3, 4], except for a new variant (P268S) in *NOD2* [5]. Hence, it is of interest to identify new susceptibility gene in IBD in Chinese Han population.

Fucosyltransferase (FUT) 2 gene is located in the q13 region of chromosome 19. The protein encoded by this gene, α-(1,2)-fucosyltransferase, is a Golgi stack membrane protein involved in the creation of a precursor of the H antigen, which forms the basis of A and B antigen synthesis. The ABH antigens are the antigens widely expressed in the stomach and small intestine. However, the expression of ABH antigens decreases progressively from the proximal to the distal colon and almost disappears in the rectum in the gastrointestinal (GI) tract [6]. Numerous studies have showed that human histoblood group antigens (HBGA), namely, ABH antigens and Lewis antigens, serve as receptors for norovirus capsid protein attachment and play a critical role in infection [7]. ABH antigens also function as receptors for *Campylobacter jejuni* [8] and rotavirus [9]. Moreover, these antigens can act as a carbon source providing energy for the metabolism of certain bacteria (e.g., the *Escherichia coli*) [10].

It has been suggested that *FUT2* gene polymorphisms may affect the predisposition of celiac disease [11], type 1 diabetes [12], and primary sclerosing cholangitis [13]. McGovern et al. reported in Caucasian population that FUT2 nonsecretor status is associated with Crohn's disease [14].

TABLE 1: Demographic characteristics of IBD patients and the controls.

Characteristics	UC	CD	Controls	P value
Total number	396	275	502	
Sex (female/male)	164/232	121/154	226/276	0.549
Age (years) [mean (SD)]	38.98 (16.01)	36.23 (15.25)	37.05 (14.99)	0.051
Age of onset (years) [mean (SD)]	33.04 (13.81)	31.20 (15.67)		0.109
Smoker/nonsmoker	69/327	56/219	82/420	0.376

UC, ulcerative colitis. CD, Crohn's disease. SD, standard deviation. P values were calculated by t-test or chi-squared test.

The role of *FUT2* gene in UC has also been investigated, but the results seem to lack consistency [11, 15]. Therefore, this study aimed to explore the relationship between *FUT2* gene polymorphism and IBD susceptibility in the Chinese population, which might provide a genetic basis for the mechanism of IBD and find potential new therapeutic targets.

2. Materials and Methods

2.1. Study Subjects. From March 2012 to March 2014, a total of 671 IBD patients, including 396 UC patients and 275 CD patients, were recruited from The Second Affiliated Hospital of Wenzhou Medical University, The First Affiliated Hospital of Wenzhou Medical University, Wenzhou Central Hospital, and Wenzhou People's Hospital in Wenzhou city, Zhejiang province of Southeast China. The diagnoses of UC and CD were made by means of endoscope, in collaboration with clinical, histopathological, and radiologic findings according to Lennard-Jones Criteria [16]. The severity of UC was evaluated by Truelove and Witt Activity Index [17]. The lesion location and behavior were evaluated on the basis of the Montreal Classification [16]. A total of 502 age- and sex-matched healthy controls were collected at the Health Examination Center of The Second Affiliated Hospital of Wenzhou Medical University, after excluding autoimmune diseases, tumors, and IBD family history. The study protocol was in line with the Treaty of Helsinki and was approved by Ethics Committees of the three hospitals mentioned above. The written informed consent was obtained.

2.2. Genomic DNA Extraction and Genotyping Analysis. Approximately 3 mL of the peripheral blood was obtained from each subject into an EDTA tube. DNeasy Blood & Tissue Kit (Qiagen GmbH) was applied for the extraction of genomic DNA from the peripheral blood according to the manufacturer's instructions. Then the genomic DNA was diluted to a concentration of 10 ng/μL and stored at 4°C for subsequent identification of genetic mutations.

The amplification primers of *FUT2* were designed as follows: $5'$ TCAACATCAAAGGCACTGGGACC $3'$ (forward) and $5'$ TGGCGGAGGTGGTGGTAGAA $3'$ (reverse). A multiplex SNaPshot assay (Applied Biosystems, California, USA) was employed to determine the genotypes. Firstly, 10 ng of genomic DNA was added to a 10 μL PCR mixture containing 20 μmol dNTPs (Promega, Wisconsin, USA), 0.5 U of FastStart Taq DNA polymerase (Roche, Basel, Switzerland), 1 μL 10x PCR buffer with $MgCl_2$ (15 mmol/L) (Roche, Basel,

Switzerland), and amplification primers with a terminal concentration of 0.1 μmol/L. The thermal cycler conditions of multiplex PCR amplification were as follows: initial denaturation at 95°C for 5 min and amplification for 35 cycles at 95°C for 30 s, 65°C for 30 s, and 72°C for 1 min, followed by a final elongation step at 72°C for 10 min. Subsequently, the PCR products were examined by electrophoresis in a 2.5% agarose gel. Secondly, we purified the PCR products using a mix of 2 U of Exonuclease I (TaKaRa, Dalian, China) and 1.5 U of shrimp alkaline phosphatase (SAP) (New England Biolabs, Massachusetts, USA) at 37°C for 80 min and then 85°C for 15 min. Thirdly, the multiplex SNaPshot sequencing reactions were performed in a final volume of 7 μL containing 2 μL of purified multiple PCR products, 1 μL of SNaPshot Multiplex Mix, 1 μL of 5x sequencing buffer (Applied Biosystems), and 3 μL of SNaPshot sequencing primers (C357T: **18T**-TGGCAGAACTACCACCTGAA; A385T: **38T**-TGGAGGAGGAATACCGCCAC; G428A: CACCGGCTAC-CCCTGCTCCT). The thermal cycler conditions were an initial denaturation at 96°C for 1 min followed by 25 cycles at 96°C for 10 s, 52°C for 5 s, and 60°C for 30 s. Then the depuration of product was performed with 1 U of SAP at 37°C for 60 min and 75°C for 15 min. Finally, 1.5 μL of SNaPshot products was genotyped in the platform of ABI 3730 Genetic Analyzer before they were mixed with 8 μL of HiDi™ formamide and 0.5 μL of GeneScan-120LIZ size standard (Applied Biosystems). Data were analyzed by GeneMapper 4.0 (Applied Biosystems). In order to guarantee the quality of the study, about 3 percent of the samples were randomly selected and regenotyped by direct sequencing. Consequently, the results from regenotyping and SNaPshot were in complete accordance with the originals.

2.3. Statistical Analysis. The data were analyzed by statistical software SPSS 17.0. The *chi-square* test (χ^2) was applied to analyze the accordance with Hardy-Weinberg equilibrium and the differences in the distribution of alleles and genotypes. Software Haploview 4.2 was employed to analyze the linkage disequilibrium and haplotype. A two-tailed P value less than 0.05 was considered significant.

3. Results

3.1. Characteristics of IBD Patients and Controls. The demographic data of UC patients, CD patients, and the controls are presented in Table 1. The 396 UC patients were composed of 250 patients with distal colitis and 146 with extensive colitis

TABLE 2: FUT2 gene polymorphisms in patients with inflammatory bowel disease (IBD) and the controls.

FUT2	Controls	UC	CD	UC versus Controls		CD versus Controls	
	n (%)	n (%)	n (%)	OR (95% CI)	P	OR (95% CI)	P
C357T							
TT	379	292	217	1		1	
TC (additive model)	112	91	57	1.055 (0.759–1.463)	0.742	0.889 (0.608–1.291)	0.521
CC (additive model)	11	13	1	1.534 (0.624–3.839)	0.302	0.159 (0.004–0.996)	0.045
Dominant model (TC+CC versus TT)				1.097 (0.811–1.485)	0.547	0.824 (0.578–1.173)	0.282
Recessive model (CC versus TT+TC)				1.515 (0.671–3.419)	0.314	0.824 (0.578–1.173)	0.282
Allele frequency model (C allele versus T allele)				1.125 (0.861–1.471)	0.387	0.780 (0.563–1.080)	0.134
A385T							
AA	150	122	80	1		1	
AT (additive model)	269	204	119	0.932 (0.691–1.259)	0.648	0.829 (0.586–1.1773)	0.290
TT (additive model)	83	70	76	1.037 (0.697–1.544)	0.858	**1.717 (1.136–2.594)**	**0.010**
Dominant model (AT+TT versus AA)				0.957 (0.719–1.274)	0.764	1.039 (0.752–1.435)	0.818
Recessive model (TT versus AA+AT)				1.084 (0.764–1.537)	0.651	**0.519 (0.364–0.739)**	**0.000**
Allele frequency model (T allele versus A allele)				1.004 (0.832–1.212)	0.964	**1.271 (1.031–1.565)**	**0.024**
G428A							
GG	497	392	266	1		1	
GA (additive model)	5	4	9	1.014 (0.271–3.802)	0.983	**3.363 (1.116–10.137)**	**0.044**
AA (additive model)	0	0	0	NA		NA	
Dominant model (GA+AA versus GG)				1.014 (0.271–3.802)	0.983	**3.363 (1.116–10.137)**	**0.044**
Recessive model (AA versus GG+GA)				NA		NA	
Allele frequency model (A allele versus G allele)				1.014 (0.271–3.789)	1.000	**3.324 (1.108–9.968)**	**0.023**

P value, OR, and 95% CI were calculated by chi-squared test. Threshold of P value is 0.05. P values of statistical significance are in bold. NA, not calculated due to low frequencies. CI, confidence interval; OR, odds ratio. The first row of each comparison group was set as reference.

in terms of lesion location, while in terms of disease severity they included 225 mild colitis, 117 intermediate colitis, and 54 severe colitis. There were 101 colonic CD, 90 ileocolonic CD, and 84 ileal CD involved in the study. The behavior of CD was composed of 113 nonstricturing, nonpenetrating CD, 71 stricturing CD, and 91 penetrating CD.

3.2. Comparison of FUT2 Gene Polymorphisms between UC Patients, CD Patients, and the Controls.

FUT2 gene polymorphisms of the IBD patients and the controls were explored. The distributions of the genotypes of FUT2 in UC patients, CD patients, and the controls are in accordance with the law of Hardy-Weinberg equilibrium by χ^2 test (all $P > 0.05$). There were no statistical differences for the allele and genotype frequencies of FUT2 gene in UC patients compared to the controls (all $P > 0.05$) (Table 2). However, mutant allele and genotype of FUT2 A385T were significantly increased in CD patients (49.27% versus 43.33%, $P = 0.024$, OR = 1.271, and 95% CI = 1.031–1.565; 27.64% versus 16.53%, $P < 0.001$, OR = 1.927, and 95% CI = 1.353–2.747, resp.) (Table 2). The same conclusion can be drawn from the polymorphism site G428A (1.64% versus 0.50%, $P - 0.023$, OR - 3.324, and 95% CI = 1.108–9.968; 3.27% versus 1.00%, $P = 0.044$, OR = 1.116–10.137, and 95% CI = 1.116–10.137, resp.).

3.3. Haplotype Analysis of FUT2 Gene in IBD Patients and the Controls.

In this study, we further applied Haploview 4.2 software for linkage disequilibrium (LD) and haplotype

TABLE 3: Haplotypes of FUT2 gene in patients with IBD and the controls.

Haplotypes	TA	TT	CA
Patients with UC (%)	42	43	14
Patients with CD (%)	41	49[#]	11
Controls (%)	44	43	13

[#] P value = 0.020, OR = 1.277, and 95% CI = 1.036–1.573.

analyses of FUT2 (C357T, A385T, and G428A). As shown in Table 3, no statistical difference in the frequencies of the haplotypes exists between UC patients and the controls ($P > 0.05$). However, compared to healthy controls, the frequency of haplotype TT, which was formed by C357T and A385T (Figure 1), was significantly increased in patients with CD ($P = 0.020$, OR = 1.277, and 95% CI = 1.036–1.573).

3.4. Relationship of FUT2 Gene Polymorphisms with the Clinical Pathogenic Characteristics of IBD Patients.

By stratified analysis, we further explored the association of FUT2 gene polymorphisms with the clinical features of UC patients and CD patients. In UC patients, the mutant alleles and genotypes of FUT2 (C357T, A385T, and G428A) did not statistically differ between patients with extensive colitis and distal colitis. Additionally, no significant association was observed between FUT2 gene polymorphisms and severity of the disease in UC patients (data not shown).

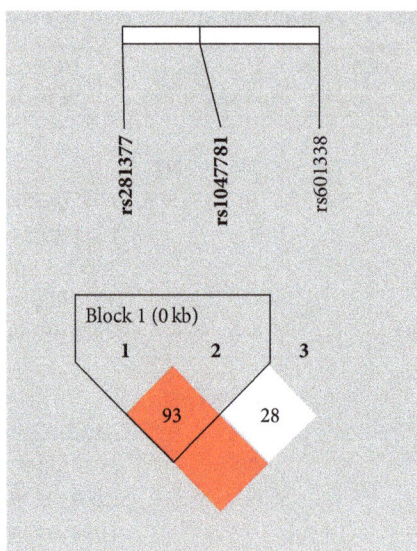

FIGURE 1: The linkage disequilibrium patterns of *FUT2* gene in Han population from Southeast China. The number in a square represents D′ value for each of the two single-nucleotide polymorphisms (SNPs). Dark color of a square indicates that there is a strong connection between the two SNPs.

In CD patients, the mutant allele (T) and genotype (AT+TT) of *FUT2* A385T were less prevalent in patients with ileocolonic CD than in colonic CD (41.67% versus 59.41%, $P = 0.001$, OR = 0.488, and 95% CI = 0.324–0.734; 63.33% versus 83.17%, $P = 0.002$, OR = 0.350, and 95% CI = 0.178–0.686, resp.) (Table 4). The frequencies of mutant allele and genotype in *FUT2* A385T were also lower in patients with ileal CD compared to colonic CD (45.24% versus 59.41%, $P = 0.007$, OR = 0.564, and 95% CI = 0.373–0.854; 64.29% versus 83.17%, $P = 0.004$, OR = 0.364, and 95% CI = 0.183–0.724, resp.) (Table 4). In terms of disease behavior of CD, nevertheless, the frequencies of mutant allele and genotype of *FUT2* polymorphisms showed no difference among stricturing, penetrating and nonstricturing, and nonpenetrating type of CD (data not shown).

4. Discussion

As a group of chronic nonspecific intestinal inflammatory disease, IBD is mainly composed of UC and CD. UC is more common in domestic China with a growing incidence rate [1]. The pathogenesis of IBD is not yet clear. Nowadays, most research suggests that the incidence of IBD could be affected by the genetic, environmental, and immune factors or by the intestinal mucosal barrier, intestinal flora, and other factors [18]. The distribution of intestinal bacteria in human is controlled by host genes to some extent. At present, *FUT2* gene is considered to be one of the important genetic factors affecting the intestinal flora [19]. Although one study involving 1503 individuals failed to confirm the association of gut microbiome composition with ABO or secretor status [20], the influence of FUT2 genotype on the gut microbiota has been highlighted not only in healthy individuals but also in patients with Crohn's disease [19, 21, 22].

Expressed mainly in the intestinal tissue, the alpha-(1,2)-fucosyltransferase *FUT2* plays an important role in the formation of the ABH tissue blood group antigen in the intestine. Blood group precursor becomes H antigen after fucosylation by *FUT2* [7]. In the presence of alpha3N-acetylgalactosamine transferase encoded by Gene A, or D-galactosyl transferase encoded by Gene B, H antigen would further become A antigen or B antigen, which together compose the ABH blood group antigen in vivo [7]. Appreciably, ABH blood group antigen is regulated by *FUT2* gene. If ABH blood group antigen is expressed in the saliva, mucous membrane tissue, or secretion of an individual, the phenotype is called ABH secretory type. If not, it is named ABH nonsecretory type. As *FUT2* gene is polymorphic, nonfunctional *FUT2* gene leads to absence of fucosylation activity. The most common *FUT2* nonfunctional locus in the European Caucasian population is G428A [23], while, in the Chinese population, the most common functional site of *FUT2* is A385T [24]. Besides, silent mutation C357T is also commonly found in Chinese nonsecretors [24]. This divergence indicates that the polymorphism of *FUT2* gene differs among races.

In this study, the distribution of *FUT2* genotypes in the control group was consistent with the Hardy-Weinberg equilibrium law ($P > 0.05$). Mutant allele and genotype of *FUT2* (A385T and G428A) and mutant haplotype TT, formed with *FUT2* (C357T and A385T), were increased in the CD patients compared to the controls, indicating that loss-of-function of *FUT2* gene increased the susceptibility of CD. The results were in line with those from McGovern et al., which suggested that the nonsecretors caused by *FUT2* gene polymorphisms increase of susceptibility of CD [14]. Forni et al. also found that nonsecretor status was associated with CD in Belgian population but not Italian population [25]. Our study also suggested that, compared to patients with

TABLE 4: Association of *FUT2* gene polymorphisms with the location of CD patients.

FUT2	Colonic	Ileocolonic	Ileal	Ileocolonic versus Colonic OR (95% CI)	P value	Ileal versus Colonic OR (95% CI)	P value
C357T							
TT	77	71	69	1		1	
TC (additive model)	23	19	15	0.896 (0.450–1.782)	0.754	0.728 (0.352–1.506)	0.391
CC (additive model)	1	0	0	0.987 (0.963–1.012)	1.000	0.987 (0.963–1.012)	1.000
Dominant model (TC+CC versus TT)				0.859 (0.434–1.699)	0.661	0.697 (0.339–1.436)	0.327
Recessive model (CC versus TT+TC)				0.990 (0.970–1.010)	1.000	0.990 (0.971–1.010)	1.000
Allele frequency model (C allele versus T allele)				0.836 (0.443–1.574)	0.578	0.694 (0.353–1.364)	0.288
A385T							
AA	17	33	30	1		1	
AT (additive model)	48	39	32	**0.419 (0.203–0.861)**	**0.017**	**0.378 (0.179–0.795)**	**0.009**
TT (additive model)	36	18	22	**0.258 (0.114–0.58)**	**0.001**	**0.345 (0.156–0.768)**	**0.008**
Dominant model (AT+TT versus AA)				**0.350 (0.178–0.686)**	**0.002**	**0.364 (0.183–0.724)**	**0.004**
Recessive model (TT versus AA+AT)				**0.451 (0.234–0.871)**	**0.017**	0.641 (0.340–1.208)	0.168
Allele frequency model (T allele versus A allele)				**0.488 (0.324–0.734)**	**0.001**	**0.564 (0.373–0.854)**	**0.007**
G428A							
GG	98	86	82	1		1	
GA (additive model)	3	4	2	1.519 (0.331–6.980)	0.709	0.797 (0.130–4.884)	1.000
AA (additive model)	0	0	0		NA		NA
Dominant model (GA+AA versus GG)				1.519 (0.331–6.980)	0.709	0.797 (0.130–4.884)	1.000
Recessive model (AA versus GG+GA)					NA		NA
Allele frequency model (A allele versus G allele)				1.508 (0.333–6.829)	0.711	0.799 (0.132–4.840)	1.000

Conducted by using unconditional logistic regression analyses, colonic colitis was set as reference compared to ileocolonic colitis and ileal colitis. Variables also included sex, age of onset, and behavior of disease. The first row of each comparison group was set as reference.

colonic CD, frequencies of mutant allele and genotype of *FUT2* A385T were significantly decreased in patients with ileocolonic and ileal CD. Similarly, a study on Japanese population showed that FUT2 secretor status was associated with colonic-type CD and that abnormal expression of blood type antigens was presented only in colonic CD [26]. These findings indicate that the influence of FUT2 gene on CD might be linked to the location of CD. Interestingly, intestinal microbiota are mainly present in the colon and reach their highest biomass in the distal gut [27]. Furthermore, it has been revealed that the expression of Lewis b decreased progressively from proximal to distal colon and disappeared in rectum [6]. We inferred that FUT2 gene might increase the predisposition of colonic CD through its potential influence on the intestinal microbiota.

However, there was no significant difference between the controls and the UC patients in the three *FUT2* mutant alleles or genotype frequencies (all $P > 0.05$). The frequencies of the haplotype between the controls and the UC patients were not significantly different either ($P > 0.05$). Mutant alleles of *FUT2* (C357T, A385T, and G428A) were not significantly different either between the distal colitis group and the extensive colitis group ($P > 0.05$). This is inconsistent with the results from another study, in which the *FUT2* G428A mutant genotype (AA+GA) in the Finland population increased the susceptibility to UC [11]. In addition, studies in China showed that the *FUT2* gene A385T polymorphism is

not associated with the susceptibility to UC in the Chinese Han nationality, but the functional mutations of C357T and G428A are in accordance with the susceptibility to IBD of the Han nationality [15]. Thus, it can be inferred that the effect of *FUT2* gene polymorphism on susceptibility to IBD may be closely related to the ethnic differences. In the Chinese Han population, *FUT2* A385T polymorphism is the most common site in the gene, which determines the secretion of ABH antigens.

In conclusion, our study revealed that *FUT2* gene polymorphisms and haplotypes were associated with the susceptibility to CD but not UC.

Competing Interests

The authors declare that they have no competing interests.

Acknowledgments

The project was supported by grants from the Science and Technology Bureau of Wenzhou (Grant no. Y20140533).

References

[1] S. C. Ng, "Epidemiology of inflammatory bowel disease: focus on Asia," *Best Practice and Research: Clinical Gastroenterology*, vol. 28, no. 3, pp. 363–372, 2014.

[2] J. Burisch and P. Munkholm, "The epidemiology of inflammatory bowel disease," *Scandinavian Journal of Gastroenterology*, vol. 50, no. 8, pp. 942–951, 2015.

[3] J. H. Cheon, "Genetics of inflammatory bowel diseases: a comparison between Western and Eastern perspectives," *Journal of Gastroenterology and Hepatology*, vol. 28, no. 2, pp. 220–226, 2013.

[4] L. Jostins, S. Ripke, R. K. Weersma et al., "Host-microbe interactions have shaped the genetic architecture of inflammatory bowel disease," *Nature*, vol. 491, no. 7422, pp. 119–124, 2012.

[5] S. C. Ng, K. K. F. Tsoi, M. A. Kamm et al., "Genetics of inflammatory bowel disease in Asia: systematic review and meta–analysis ," *Inflammatory Bowel Diseases*, vol. 18, no. 6, pp. 1164–1176, 2012.

[6] M. Yuan, S. H. Itzkowitz, Y. S. Kim et al., "Distribution of blood group antigens A, B, H, Lewis A and Lewis B in human normal, fetal, and malignant colonic tissue," *Cancer Research*, vol. 45, no. 9, pp. 4499–4511, 1985.

[7] H. Shirato, "Norovirus and histo-blood group antigens," *Japanese Journal of Infectious Diseases*, vol. 64, no. 2, pp. 95–103, 2011.

[8] G. M. Ruiz-Palacios, L. E. Cervantes, P. Ramos, B. Chavez-Munguia, and D. S. Newburg, "Campylobacter jejuni binds intestinal H(O) antigen (Fucα1, 2Galβ1, 4GlcNAc), and fucosyloligosaccharides of human milk inhibit its binding and infection," *Journal of Biological Chemistry*, vol. 278, no. 16, pp. 14112–14120, 2003.

[9] L. Hu, S. E. Crawford, R. Czako et al., "Cell attachment protein VP8* of a human rotavirus specifically interacts with A-type histo-blood group antigen," *Nature*, vol. 485, no. 7397, pp. 256–259, 2012.

[10] A. R. Pacheco, M. M. Curtis, C. G. Moreira, V. Sperandio, and J. M. Ritchie, "Fucose sensing regulates bacterial intestinal colonization," *Nature*, vol. 492, no. 7427, pp. 113–117, 2012.

[11] A. S. Parmar, N. Alakulppi, P. Paavola-Sakki et al., "Association study of FUT2 (rs601338) with celiac disease and inflammatory bowel disease in the Finnish population," *Tissue Antigens*, vol. 80, no. 6, pp. 488–493, 2012.

[12] D. J. Smyth, J. D. Cooper, J. M. M. Howson et al., "FUT2 non-secretor status links type 1 diabetes susceptibility and resistance to infection," *Diabetes*, vol. 60, no. 11, pp. 3081–3084, 2011.

[13] T. Folseraas, E. Melum, P. Rausch et al., "Extended analysis of a genome-wide association study in primary sclerosing cholangitis detects multiple novel risk loci," *Journal of Hepatology*, vol. 57, no. 2, pp. 366–375, 2012.

[14] D. P. B. McGovern, M. R. Jones, K. D. Taylor et al., "*Fucosyltransferase 2 (FUT2)* non-secretor status is associated with Crohn's disease," *Human Molecular Genetics*, vol. 19, no. 17, pp. 3468–3476, 2010.

[15] A. Aheman, H.-S. Luo, and F. Gao, "Association of fucosyltransferase 2 gene variants with ulcerative colitis in Han and Uyghur patients in China," *World Journal of Gastroenterology*, vol. 18, no. 34, pp. 4758–4764, 2012.

[16] J. Satsangi, M. S. Silverberg, S. Vermeire, and J.-F. Colombel, "The Montreal classification of inflammatory bowel disease: controversies, consensus, and implications," *Gut*, vol. 55, no. 6, pp. 749–753, 2006.

[17] S. C. Truelove, "Cortisone in ulcerative colitis final report on a therapeutic trial," *British Medical Journal*, vol. 2, no. 4947, pp. 1041–1048, 1955.

[18] C. Abraham and J. H. Cho, "Inflammatory bowel disease," *The New England Journal of Medicine*, vol. 361, no. 21, pp. 2066–2078, 2009.

[19] P. Wacklin, J. Tuimala, J. Nikkilä et al., "Faecal microbiota composition in adults is associated with the FUT2 gene determining the secretor status," *PLoS ONE*, vol. 9, no. 4, Article ID e94863, 2014.

[20] E. R. Davenport, J. K. Goodrich, J. T. Bell, T. D. Spector, R. E. Ley, and A. G. Clark, "ABO antigen and secretor statuses are not associated with gut microbiota composition in 1,500 twins," *BMC Genomics*, vol. 17, no. 1, article 941, 2016.

[21] P. Rausch, A. Rehman, S. Künzel et al., "Colonic mucosa-associated microbiota is influenced by an interaction of crohn disease and FUT2 (Secretor) genotype," *Proceedings of the National Academy of Sciences of the United States of America*, vol. 108, no. 47, pp. 19030–19035, 2011.

[22] M. Tong, I. McHardy, P. Ruegger et al., "Reprograming of gut microbiome energy metabolism by the FUT2 Crohn's disease risk polymorphism," *ISME Journal*, vol. 8, no. 11, pp. 2193–2206, 2014.

[23] R. J. Kelly, S. Rouquier, D. Giorgi, G. G. Lennon, and J. B. Lowe, "Sequence and expression of a candidate for the human Secretor blood group α(1,2)fucosyltransferase gene (FUT2). Homozygosity for an enzyme- inactivating nonsense mutation commonly correlates with the non-secretor phenotype," *Journal of Biological Chemistry*, vol. 270, no. 9, pp. 4640–4649, 1995.

[24] S. P. Yip, S. K. Lai, and M. L. Wong, "Systematic sequence analysis of the human fucosyltransferase 2 (FUT2) gene identifies novel sequence variations and alleles," *Transfusion*, vol. 47, no. 8, pp. 1369–1380, 2007.

[25] D. Forni, I. Cleynen, M. Ferrante et al., "ABO histo-blood group might modulate predisposition to Crohn's disease and affect disease behavior," *Journal of Crohn's and Colitis*, vol. 8, no. 6, pp. 489–494, 2014.

[26] J. Miyoshi, T. Yajima, S. Okamoto et al., "Ectopic expression of blood type antigens in inflamed mucosa with higher incidence of FUT2 secretor status in colonic Crohn's disease," *Journal of Gastroenterology*, vol. 46, no. 9, pp. 1056–1063, 2011.

[27] J. K. Goodrich, E. R. Davenport, J. L. Waters, A. G. Clark, and R. E. Ley, "Cross-species comparisons of host genetic associations with the microbiome," *Science*, vol. 352, no. 6285, pp. 532–535, 2016.

20

Clinicopathological Features and Prognostic Factors of Colorectal Neuroendocrine Neoplasms

Mengjie Jiang,[1] **Yinuo Tan,**[2] **Xiaofen Li,**[1] **Jianfei Fu,**[3,4] **Hanguang Hu,**[1] **Xianyun Ye,**[1] **Ying Cao,**[1] **Jinghong Xu,**[5] **and Ying Yuan**[1]

[1]*Department of Medical Oncology, The Second Affiliated Hospital, Zhejiang University School of Medicine, Hangzhou, Zhejiang Province, China*
[2]*Department of Surgical Oncology, The Second Affiliated Hospital, Zhejiang University School of Medicine, Hangzhou, Zhejiang Province, China*
[3]*Cancer Institute (Key Laboratory of Cancer Prevention and Intervention, Chinese National Ministry of Education; Key Laboratory of Molecular Biology in Medical Sciences, Zhejiang Province, China), The Second Affiliated Hospital, Zhejiang University School of Medicine, Hangzhou, Zhejiang Province, China*
[4]*Department of Oncology, Jinhua Central Hospital (Jinhua Hospital of Zhejiang University School of Medicine), Jinhua, Zhejiang Province, China*
[5]*Department of Pathology, The Second Affiliated Hospital, Zhejiang University School of Medicine, Hangzhou, Zhejiang Province, China*

Correspondence should be addressed to Ying Yuan; yuanying1999@zju.edu.cn

Academic Editor: Laura Lorenzon

Background. Limited research is available regarding colorectal NENs and the prognostic factors remain controversial. *Materials and Methods.* A total of 68 patients with colorectal NENs were studied retrospectively. Clinical characteristics and prognosis between colonic and rectal NENs were compared. The Cox regression models were used to evaluate the predictive capacity. *Results.* Of the 68 colorectal NENs patients, 43 (63.2%) had rectal NENs, and 25 (36.8%) had colonic NENs. Compared with rectal NENs, colonic NENs more frequently exhibited larger tumor size ($P < 0.0001$) and distant metastasis ($P < 0.0001$). Colonic NENs had a worse prognosis ($P = 0.027$), with 5-year overall survival rates of 66.7% versus 88.1%. NET, NEC, and MANEC were noted in 61.8%, 23.5%, and 14.7% of patients, respectively. Multivariate analyses revealed that tumor location was not an independent prognostic factor ($P = 0.081$), but tumor size ($P = 0.037$) and pathological classification ($P = 0.012$) were independent prognostic factors. *Conclusion.* Significant differences exist between colonic and rectal NENs. Multivariate analysis indicated that tumor size and pathological classification were associated with prognosis. Tumor location was not an independent factor. The worse outcome of colonic NENs observed in clinical practice might be due not only to the biological differences, but also to larger tumor size in colonic NENs caused by the delayed diagnosis.

1. Introduction

Neuroendocrine neoplasms (NENs) consist of a spectrum of malignancies that arise from neuroendocrine cells, which are located throughout the body. NENs are a group of fairly rare tumors with obvious heterogeneity. These tumors were formerly referred to as "carcinoid," which means "carcinoma-like."

Based on the current literature, the worldwide incidence of NENs seems to have increased markedly [1–4]. According to the Surveillance Epidemiology and End Results (SEER) database of the United States, the annual incidence of NENs has increased nearly fivefold from 1973 (1.09/100,000) to 2004 (5.25/100,000) [5]. More than half of all NENs are gastroenteropancreatic NENs (GEP-NENs), with an annual incidence of 3.65–4.7/100,000 in the United States [5–7].

The annual incidence of colonic NENs increased from 0.02/100,000 to 0.2/100,1000 and rectal NENs increased from 0.2/100,000 to 0.86/100,000 [8]. Widespread endoscopic screening, increased awareness of neuroendocrine histology, and improved data capture likely have contributed to this trend [4, 5, 9–11]. The most common primary site of colonic NENs is the cecum, followed by sigmoid colon and ascending colon. Rectal NENs occurred at a markedly higher frequency among Asian population than among white patients [5, 8, 12, 13].

The nomenclature and classification of NENs have always been a dispute, which are lack of uniform standard. Traditionally, NENs were classified based on the embryonic origins as foregut, midgut, and hindgut tumors. However, recent attempts have been made to change the nomenclature according to primary sites [8]. The World Health Organization (WHO) classifies NENs of the colon and rectum together as a single entity. According to the 2010 WHO classification, NENs are classified as neuroendocrine tumor (NET), neuroendocrine carcinoma (NEC), or mixed adenoneuroendocrine carcinoma (MANEC). Furthermore, NET/NEC are graded into three levels based on different definitions of proliferation using the mitotic count and/or the Ki-67 index: Grade 1 (G1), mitotic count < 2 per 10 high-power fields (HPF) and/or Ki-67 ≤ 2%; Grade 2 (G2), mitotic count 2–20 per 10 HPF and/or Ki-67 3 to 20%; Grade 3 (G3), mitotic count > 20 per 10 HPF and/or Ki-67 > 20% [8, 14].

It is generally accepted that tumor size and pathological classification are associated with prognosis [5, 12, 14, 15]. However, the impact of tumor location on the outcome of colorectal NENs remains controversial. Clinical practice demonstrated a better outcome in rectal NENs compared with colonic NENs, but whether tumor location is an independent prognostic factor remains unknown. It is not clear whether differences in prognosis between colonic NENs and rectal NENs are due to inherent distinctions between these conditions. Given the significant differences in prognosis between colonic NENs and rectal NENs, should different treatments be administered to these two groups?

Many American and European studies have reported the epidemiology, clinical manifestations, pathology, management, and survival of GEP-NENs [5, 7, 9], but there is a lack of data in Asian population, especially in China. And the research about colorectal NENs is rare because of the low incidence. Therefore, the objective of the present study was to perform an epidemiological and prognosis research of colorectal NENs in a Chinese population [16]. We collected and retrospectively analyzed the data from colorectal NEN patients registered at the Second Affiliated Hospital, Zhejiang University School of Medicine, from March 2001 to March 2014 to investigate the clinicopathological characteristics and prognostic factors of colorectal NENs.

2. Materials and Methods

A total of 68 colorectal NENs patients who were treated in the Second Affiliated Hospital, Zhejiang University School of Medicine, between March 2001 and March 2014 were included in this retrospective study. All of the cases were confirmed by pathology. To standardize the pathological diagnosis, the same pathologist reviewed all slides. The hospital's ethics committee approved this study with written informed consent. Data obtained from the patients included demographic (e.g., age, gender, and diagnosed time), clinical (e.g., symptoms at presentation, tumor location, treatment, and survival time), and pathological data (e.g., tumor size, depth of invasion, lymph nodes status, distant metastasis, pathological classification, and Ki-67 index).

Tumors were restaged according to the American Joint Committee on Cancer (AJCC) 7th Tumor, Lymph Node and Metastasis (TNM) staging system. The tumor location was described as colon or rectum. The rectum was defined as being 15 centimeters from the anal verge. Both the sigmorectal junction and ileocecal junction were classified as the colon. Classification and grading were based on morphological criteria and tumor proliferative activity according to the 2010 WHO classification. In treatment, patients were classified as undergoing regional surgery, endoscopic radical surgery, or best supportive care. The regional surgeries encompass anterior resection, abdominal perineal resection, and transanal endoscopic microsurgery (TEM), and endoscopic radical surgeries encompass endoscopic mucosal resection (EMR) and endoscopic submucosal dissection (ESD). Best supportive care means cancer pain control, nutritional support, and symptomatic treatment.

Specific staff members in the oncology institution were responsible for collecting data from patients and subsequently contacting with patients. Follow-up was conducted by a combination of physical examination, colonoscopy, and computed tomography at either six-monthly or yearly intervals. Overall survival was calculated from the time of the patient's final diagnosis to their death caused by colorectal NENs. Death attributed to other causes or patients lost to follow-up were defined as censored observation.

Data of all categorical variables were summarized using frequencies and percentages. Comparisons between groups were performed using Pearson's chi-square or Fisher's exact tests. Survival curves were generated using Kaplan-Meier methods, and the log-rank test was performed to evaluate the survival difference. Adjusted relative ratios (RRs) along with 95% confidence intervals (CI) were calculated using Cox proportional hazards regression models. When the two-side P value was less than 0.05, the difference was considered statistically significant. SPSS 16.0 statistics software (SPSS Chicago IL, USA) was used for data analysis.

3. Results

3.1. Clinicopathological Features of the 68 Patients. The current cohort represented 68 adult patients with colorectal NENs. Of these patients, 43 (63.2%) had rectal NENs, and 25 (36.8%) had colonic NENs. All the patients were Han Chinese. Additionally, 44 (64.7%) patients were male, and 24 (35.3%) were female. The male-to-female ratio was 1.8 : 1. The average age was 55.7 years old (range, 20 to 82 years old). Among all the patients, 25 (36.8%) patients presented with abdominal pain, 11 (16.2%) with hematochezia, 4 (5.8%) with an alteration in stool property, 3 (4.4%) with an alteration in bowel habit, and 1 (1.5%) with unexplained weight loss. The remaining 24 (35.3%) cases were an incidental finding without obvious symptoms. None of the patients presented with carcinoid syndrome (e.g., hot flash, watery diarrhea, or palpitation). No synchronic NEN was noted in other parts of the body. For rectal NENs, the median distance from the anal verge was 7.0 cm (range, 2 to 15 cm).

All 68 patients were diagnosed via histopathology. The median diameter on histological analysis was 10 mm (range, 2 to 200 mm). Moreover, 30 lesions (44.1%) were smaller than 10 mm in diameter, 8 lesions (11.8%) ranged from 11 to 20 mm, and 30 lesions (44.1%) were larger than 20 mm. According to the 2010 WHO classification, 42 of 68 (61.8%) cases were classified as NET, 16 (23.5%) as NEC, and 10 (14.7%) as MANEC. Some pathology reports ($n = 19$) did not present the Ki-67 index. According to the available data ($n = 49$), the Ki-67 indices of 27 (39.7%) patients were ≤2%, 6 (8.8%) ranged from 3% to 20%, and 16 (23.5%) were >20%. Mitotic rates were not reported in most pathology reports.

3.2. Distinctions between Colonic NENs and Rectal NENs.

Significant differences were noted between colonic NENs and rectal NENs in clinical practice. Rectal NENs exhibited increased morbidity compared with colonic NENs. The latter cecum was the most common site involved followed by the ascending colon and sigmoid colon. In addition, rectal NENs were often diagnosed in patients of a relatively younger age ($P = 0.01$).

Rectal NENs were typically smaller than colonic tumors ($P < 0.0001$) and always located on the anterior or lateral rectal wall. A significant difference was noted between colonic NENs and rectal NENs regarding pathological classification ($P = 0.001$). More rectal NENs were classified as well-differentiated NET, whereas more colonic NENs were poorly differentiated NEC/MANEC. A similar trend was observed regarding tumor stage and tumor grade; namely, colonic NENs were often diagnosed at later stage ($P < 0.0001$) and higher grade. Compared with rectal NENs, colonic NENs were more likely metastatic when diagnosed. A total of 18 (26.5%) patients had metastases at the time of diagnosis. Of these patients, 13 had colonic NENs. Metastases were often noted in the liver, lymph nodes, and mesenteric peritoneum.

In summation, colonic NENs were relatively scarce compared with rectal NENs but occurred at a markedly increased frequency with larger tumor size, poorly differentiated classification, and distant metastases. The detailed distinctions between rectal NENs and colonic NENs are provided in Table 1.

3.3. Therapy.

The majority of the patients ($n = 52$) underwent regional surgery with curative intent ($n = 47$) or for palliative purposes ($n = 5$). A total of 4 patients with metastatic disease underwent resection of their metastatic lesions, including liver metastasis, gallbladder metastasis, and adnexa metastasis. A total of 15 patients underwent endoscopic radical surgery, among which 12 patients underwent complete excision with a negative margin and 3 patients were with a positive margin; no specimens were fragmented. Only one patient pathologically diagnosed via endoscopic

biopsy did not undergo surgical operation due to the presence of widespread metastases and poor physical condition. He received best supportive care exclusively. There are 3 patients who took preoperative chemotherapy and 5 patients took postoperative adjuvant chemotherapy. Palliative chemotherapy was administered to 5 patients. The chemotherapy regimens included oxaliplatin-fluorouracil ($n = 2$), platinum-etoposide ($n = 2$), and irinotecan-fluorouracil ($n = 1$). None of the patients received radiotherapy and targeted therapy.

3.4. Survival and Prognostic Factors.

The cut-off date of follow-up was September 2014. In total, 63 of 68 patients received complete follow-up with a median duration of 4 years (range, 0.5 to 13 years). The 1-year, 3-year, and 5-year survival rates of the entire cohort were 89.7%, 85.3%, and 82.4%, respectively.

3.5. Univariate Analyses of Outcome.

Regarding the impact of tumor location on outcome, univariate analysis indicated that the colonic NENs exhibited worse outcomes compared with rectal NENs. The 5-year overall survival rates were 66.7% and 88.1% for colonic NENs and rectal NENs subgroups, respectively, and a significant difference was noted ($P = 0.03$) (Figure 1(a)).

Additionally, tumor size, pathological classification, tumor infiltration (T-classification), lymph nodes status (N-classification), and distant metastasis (M-classification) could predict the outcome, whereas the age or the gender could not. Larger tumor size, poorly differentiated pathological classification (NEC/MANEC), T-classification (T3/T4), N-classification (N1), and M-classification (M1) were associated with dismal prognoses ($P < 0.05$). The 5-year survival rate was 33.3% in patients with distant metastases and 95.8% in patients without distant metastases (Figure 1).

3.6. Multivariate Analyses of Outcome.

All factors associated with survival based on univariate analysis and various innate factors, such as gender and age, were included in the Cox model. In the multivariate analysis, tumor size, pathological classification, age, T-classification, and M-classification were independent prognostic factors ($P < 0.05$) (Table 2).

In the multivariate analysis, after adjusting for covariates, including gender, age, pathological classification, T-classification, N-classification, and M-classification, tumor location was no longer an independent factor for the prognosis of colorectal NENs ($P = 0.08$) (Table 2).

4. Discussion

The current study described the clinicopathology and assessed the prognostic factors among 68 cases of Chinese colorectal NENs. During the same period, 2460 colorectal adenocarcinoma patients registered to our center with complete follow-up information [17]. Colorectal NENs accounted for 2.8% of all the colorectal cancer patients. In clinical practice, colonic NENs usually present late, as large tumors, often with extensive metastatic disease and poor outcome. However, after multivariate analysis, we found that tumor size

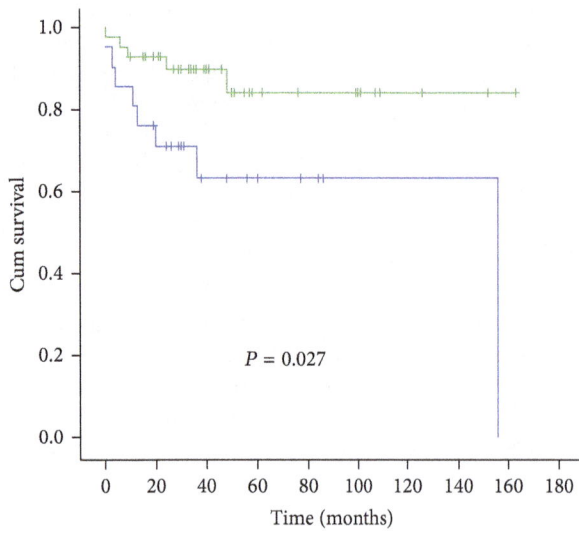

Number at risk

Colon	21	15	7	5	3	1	1	1	0	0
Rectum	42	33	19	10	8	7	3	2	1	0

Location

◻ Colon
◻ Rectum

(a)

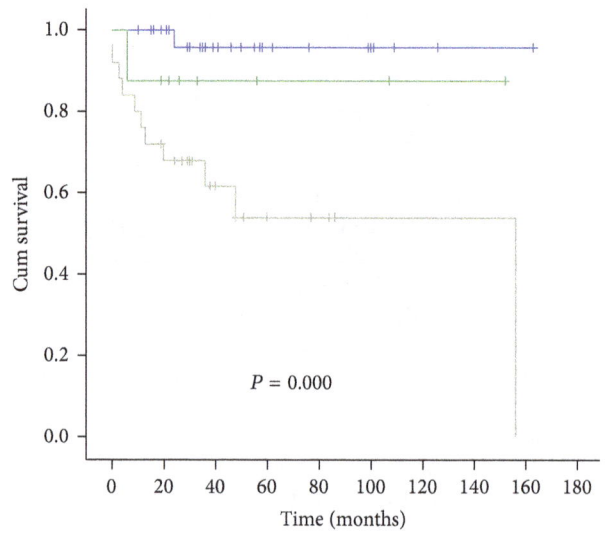

Number at risk

1–10 mm	30	30	14	8	6	4	2	1	1	0
11–20 mm	8	6	3	2	2	2	1	1	0	0
≥21 mm	25	16	8	4	3	1	1	1	0	0

Size

◻ 1–10 mm   ◻ ≥21 mm
◻ 11–20 mm

(b)

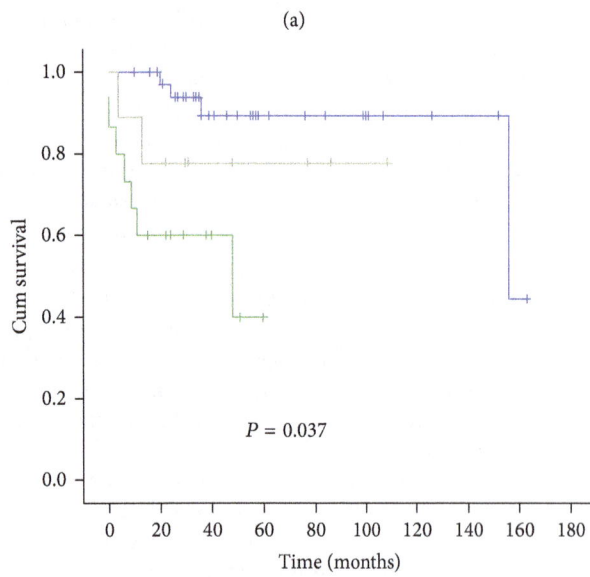

Number at risk

NET	39	32	18	11	9	6	4	3	1	0
NEC	15	8	3	0	0	0	0	0	0	0
MANEC	9	7	4	3	2	1	0	0	0	0

Classification

◻ NET   ◻ MANEC
◻ NEC

(c)

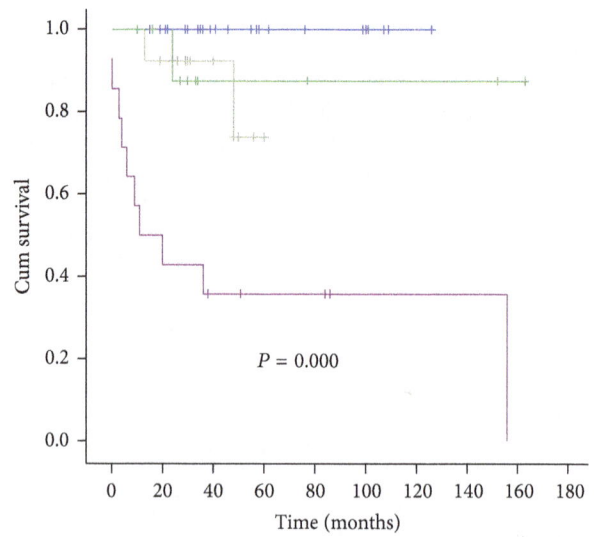

Number at risk

T1	26	26	26	26	26	26	26	26	26	26
T2	10	7	3	3	2	2	2	2	1	0
T3	13	11	6	1	0	0	0	0	0	0
T4	14	7	4	3	3	1	1	1	0	0

T-stage

◻ T1   ◻ T3
◻ T2   ◻ T4

(d)

FIGURE 1: Continued.

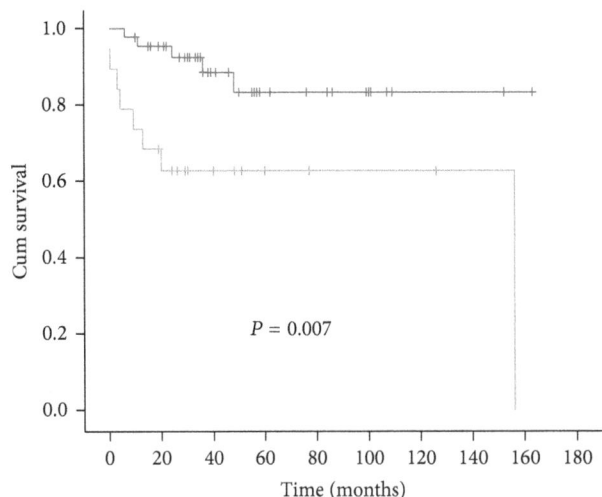

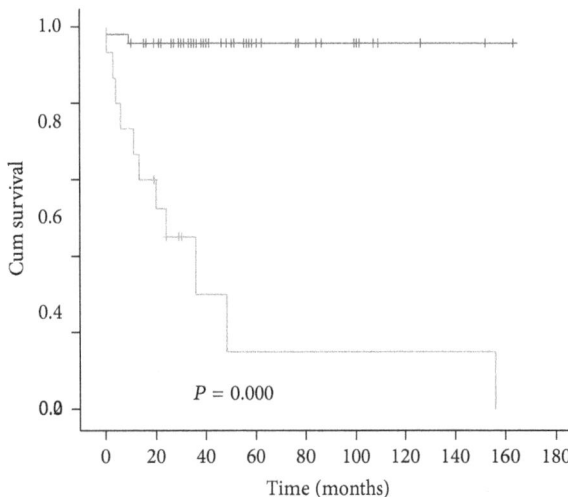

Number at risk									
N0	44	36	19	11	9	5	2	2	1	0
N1	19	11	6	3	2	2	2	1	0	0

N-stage
⌐ N0
⌐ N1

(e)

Number at risk									
M0	48	40	24	14	10	7	3	2	1	0
M1	15	8	2	1	1	1	1	0	0	0

M-stage
⌐ M0
⌐ M1

(f)

FIGURE 1: (a) Overall survival based on tumor location. (b) Overall survival based on tumor size. (c) Overall survival based on pathological classification. (d) Overall survival based on T-classification. (e) Overall survival based on N-classification. (f) Overall survival based on M-classification.

and pathological classification were independent prognostic factors, whereas tumor location was not.

Limited research is available regarding NENs, especially colorectal NENs. The rarity of NENs and lack of union definition are impediments to large-scale clinical trials and development of accepted guidelines for management. Although large population-based studies of gastrointestinal carcinoids have been conducted in the US, these studies did not focus on colorectal NENs or analyze the exact prognostic factors [5, 7, 9].

The inconsistent findings were noted among studies of NENs from different areas [5, 7, 9, 12, 14, 15]. Firstly, the proportion of rectal NENs varied widely. The current study revealed that 63.2% of colorectal NENs were located in the rectum. Our results were not consistent with previous report from Japan in which 304 of 345 (90%) cases of colorectal carcinoids originated from the rectum [12]. According to the SEER database [9], rectal carcinoids accounted for 31.6% of all the NENs in large intestine. In previous Chinese studies, Wang et al. [15] and Zhang et al. [14] collected clinical and pathological data from 178 and 168 patients diagnosed with gastroenteropancreatic neuroendocrine neoplasms (GEP-NENs), respectively, for analysis; these studies involve the largest NENs samples in China to date. Wang et al. [15] reported that the most common primary site was the pancreas (62/178, 34.8%) followed by rectum (36/178, 20.2%), stomach (25/178, 14.0%), duodenum (13/178, 7.3%),

and unknown primary site (12/178, 6.7%). The ratio of colorectal NENs was only 20.8% (37/178). However, Zhang et al. [14] found that the rectum was the most common site of involvement (58.93%) followed by pancreas (13.69%), stomach (9.52%), duodenum (2.38%), colon (4.76%), and appendix (4.76%). In his study, colorectal NEN accounted for 63.69% of all patients. It is possible that some colonic carcinoids registered in SEER data were misdiagnosed and were actually poorly differentiated adenocarcinomas or undifferentiated carcinomas. Another possibility is the existence of an obviously increased frequency of both NENs and adenocarcinomas in right-sided colons with the westernized lifestyle [11, 18, 19]. In addition, the inconsistencies may be due to racial and geographical disparities. Overall, rectal NENs appear to be more common in the Asian population. In contrast, the prevalence of colonic and appendiceal NENs appears to be considerably increased among the Caucasian population.

In addition, a distinction in the aspect of distant metastasis was noted between colonic and rectal NENs. In the SEER database, 45% of colonic NENs were localized when diagnosed [9]. In a Japanese series, this ratio was 65% [12]. In current study, 48% of colonic NENs were localized when diagnosed. On the other hand, the majority of rectal NENs were localized at diagnosis. The ratios of metastatic rectal NEN patients were 5% in the SEER database [9], 8% in the Japanese registry [12], and 11.6% in the current study. Given

TABLE 1: The clinicopathological characteristics of 68 colorectal neuroendocrine neoplasm patients.

Variance	Rectal NEN ($n = 43$) (patients [%])	Colonic NEN ($n = 25$) (patients [%])	P
Gender			NS
Male	26 (60.5)	18 (72.0)	
Female	17 (39.5)	7 (28.0)	
Age			0.012
≤60	31 (72.1)	10 (40.0)	
>60	12 (27.9)	15 (60.0)	
Size (mm)			0.000
1–10	30 (69.8)	0 (0)	
11–20	6 (13.9)	2 (8.0)	
≥21	7 (16.3)	23 (92.0)	
T-classification*			0.000
T1	26 (60.5)	0 (0)	
T2	9 (20.9)	1 (4.0)	
T3	4 (9.3)	12 (48.0)	
T4	4 (9.3)	12 (48.0)	
N-classification*			0.000
N0	37 (86.0)	10 (40.0)	
N1	6 (14.0)	15 (60.0)	
M-classification*			0.000
M0	38 (88.4)	12 (48.0)	
M1	5 (11.6)	13 (52.0)	
Stage			0.000
I	25 (58.1)	0 (0)	
II	9 (21.0)	4 (16.0)	
III	4 (9.3)	8 (32.0)	
IV	5 (11.6)	13 (52.0)	
Pathology#			0.001
NET	33 (76.7)	9 (36.0)	
NEC	8 (18.6)	8 (32.0)	
MANEC	2 (4.7)	8 (32.0)	
Ki-67 index (%)			NS
≤2	20 (46.5)	7 (28.0)	
3–20	4 (9.3)	2 (8.0)	
>20	8 (18.6)	8 (32.0)	
Unclear	11 (25.6)	8 (32.0)	

*T-classification, N-classification, M-classification, and stages I, II, III, and IV according to the 7th AJCC TNM staging system.
#Pathological classification according to WHO 2010.

TABLE 2: Univariate and multivariate analysis (Cox proportional hazard model) of prognostic factors for 63 colorectal neuroendocrine neoplasm patients with complete follow-ups.

Variables (reference)	Univariate analysis			Multivariate analysis		
	RR	95% CI	P	RR	95% CI	P
Age (≤60 years old)	1.116	0.363–3.426	0.848	0.136	0.024–0.776	0.025
Gender (male)	0.947	0.285–3.147	0.929	1.533	0.389–6.045	0.541
Location (colon)	0.303	0.099–0.931	0.037	4.121	0.838–20.267	0.081
Size (≤10 mm)	3.801	1.491–9.692	0.005	0.088	0.009–0.859	0.037
Pathology (NET)	1.930	1.010–3.689	0.047	4.338	1.376–13.681	0.012
T-classification (T1)	4.730	1.946–11.502	0.001	25.326	3.919–163.668	0.001
N-classification (N0)	4.217	1.368–13.000	0.012	4.331	0.796–23.565	0.090
M-classification (M0)	24.761	5.357–114.441	0.000	33.791	4.486–254.524	0.001

RR: relative risk. CI: confident index.

that distant metastasis was one of the strongest prognostic factors of outcome [12, 20–24], differences in overall survival were also noted between colonic NENs and rectal NENs. In the SEER database, colonic NEN patients exhibited the worst prognosis among all GEP-NENs patients, with a 5-year overall survival rate of 41.6%. Rectal NENs appear to exhibit a low propensity to metastasize and thus are associated with a favorable prognosis, with a 5-year overall survival rate of 88.3% [9]. In current study, the 5-year survival rate for colonic NENs was 66.7%, and 5-year survival for rectal NENs was 88.1%, which was similar to that reported in the SEER database. In Wang et al.'s study, the 1-, 3-, and 5-year survival rates for GEP-NENs were 74.4%, 66.7%, and 54.5% [15], respectively, lower than the current study with a 5-year overall survival rate of 82.4% for colorectal NENs. This disparity was because the current cohort was exclusively composed of NENs originating from the colon and rectum, whereas the previous two studies contained GEP-NENs originating from any part of the digestive system.

Regarding the most important prognostic factors, each study did not arrive at exactly the same answer. Konishi et al. [12] studied 345 colorectal NENs cases and revealed that tumor site in the colon was statistically correlated with distant metastasis. However, after multivariate analysis, the independent risk factors for distant metastasis only included tumor size $\geq$ 21 mm and venous invasion. Tumor location was not an independent prognostic factor, and this finding is similar to the current results. Wang et al. [15] observed that NET/G1 patients without distant metastasis exhibited enhanced survival compared with patients with other types of NENs, thus suggesting that pathological classification, tumor grade, and distant metastasis were prognostic factors. However, the age, gender, and primary tumor location had little impact on overall survival. According to the study of Zhang et al. [14], the univariate analysis revealed that gender and tumor size were related to survival but did not translate into independent risk factors for survival according to the Cox regression model. Age and pathological classification were the only independent prognostic factors for overall survival ($P = 0.02$ and $P = 0.04$, resp.). Tumor location was not associated with prognosis ($P = 0.11$). In the current study, gender was not associated with prognosis, but tumor size and pathological classification were independent prognostic factors. Tumor location was associated with prognosis in the univariate analysis but not in the multivariate analysis. Given that numerous previous studies confirmed that GEP-NENs comprise a heterogeneous group in relation to their primary locations [2, 5, 9, 25], NENs originating from different sites should not be categorized in the same class. In previous Chinese studies of NENs, colorectal NENs were consistently grouped with GEP-NENs and underrepresented. Our study exclusively assessed colonic and rectal NENs, thus increasing the reliability of our study.

Tumor location was statistically significant in univariate analysis but not in multivariate analysis. Both univariate and multivariate analyses indicated that tumor size and pathological classification were independent factors for the prognosis of colorectal NENs. Based on the above results, we hypothesize that the worse outcome of colonic NENs

observed in clinical practice might be due not only to the biological differences, but also to larger tumor size in colonic NENs caused by the delayed diagnosis. In other words, the association between tumor location and overall survival was influenced by tumor size and pathological classification. The diagnosis of colonic NENs at late stages was probably due to the lack of early performance and difficulty accessing high-quality endoscopy. Early detection enables tumor treatment at an earlier stage without distant metastasis, which is the key to achieving curative resection and prolonging survival. In summary, extending enteroscopy and the exploration of novel diagnostic methods were of the most importance to improve the prognosis of colonic NENs [26, 27].

Ki-67 is a kind of nucleus antigen reflecting cell proliferation, which closely associated with tumor proliferation, infiltration, metastasis potentiality, and prognosis. Previous researches have indicated that higher Ki-67 index showed worse prognosis in GEP-NENs [28, 29]. Some studies with small sample sizes of colorectal NENs also presented similar results. Based on the above main findings, ENETS Consensus Guidelines put forward that NENs could be graded as G1, G2, and G3 according to the Ki-67 index (G1, Ki-67 $\leq$ 2%; G2, Ki-67 3 to 20%; G3, Ki-67 > 20%) [8]. We could not evaluate the prognostic value of Ki-67 index due to incompleteness of data. In available data, the G1/G2 NET were in the majority, which was accordant to the related researches overseas.

Several limitations in this study should be noted. First, our data were retrospectively collected from single medical center, and this method carries an inherent risk of bias. Our data only included the Chinese population, and it is not clear whether the results could be generalized to populations worldwide. Second, additional known risk factors that could predict survival were not evaluated, including histological growth pattern, mitotic rate, Ki-67 index, and immuno-histochemistry markers, such as chromogranin A (CgA) and synaptophysin (Syn) [21, 30–33]. Finally, our analysis did not adjust for treatment approaches that may impact outcomes [34]. To elucidate these questions, multicenter prospective studies with large samples are needed. Despite these limitations, we believe that current study reflects the actual distribution, clinical features, and prognostic factors of colorectal NENs in the Chinese population.

5. Conclusion

Significant differences in clinicopathological feature and outcome exist between colonic and rectal NENs. Multivariate analysis indicated that tumor size and pathological classification were associated with the prognosis. However, tumor location was not an independent factor. The worse outcome of colonic NENs observed in clinical practice might be due not only to the biological differences, but also to larger tumor size in colonic NENs caused by the delayed diagnosis.

Competing Interests

The authors declare that they have no competing interests.

Authors' Contributions

Mengjie Jiang, Yinuo Tan, and Xiaofen Li are co-first authors; they contributed equally to the work; Ying Yuan and Mengjie Jiang made substantial contribution to the conception and design of this study; Mengjie Jiang, Yinuo Tan, Xiaofen Li, Jianfei Fu, Hanguang Hu, Xianyun Ye, and Ying Cao collected, analyzed, and interpreted the data; pathologist Jinghong Xu read the pathological section. Mengjie Jiang, Yinuo Tan, and Xiaofen Li wrote the manuscript; Ying Yuan gave final approval to submit the manuscript for publication; Mengjie Jiang submitted the manuscript for publication.

Acknowledgments

The research was supported by (1) Key Projects in the National Science & Technology Pillar Program during the Twelfth Five-Year Plan Period (2014BAI09B07); (2) Training Program of the Major Research Plan of the National Natural Science Foundation of China (91229104); (3) the National High Technology Research and Development Program of China (863 Program) (2012AA02A506); (4) the National Science and Technology Major Project (2011ZX09307-001-05); (5) the National High Technology Research and Development Program of China (863 Program) (2012AA02A204).

References

[1] M. Fraenkel, M. Kim, A. Faggiano, W. W. de Herder, and G. D. Valk, "Incidence of gastroenteropancreatic neuroendocrine tumours: a systematic review of the literature," *Endocrine-Related Cancer*, vol. 21, no. 3, pp. R153–R163, 2014.

[2] H. Scherübl, B. Streller, R. Stabenow et al., "Clinically detected gastroenteropancreatic neuroendocrine tumors are on the rise: epidemiological changes in Germany," *World Journal of Gastroenterology*, vol. 19, no. 47, pp. 9012–9019, 2013.

[3] M. Fraenkel, M. K. Kim, A. Faggiano, and G. D. Valk, "Epidemiology of gastroenteropancreatic neuroendocrine tumours," *Best Practice & Research: Clinical Gastroenterology*, vol. 26, no. 6, pp. 691–703, 2012.

[4] J. Hallet, C. H. L. Law, M. Cukier, R. Saskin, N. Liu, and S. Singh, "Exploring the rising incidence of neuroendocrine tumors: a population-based analysis of epidemiology, metastatic presentation, and outcomes," *Cancer*, vol. 121, no. 4, pp. 589–597, 2015.

[5] J. C. Yao, M. Hassan, A. Phan et al., "One hundred years after 'carcinoid': epidemiology of and prognostic factors for neuroendocrine tumors in 35,825 cases in the United States," *Journal of Clinical Oncology*, vol. 26, no. 18, pp. 3063–3072, 2008.

[6] B. Lawrence, B. I. Gustafsson, A. Chan, B. Svejda, M. Kidd, and I. M. Modlin, "The epidemiology of gastroenteropancreatic neuroendocrine tumors," *Endocrinology and Metabolism Clinics of North America*, vol. 40, no. 1, pp. 1–18, 2011.

[7] M. A. Maggard, J. B. O'Connell, and C. Y. Ko, "Updated population-based review of carcinoid tumors," *Annals of Surgery*, vol. 240, no. 1, pp. 117–122, 2004.

[8] M. Caplin, A. Sundin, O. Nillson et al., "ENETS consensus guidelines for the management of patients with digestive neuroendocrine neoplasms: colorectal neuroendocrine neoplasms," *Neuroendocrinology*, vol. 95, no. 2, pp. 88–97, 2012.

[9] I. M. Modlin, K. D. Lye, and M. Kidd, "A 5-decade analysis of 13,715 carcinoid tumors," *Cancer*, vol. 97, no. 4, pp. 934–959, 2003.

[10] I. M. Modlin, I. Latich, M. Zikusoka, M. Kidd, G. Eick, and A. K. C. Chan, "Gastrointestinal carcinoids: the evolution of diagnostic strategies," *Journal of Clinical Gastroenterology*, vol. 40, no. 7, pp. 572–582, 2006.

[11] O. S. Lin, R. A. Kozarek, and J. M. Cha, "Impact of sigmoidoscopy and colonoscopy on colorectal cancer incidence and mortality: an evidence-based review of published prospective and retrospective studies," *Intestinal Research*, vol. 12, no. 4, pp. 268–274, 2014.

[12] T. Konishi, T. Watanabe, J. Kishimoto, K. Kotake, T. Muto, and H. Nagawa, "Prognosis and risk factors of metastasis in colorectal carcinoids: results of a nationwide registry over 15 years," *Gut*, vol. 56, no. 6, pp. 863–868, 2007.

[13] T. Ito, H. Sasano, M. Tanaka et al., "Epidemiological study of gastroenteropancreatic neuroendocrine tumors in Japan," *Journal of Gastroenterology*, vol. 45, no. 2, pp. 234–243, 2010.

[14] X. Zhang, L. Ma, H. Bao, J. Zhang, Z. Wang, and P. Gong, "Clinical, pathological and prognostic characteristics of gastroenteropancreatic neuroendocrine neoplasms in China: a retrospective study," *BMC Endocrine Disorders*, vol. 14, article no. 54, 2014.

[15] Y.-H. Wang, Y. Lin, L. Xue, J.-H. Wang, M.-H. Chen, and J. Chen, "Relationship between clinical characteristics and survival of gastroenteropancreatic neuroendocrine neoplasms: a single-institution analysis (1995–2012) in South China," *BMC Endocrine Disorders*, vol. 12, article 30, 2012.

[16] N. Reed, *ENETS conference for the diagnosis and treatment of neuroendocrine tumor disease*, vol. 103, S. Karger AG, Barcelona, Spain, 2016.

[17] J. Fu, J. Yang, Y. Tan et al., "Young patients (≤ 35 years old) with colorectal cancer have worse outcomes due to more advanced disease: a 30-year retrospective review," *Medicine*, vol. 93, no. 23, p. e135, 2014.

[18] S. L. Stewart, J. M. Wike, I. Kato, D. R. Lewis, and F. Michaud, "A population-based study of colorectal cancer histology in the United States, 1998–2001," *Cancer*, vol. 107, supplement 5, pp. 1128–1141, 2006.

[19] H. Shen, J. Yang, Q. Huang et al., "Different treatment strategies and molecular features between right-sided and left-sided colon cancers," *World Journal of Gastroenterology*, vol. 21, no. 21, pp. 6470–6478, 2015.

[20] X. Jiao, Y. Li, H. Wang, S. Liu, D. Zhang, and Y. Zhou, "Clinicopathological features and survival analysis of gastroenteropancreatic neuroendocrine neoplasms: a retrospective study in a single center of China," *Chinese Journal of Cancer Research*, vol. 27, no. 3, pp. 258–266, 2015.

[21] M. P. de Miguel Novoa, F. Fernández Capel, J. V. Redondo Sedano et al., "Gastroenteropancreatic neuroendocrine tumors: clinical characteristics, diagnosis and prognosis at Hospital Universitario Clínico San Carlos (Madrid)," *Endocrinologia y Nutricion*, vol. 61, no. 5, pp. 234–241, 2014.

[22] H.-K. Hu, N.-W. Ke, A. Li, X.-J. Du, Q. Guo, and W.-M. Hu, "Clinical characteristics and prognostic factors of gastroenteropancreatic neuroendocrine tumors: a single center experience in China," *Hepato-Gastroenterology*, vol. 62, no. 137, pp. 178–183, 2015.

[23] E. Lewkowicz, M. Trofimiuk-Müldner, K. Wysocka et al., "Gastroenteropancreatic neuroendocrine neoplasms: a 10-year

experience of a single center," *Polskie Archiwum Medycyny Wewnetrznej*, vol. 125, no. 5, pp. 337–346, 2015.

[24] X. Wang, Z.-F. Song, W.-X. Yao, C.-C. Pan, M.-F. Xiang, and H. Wang, "Clinicopathological features and multivariate analysis of prognostic factors for patients with gastroenteropancreatic neuroendocrine tumors," *Zhonghua Yi Xue Za Zhi*, vol. 93, no. 18, pp. 1411–1414, 2013.

[25] B. Yucel, N. A. K. Babacan, T. Kacan et al., "Survival analysis and prognostic factors for neuroendocrine tumors in Turkey," *Asian Pacific journal of cancer prevention : APJCP*, vol. 14, no. 11, pp. 6687–6692, 2014.

[26] I. M. Modlin, I. Drozdov, D. Alaimo et al., "A multianalyte PCR blood test outperforms single analyte ELISAs (chromogranin A, pancreastatin, neurokinin A) for neuroendocrine tumor detection," *Endocrine-Related Cancer*, vol. 21, no. 4, pp. 615–628, 2014.

[27] C. Vicentini, M. Fassan, E. D'Angelo et al., "Clinical application of microRNA testing in neuroendocrine tumors of the gastrointestinal tract," *Molecules*, vol. 19, no. 2, pp. 2458–2468, 2014.

[28] Y.-J. Boo, S.-S. Park, J.-H. Kim, Y.-J. Mok, S.-J. Kim, and C.-S. Kim, "Gastric neuroendocrine carcinoma: clinicopathologic review and immunohistochemical study of E-cadherin and Ki-67 as prognostic markers," *Journal of Surgical Oncology*, vol. 95, no. 2, pp. 110–117, 2007.

[29] H. C. Miller, P. Drymousis, R. Flora, R. Goldin, D. Spalding, and A. Frilling, "Role of ki-67 proliferation index in the assessment of patients with neuroendocrine neoplasias regarding the stage of disease," *World Journal of Surgery*, vol. 38, no. 6, pp. 1353–1361, 2014.

[30] S. Massironi, R. E. Rossi, G. Casazza et al., "Chromogranin a in diagnosing and monitoring patients with gastroenteropancreatic neuroendocrine neoplasms: a large series from a single institution," *Neuroendocrinology*, vol. 100, pp. 240–249, 2014.

[31] M. Stridsberg, K. Oberg, Q. Li, U. Engstrom, and G. Lundqvist, "Measurements of chromogranin A, chromogranin B (secretogranin I), chromogranin C (secretogranin II) and pancreastatin in plasma and urine from patients with carcinoid tumours and endocrine pancreatic tumours," *The Journal of Endocrinology*, vol. 144, no. 1, pp. 49–59, 1995.

[32] J. Jernman, J. Hagström, H. Mäenpää et al., "Expression of stem cell-associated marker HES77 in rectal neuroendocrine tumors," *Anticancer Research*, vol. 35, no. 7, pp. 3767–3772, 2015.

[33] Y.-H. Wang, Q.-C. Yang, Y. Lin, L. Xue, M.-H. Chen, and J. Chen, "Chromogranin a as a marker for diagnosis, treatment, and survival in patients with gastroenteropancreatic neuroendocrine neoplasm," *Medicine*, vol. 93, no. 27, article 247, 2014.

[34] S. Pusceddu, F. De Braud, F. Festinese et al., "Evolution in the treatment of gastroenteropancreatic-neuroendocrine neoplasms, focus on systemic therapeutic options: a systematic review," *Future Oncology*, vol. 11, no. 13, pp. 1947–1959, 2015.

21

Cerebral Hemodynamics and Cognitive Function in Cirrhotic Patients with Hepatic Encephalopathy

Yuqing Zhou,[1,2] Qian Dong,[3] Rong Zhang,[1,3] Shunfeng Zhou,[1,2] Linqiang Li,[1,2] Keran Cheng,[1,2] Rui Kong,[1,2] Qiang Yu,[1,3] Shizan Xu,[1,3] Jingjing Li,[1] Sainan Li,[1] Jiao Feng,[1] Liwei Wu,[1] Tong Liu,[1] Xiya Lu,[1] Kan Chen,[1] Yujing Xia,[1] Jie Lu,[1] Yingqun Zhou,[1] and Chuanyong Guo[1]

[1]Department of Gastroenterology, Shanghai Tenth People's Hospital, School of Medicine, Tongji University, Shanghai 200072, China
[2]The School of Medicine of Soochow University, Suzhou 215006, China
[3]The Shanghai Tenth Hospital, School of Clinical Medicine of Nanjing Medical University, Shanghai 200072, China

Correspondence should be addressed to Yingqun Zhou; yqzh02@163.com and Chuanyong Guo; guochuanyong@hotmail.com

Academic Editor: Paul Enck

Aims. To investigate cerebral hemodynamics in cirrhotic patients with HE and to observe effects of treatment in cerebral hemodynamics and correlations among ammonia, cerebral hemodynamics, and cognitive function. *Methods.* There were four groups: healthy controls (group 1), cirrhosis without HE (group 2), cirrhosis with MHE (group 3), and cirrhosis with OHE (group 4). Ammonia and cerebral hemodynamics (by TCD) were assessed. Patients in group 3 were subsequently randomized to two subgroups: the control (group A) and the treated (group B, treated with lactulose for two months), and they were retested for ammonia and TCD after treatment. Results. Ammonia, V_m, V_d, PI, and RI were statistically different before treatment, and ammonia, PI, and RI levels paralleled the severity of HE ($P < 0.05$). In group B, V_d increased and ammonia, PI, and RI declined following treatment ($P < 0.05$), while there were no differences in group A ($P > 0.05$). Correlations were found between ammonia and V_d, PI, RI, NCT-A, and DST and also found between V_d, PI, RI, and NCT-A and DST ($P < 0.05$). *Conclusions.* This study revealed that cerebral hemodynamics were related to the severity of HE and cerebral autoregulation was impaired. There were tight correlations among ammonia, cerebral hemodynamics, and cognitive function, and, following treatment, cerebral hemodynamics improved.

1. Introduction

Hepatic encephalopathy (HE) refers to a clinical syndrome associated with a wide spectrum of neurological or psychiatric abnormalities based on metabolic disorders, which is caused by serious acute/chronic liver dysfunction and/or portal-systemic shunt [1]. HE is associated with a poor prognosis, with a 1-year survival rate of less than 50%, which decreases to less than 25% 3 years following diagnosis [2]. HE includes the subtypes minimal hepatic encephalopathy (MHE) and overt hepatic encephalopathy (OHE). It has been reported that the incidence of MHE in patients with chronic liver diseases is up to 50% [3], with more than 50% of patients diagnosed with MHE reported to develop OHE within 30 months [4]. Patients with MHE do not present with obvious clinical symptoms, demonstrating subtle abnormalities in intelligence, neurological function, and cerebral blood flow by fine intelligence tests or electroneurophysiological examinations [5], and patients with OHE do present with obvious clinical symptoms such as changes in temperament, sleepiness, and even coma. The occurrence of HE increases the length of hospital stay, readmission rates, and risk of death and is associated with substantial personal and economic burden on their family and society [6].

Transcranial Doppler (TCD) is a simple, reproducible, and noninvasive method used to detect continuous, long-term hemodynamics and blood physiological parameters in the major intracranial artery including the middle cerebral artery (MCA) at the base of the skull. Cerebral blood flow and metabolism are closely related to cerebral function

TABLE 1: Cirrhotic patient demographics.

Variables	Mean/proportion
Age (year)	58.91 ± 8.59
Sex (M/F)	54/38
Educational years	9.74 ± 3.17
Etiology	
B viral hepatitis cirrhosis	40 (43.5%)
C viral hepatitis cirrhosis	3 (3.2%)
Primary biliary cirrhosis	7 (7.6%)
Autoimmune hepatitis cirrhosis	8 (8.7%)
Schistosomiasis cirrhosis	8 (8.7%)
Cryptogenic cirrhosis	26 (28.3%)
Child-Pugh grading	
Grade A	24 (26.1%)
Grade B	36 (39.1%)
Grade C	32 (34.8%)
Child-Pugh scores	8.87 ± 2.40

Table 1 presents cirrhotic patient demographics including age, sex, educational years, etiology, Child-Pugh grading, and Child-Pugh scores before treatment. Data derived from descriptive statistical analysis were presented as percentages for categorical variables and mean ± SD for continuous data.

and indirectly affect cognitive function [7]. In the present study, TCD was used to observe the changes of cerebral hemodynamics in healthy people and cirrhotic patients. Concurrently, we assessed the improvements of cerebral hemodynamics in patients with MHE after two-month oral treatment by lactulose, in order to provide an important basis for the clinical development, diagnosis, and treatment of HE.

2. Materials and Methods

2.1. Patient Demographics. From August 2015 to April 2016, 92 inpatients and outpatients with cirrhosis of Shanghai Tenth People's Hospital were enrolled in the study. They were aged between 37 and 76 years and included 54 males and 38 females with between 3 and 16 years of education. In etiology, there were 40 cases with B viral hepatitis cirrhosis, 3 cases with C viral hepatitis cirrhosis, 7 cases with primary biliary cirrhosis, 8 cases with autoimmune hepatitis cirrhosis, 8 cases with schistosomiasis cirrhosis, and 26 cases with cryptogenic cirrhosis. Simultaneously, we determined their grades (24 cases of grade A, 36 cases of grade B, and 32 cases of grade C) and scores of Child-Pugh [8] (Table 1). The diagnosis of cirrhosis was made by experienced clinicians and based on clinical signs and symptoms, laboratory tests, and imaging such as ultrasound, CT, and MRI. The diagnosis was consistent with "The Guideline of Prevention and Treatment for Chronic Hepatitis B (2010 version)" [9]. Additionally, 40 healthy volunteers served as controls and were matched with cirrhosis patients according to age (between 35 and 71 years of age), sex (24 males and 16 females), and educational level (between 3 and 16 years of education). The controls had no history of liver diseases, exhibiting normal liver function and morphology. Written informed consent was obtained from all subjects.

Patients with the following conditions were excluded from the study: diseases of the central nervous system (CNS) such as cerebral hemorrhage, cerebral infarction, or mental illnesses. Similarly, patients with alcoholic cirrhosis or drinking history in the past three months were excluded as long-term drinking can cause alcoholic cirrhosis and can also lead to alcoholism encephalopathy, both of which may cause abnormity in TCD. A clinical history of fever in the past one week; fluid, electrolyte, and acid-base disequilibrium in the past two weeks; gastrointestinal bleeding and hemoglobin less than 90 g/L in the past two weeks; taking lactulose, probiotics, and rifaximin in the past two months; taking neuropsychiatric drugs in the past one month; diagnoses of heart diseases, lung diseases, kidney diseases, hypertension, or diabetes; and illiteracy were also grounds for exclusion.

2.2. Groups. All subjects were divided into four groups: healthy controls (*n* = 40, group 1), cirrhosis without HE (*n* = 52, group 2), cirrhosis with MHE (*n* = 21, group 3), and cirrhosis with OHE (*n* = 19, group 4). After completion of all the examinations on the day of selection, patients in group 3 were randomized into one of the two subgroups, the control group (*n* = 10, group A) which were given standard liver treatments including hepatoprotective drugs, intravenous infusion of albumin, branched chain amino acids, maintaining fluid, electrolyte and acid-base balance, and prevention of complications for two months, and the treated group (*n* = 11, group B) which were treated by lactulose oral solution (Duphalac, Solvay Pharmaceuticals B.V., Weesp, Netherlands) three times a day, 15 mL at a time, for two months in combination with standard liver treatments. This study was a retrospective, single-blind, and blank randomized controlled trial.

2.3. Study Design. Blood analysis was performed on all patients with cirrhosis and included assessment of ammonia, creatinine (Cr), total bilirubin (TBil), albumin (ALB), and prothrombin time (PT). Prior to blood collection patients were fasted for 8 hours or more, before 8 mL blood was collected. Serum specimens were used for liver and renal function tests. Anticoagulant plasma by heparin was used for ammonia tests using the VITROS-250 dry chemistry analyzer (Johnson & Johnson, New Brunswick Zwick, New Jersey, USA) and serum Cr, TBil, and ALB tested using the automatic biochemical analyzer (Beckman, Fullerton, California, USA). The levels of ammonia were retested in group A and group B following two months of treatment. Using a combination of ascites and stage of HE, we determined the grades and scores of Child-Pugh.

In order to confirm diagnosis of MHE, subjects without OHE were administered Number Connection Test-A (NCT-A) and Digit Symbol Test (DST) in a quiet environment prior to TCD examinations. Abnormal results in both tests indicated MHE diagnosis, where abnormity of NCT-A is the mean plus twice the standard deviation, while DST is the mean minus twice the standard deviation [1].

TABLE 2: Patient demographics and blood analysis before treatment among groups 1, 2, 3, and 4.

Variables	Group 1	Group 2	Group 3	Group 4	F/χ^2 value	P
Cases	40	52	21	19	—	—
Age (year)	54.32 ± 10.14	58.31 ± 9.24	59.10 ± 7.55	60.37 ± 8.05	2.587	0.056
Sex (M/F)	24/16	31/21	12/9	11/8	0.064	0.996
Educational years	9.55 ± 3.37	10.37 ± 3.33	9.19 ± 2.87	8.63 ± 2.75	1.662	0.178
Etiology					7.148	0.711
B viral hepatitis cirrhosis	—	21	11	8		
C viral hepatitis cirrhosis	—	1	1	1		
Primary biliary cirrhosis	—	3	3	1		
Autoimmune hepatitis cirrhosis	—	5	0	3		
Schistosomiasis cirrhosis	—	6	1	1		
Cryptogenic cirrhosis	—	16	5	5		
Child-Pugh grading					7.229	0.124
Grade A	—	18	4	2		
Grade B	—	21	8	7		
Grade C	—	13	9	10		
Child-Pugh scores	—	8.27 ± 2.36	9.19 ± 2.16	10.16 ± 2.27	4.965	0.009
Ammonia (μmol/L)	—	37.12 ± 15.28	63.81 ± 19.22	106.21 ± 46.14	52.154	<0.001
Cr (μmol/L)	—	86.01 ± 22.80	83.35 ± 40.11	79.14 ± 43.92	0.318	0.728
TBil (μmol/L)	—	45.78 ± 16.76	45.57 ± 14.51	42.81 ± 14.83	0.254	0.776
ALB (g/L)	—	29.62 ± 7.92	28.38 ± 5.36	31.05 ± 6.71	0.691	0.504
PT (sec)	—	3.14 ± 1.76	2.87 ± 1.74	3.25 ± 1.76	0.263	0.769
NCT-A (sec)	46.92 ± 11.80	51.31 ± 10.93	88.29 ± 9.38	—	108.840	<0.001
DST (scores)	52.35 ± 10.69	49.98 ± 9.98	23.57 ± 4.04	—	72.476	<0.001

Table 2 indicates comparison of age, sex, educational years, etiology, Child-Pugh grading, Child-Pugh scores, ammonia, Cr, TBil, ALB, PT, NCT-A, and DST among groups 1, 2, 3, and 4 before treatment. Group 1 is healthy controls group, group 2 is cirrhosis without HE group, group 3 is cirrhosis with MHE group, and group 4 is cirrhosis with OHE group. Continuous data were compared using ANOVA and categorical data were compared by a chi-square test. $P < 0.05$ means significant differences in an index among groups.

Following biochemical examinations and NCT-A and DST tests, all subjects were subjected to TCD examinations. We used TC8080 TCD diagnostic instrument (Elektromaschinenbau Ettlingen Maschinenfabrik Clasen GmbH, Ettlingen, Baden-Württemberg, Germany) to detect the right MCA by placing a 2 MHz pulsed Doppler probe on the temporal temple. An experienced clinician performed this examination. Peak systolic velocity (V_p), mean velocity (V_m), end diastolic velocity (V_d) as well as the pulsatility index (PI), which reflects cerebrovascular compliance and elasticity, and resistance index (RI), which reflects cerebrovascular diastolic, systolic, and resistant status of the right MCA, of each subject were measured. Finally, after two months of treatment, we again assessed the improvements in these indexes in group A and group B patients.

2.4. Statistical Analysis. Data derived from descriptive statistical analysis are presented as percentages for categorical variables and mean ± SD for continuous data and all data were analyzed by SPSS20.0. Measurement data were tested by the Kolmogorov-Smirnov test of normality and Levene test of homogeneity of variance. If the data conformed to normality and homogeneity of variance, they were compared using t-test or ANOVA, as appropriate. Pairwise comparisons between multiple groups were performed using SNK-q or LSD-t method of ANOVA. Alternatively, we used Mann-Whitney rank sum test (two groups) or Kruskal-Wallis test (multiple groups). Categorical data were compared by chi-square test. Correlation was analyzed by partial correlation analysis and Pearson's correlation coefficient used for bivariate normal distribution data or Spearman's rank correlation coefficient. A P value < 0.05 was considered statistically significant.

3. Results

3.1. Comparison of Patient Demographics and Blood Analysis before Treatment. In cirrhotic patients, the incidence of MHE was 22.8% compared to 20.7% in patients with OHE. The prevalence of MHE in Child-Pugh A was 19.0%, 38.1% in Child-Pugh B and the highest in Child-Pugh C at 42.9%. No statistically significant differences in age, sex, educational years, etiology of cirrhosis, Child-Pugh grading, Cr, TBil, ALB, and PT ($P > 0.05$) were observed, while there were significant differences in Child-Pugh scores (0.009) and ammonia ($P < 0.001$) in all groups before treatment (Table 2). Interestingly, ammonia levels appeared to parallel the severity of HE, as ammonia was lowest in cirrhosis patients without HE (37.12 ± 15.28), greater in MHE patients (63.81 ± 19.22), and highest in the OHE group (106.21 ± 46.14) (Figure 1).

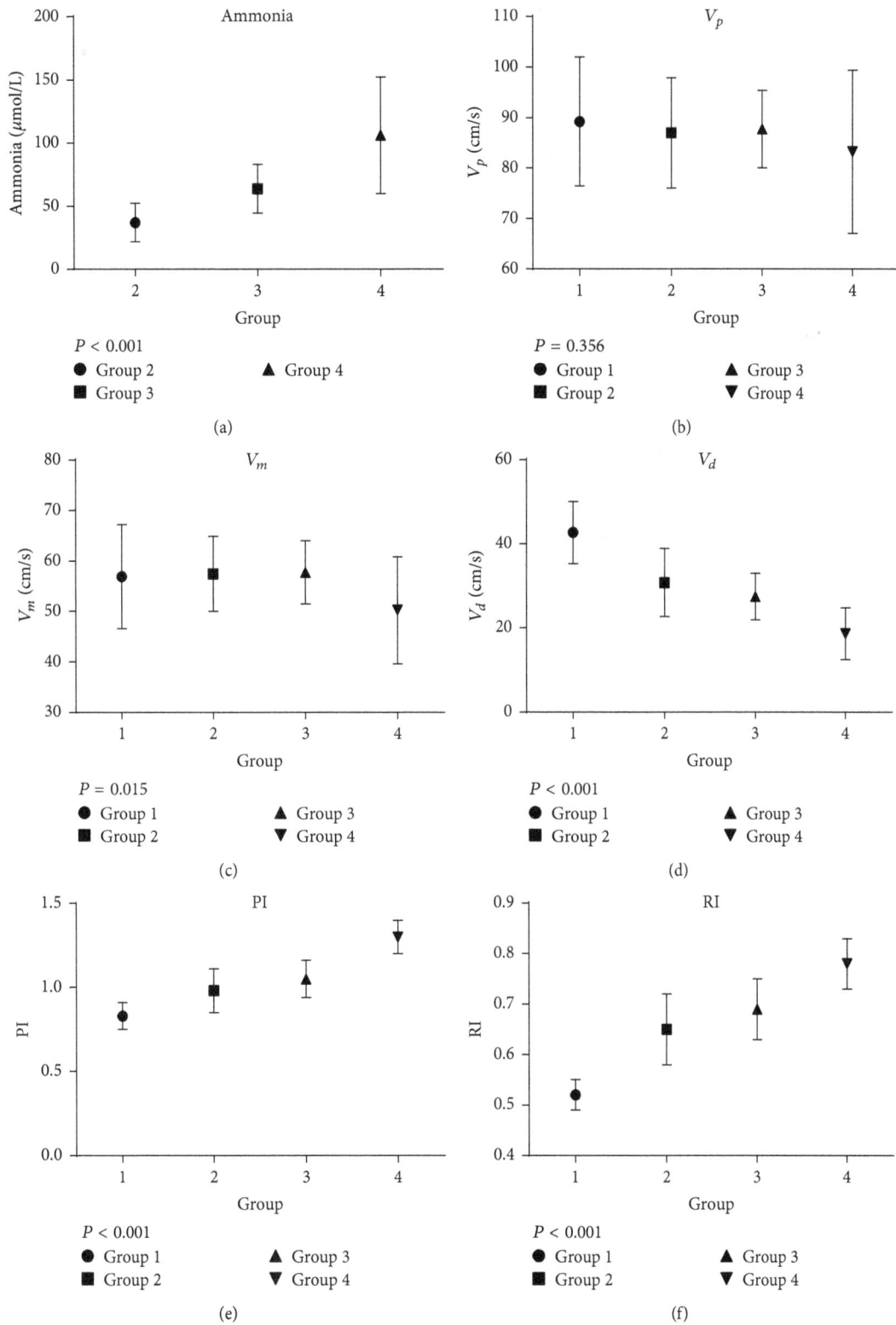

FIGURE 1: *Comparison of ammonia and TCD among groups 1, 2, 3, and 4 before treatment.* It includes the subfigures (a, b, c, d, e, and f). Subfigure (a) is comparison of ammonia among groups 2, 3, and 4. Subfigure (b) is comparison of V_p among groups 1, 2, 3, and 4. Subfigure (c) is comparison of V_m among groups 1, 2, 3, and 4. Subfigure (d) is comparison of V_d among groups 1, 2, 3, and 4. Subfigure (e) is comparison of PI among groups 1, 2, 3, and 4. Subfigure (f) is comparison of RI among groups 1, 2, 3, and 4. Group 1 is healthy controls group, group 2 is cirrhosis without HE group, group 3 is cirrhosis with MHE group, and group 4 is cirrhosis with OHE group. The data were compared using ANOVA and presented as mean ± SD. $P < 0.05$ means significant differences in an index among groups.

TABLE 3: Patient demographics and blood analysis before treatment between groups A and B.

Variables	Group A	Group B	t/χ^2 value	P
Cases	10	11	—	—
Age (year)	58.10 ± 6.67	60.00 ± 8.49	−0.566	0.578
Sex (M/F)	6/4	6/5	0.064	0.801
Educational years	9.00 ± 2.83	9.36 ± 3.04	−0.283	0.780
Etiology			2.582	0.630
B viral hepatitis cirrhosis	5	6		
C viral hepatitis cirrhosis	1	0		
Primary biliary cirrhosis	2	1		
Autoimmune hepatitis cirrhosis	0	0		
Schistosomiasis cirrhosis	0	1		
Cryptogenic cirrhosis	2	3		
Child-Pugh grading			0.565	0.754
Grade A	2	2		
Grade B	5	4		
Grade C	3	5		
Child-Pugh scores	9.10 ± 2.42	9.27 ± 2.01	−0.179	0.860
Ammonia (μmol/L)	64.30 ± 17.07	63.45 ± 21.33	0.098	0.923
Cr (μmol/L)	89.00 ± 45.63	78.22 ± 35.82	0.605	0.552
TBil (μmol/L)	42.53 ± 14.14	48.34 ± 14.94	−0.912	0.373
ALB (g/L)	29.40 ± 7.03	27.45 ± 3.33	0.824	0.420
PT (sec)	2.98 ± 2.17	2.76 ± 1.34	0.278	0.784
NCT-A (sec)	87.20 ± 7.83	89.27 ± 10.89	−0.496	0.626
DST (scores)	24.20 ± 3.36	23.00 ± 4.67	0.670	0.511

Table 3 indicates comparison of age, sex, educational years, etiology, Child-Pugh grading, Child-Pugh scores, ammonia, Cr, TBil, ALB, PT, NCT-A, and DST between groups A and B before treatment. Group A is the control group; group B is the treated group. Continuous data were compared using t-test and categorical data were compared by a chi-square test. $P < 0.05$ means significant differences in an index between two groups.

TABLE 4: Comparison of TCD before treatment.

Variables	Group 1	Group 2	Group 3	Group 4	F value	P
V_p (cm/s)	89.22 ± 12.76	86.98 ± 10.90	87.71 ± 7.67	83.26 ± 16.14	1.089	0.356
V_m (cm/s)	56.90 ± 10.29	57.42 ± 7.46	57.71 ± 6.29	50.21 ± 10.59	3.608	0.015
V_d (cm/s)	42.65 ± 7.37	30.80 ± 8.13	27.43 ± 5.52	18.63 ± 6.15	53.131	<0.001
PI	0.83 ± 0.08	0.98 ± 0.13	1.05 ± 0.11	1.30 ± 0.10	81.599	<0.001
RI	0.52 ± 0.03	0.65 ± 0.07	0.69 ± 0.06	0.78 ± 0.05	98.676	<0.001

Table 4 describes comparison of TCD including V_p, V_m, V_d, PI, and RI among groups 1, 2, 3, and 4 before treatment. Group 1 is healthy controls group, group 2 is cirrhosis without HE group, group 3 is cirrhosis with MHE group, and group 4 is cirrhosis with OHE group. Continuous data were compared using ANOVA. $P < 0.05$ means significant differences in an index among groups.

Before treatment, there were no statistically significant differences in age, sex, educational years, etiology, Child-Pugh grading, Child-Pugh scores, ammonia, Cr, TBil, ALB, PT, NCT-A, and DST between group A and group B (Table 3).

3.2. Comparison of TCD before Treatment. Prior to treatment, no significant differences were observed among group 1, group 2, group 3, and group 4 in V_p ($P = 0.356$) of right MCA, while profound differences were observed in V_m ($P = 0.015$), V_d ($P < 0.001$), PI ($P < 0.001$), and RI ($P < 0.001$) among these four groups (Table 4) (Figure 1). Pairwise comparison of V_m within groups 1 to 3 did not reveal any significant

differences; however, we observed important differences with group 4 ($P_{1,2} = 0.776$, $P_{1,3} = 0.730$, $P_{1,4} = 0.007$, $P_{2,3} = 0.898$, $P_{2,4} = 0.003$, and $P_{3,4} = 0.008$). Further pairwise comparison of V_d within all groups demonstrated statistical significance, with no significant differences observed between groups 2 and 3 ($P_{1,2} < 0.001$, $P_{1,3} < 0.001$, $P_{1,4} < 0.001$, $P_{2,3} = 0.075$, $P_{2,4} < 0.001$, and $P_{3,4} < 0.001$). Additionally, PI paralleled the severity of HE as PI was 0.83 ± 0.08 in group 1, 0.98 ± 0.13 in group 2, 1.05 ± 0.11 in group 3, and 1.30 ± 0.10 in group 4 ($P_{1,2} < 0.001$, $P_{1,3} < 0.001$, $P_{1,4} < 0.001$, $P_{2,3} = 0.024$, $P_{2,4} < 0.001$, and $P_{3,4} < 0.001$). Furthermore, the same was observed of RI (0.52 ± 0.03, 0.65 ± 0.07, 0.69 ± 0.06, 0.78 ± 0.05, $P_{1,2} < 0.001$, $P_{1,3} < 0.001$, $P_{1,4} < 0.001$, $P_{2,3} = 0.011$, $P_{2,4} < 0.001$, and $P_{3,4} < 0.001$) (Table 5).

TABLE 5: Pairwise comparison of TCD before treatment.

Variables	$P_{1,2}$	$P_{1,3}$	$P_{1,4}$	$P_{2,3}$	$P_{2,4}$	$P_{3,4}$
V_p (cm/s)	0.373	0.640	0.076	0.813	0.248	0.242
V_m (cm/s)	0.776	0.730	0.007	0.898	0.003	0.008
V_d (cm/s)	<0.001	<0.001	<0.001	0.075	<0.001	<0.001
PI	<0.001	<0.001	<0.001	0.024	<0.001	<0.001
RI	<0.001	<0.001	<0.001	0.011	<0.001	<0.001

Table 5 presents pairwise comparison of TCD including V_p, V_m, V_d, PI, and RI among groups 1, 2, 3, and 4 before treatment. $P_{1,2}$ indicates comparison between group 1 and group 2, $P_{1,3}$ means comparison between group 1 and group 3, $P_{1,4}$ compares group 1 and group 4, $P_{2,3}$ refers to a comparison between group 2 and group 3, $P_{2,4}$ indicates a comparison between group 2 and group 4, and $P_{3,4}$ means comparison between group 3 and group 4. Group 1 is healthy controls group, group 2 is cirrhosis without HE group, group 3 is cirrhosis with MHE group, and group 4 is cirrhosis with OHE group. Pairwise comparisons between multiple groups were performed using SNK-q or LSD-t method of ANOVA. $P < 0.05$ means significant differences in an index between two groups.

3.3. Comparison between Control and Treatment Groups before and after Treatment. In controls (group A), comparison of ammonia and TCD revealed no significant differences before or after treatment ($P > 0.05$) (Table 6, Figure 2). However, in the treatment group (group B) patients demonstrated a decrease in ammonia following treatment (from 63.45 ± 21.33 to 43.36 ± 10.63, $P = 0.004$). In addition, we observed that V_d increased (from 27.55 ± 6.27 to 34.09 ± 7.38, $P = 0.007$), whilst PI (from 1.06 ± 0.09 to 0.93 ± 0.12, $P = 0.008$) and RI (from 0.69 ± 0.06 to 0.63 ± 0.06, $P = 0.019$) declined. No statistically significant differences were observed in V_p or V_m ($P = 0.185$, $P = 0.143$) (Table 6, Figure 2).

3.4. Correlation Analysis among Ammonia, Cerebral Hemodynamics, and Declining Cognitive Function in Patients with MHE. In patients with MHE, there was no correlation observed between ammonia and V_m ($r = -0.286$, $P = 0.209$), but there was positive correlation between ammonia and PI ($r = 0.892$, $P < 0.001$), RI ($r = 0.742$, $P < 0.001$), and also NCT-A ($r = 0.824$, $P < 0.001$). In contrast, there was negative correlation between ammonia and V_d ($r = -0.719$, $P < 0.001$), DST ($r = -0.742$, $P < 0.001$) (Figure 3).

In patients with MHE, there was no correlation observed between V_m and NCT-A ($r = -0.321$, $P = 0.156$), DST ($r = 0.282$, $P = 0.216$); however we did detect a correlation between V_d and NCT-A ($r = -0.596$, $P = 0.004$), DST ($r = 0.589$, $P = 0.005$), which was opposite to PI ($r = 0.793$, $P < 0.001$; $r = -0.738$, $P < 0.001$) and RI ($r = 0.597$, $P = 0.004$; $r = -0.589$, $P = 0.005$) (Figure 4).

4. Discussion

To date, the pathogenesis of HE has not been fully elucidated. It has been proposed that HE is the result of multiple factors and it is widely believed that it is the collective effects by severe dysfunction of organism metabolism and toxic accumulation, amongst which elevated ammonia has emerged as one of the main pathogeneses [10, 11].

In severe liver diseases, liver dysfunction, reduced transformation, and clearance of metabolites by liver, coupled with overgenerating of ammonia, cause significant increasing of blood ammonia and it cannot be excluded from the body. Ammonia has toxic effects on the nervous system. (1) Ammonia enters the CNS through the blood-brain barrier (BBB) and astrocytes are the only cells in the brain that can metabolize ammonia [12] which play an important role in maintaining the balance of BBB, autoregulation function of CNS, and cerebral blood flow [13]. Synthetizing of glutamine by ammonia and glutamic acid results in obvious increasing of glutamine in astrocytes, causing conduction disorders of glutamatergic neurons, astrocytes swelling, cerebral edema, and intracranial hypertension [14, 15]. Long-time exposure of astrocytes in high concentration of ammonia will lead to compensatory loss of permeating substances such as taurine and inositol, so that the astrocytes become very sensitive to the edema effect caused by other HE-induced factors and then induce HE or result in sudden deterioration of HE [16–18]. (2) Ammonia can bring about energy metabolism obstacles of carbohydrate utilization, glycolysis, tricarboxylic acid cycle, and ATP synthesis and utilization and result in insufficiency of brain energy supply; thus it cannot maintain the excitement of the CNS [19]. (3) Ammonia may decrease the activity of Na^+-K^+-ATPase in CNS, weakening the function of BBB enzyme system, leading to the unblocking of toxic substances into CNS through the damaged BBB and impairing the autoregulation function of intracranial blood flow. Ammonia may also compete with K^+ for binding to Na^+-K^+-ATPase in neuronal cells and astrocytes membrane, leading to conduction disturbances of nerve impulse and astrocytes swelling or brain edema [20]. (4) Ammonia can act directly on the nerve membrane, causing postsynaptic inhibition and interference with nerve action potential. Glutamine receptors activity on the postsynaptic plate will reduce and glutamine carriers on the astrocytic membrane will inactivate, thereby leading to astrocytes swelling [21]. Over time, these cells transform into Alzheimer type II astrocytes [22, 23]. (5) In addition, ammonia can lead to imbalance of inhibitory and excitatory neurotransmitter, increasing the contents of inhibitory neurotransmitter; it will change gene expression of astrocytes structural protein, glial fibrillary acidic protein, aquaporin 4, and so forth, so that proteins maintain the normal function of the brain alter abnormally [24]; it may also increase calcium influx in astrocytes and start oxidation and nitrification stress directly, resulting in mitochondrial dysfunction and energy loss, causing inflammation and damaging intracellular signaling pathways, and ultimately leading to nervous system dysfunction [25–27].

Although our study found that there were significant differences in ammonia ($P < 0.001$) amongst all experimental groups and that ammonia paralleled the severity of HE, we demonstrate that ammonia levels had significant overlap in different grades of HE consistent with the observations in Blei and Córdoba's study [28]. This overlap may be related to the generation, absorption, and removal of ammonia which can be affected by a variety of intrahepatic and extrahepatic factors and ammonia may not be the only pathogenesis of HE [29]. Also, clinical testing and experimental studies

TABLE 6: Comparison of ammonia and TCD before and after treatment.

Variables	Group A		Group B		t_1 value	t_2 value	P_1	P_2
	Before	After	Before	After				
Ammonia (μmol/L)	64.30 ± 17.67	66.30 ± 14.19	63.45 ± 21.33	43.36 ± 10.63	−0.621	3.760	0.550	0.004
V_p (cm/s)	87.80 ± 6.48	91.20 ± 8.24	87.64 ± 8.94	90.82 ± 6.59	−1.880	−1.423	0.093	0.185
V_m (cm/s)	58.20 ± 2.82	58.60 ± 6.80	57.27 ± 8.46	63.18 ± 8.65	−0.217	−1.590	0.833	0.143
V_d (cm/s)	27.30 ± 4.90	30.40 ± 7.35	27.55 ± 6.27	34.09 ± 7.38	−1.730	−3.404	0.118	0.007
PI	1.04 ± 0.13	1.03 ± 0.13	1.06 ± 0.09	0.93 ± 0.12	0.399	3.333	0.699	0.008
RI	0.69 ± 0.06	0.66 ± 0.08	0.69 ± 0.06	0.63 ± 0.06	1.262	2.785	0.239	0.019

Table 6 indicates comparison of ammonia and TCD including V_p, V_m, V_d, PI, and RI between group A and B before and after treatment. t_1 and P_1 represent comparison before and after treatment in group A; t_2 and P_2 represent comparison before and after treatment in group B. Group A is the control group; group B is the treated group. Continuous data were compared using t-test. $P < 0.05$ means significant differences in an index before and after treatment.

have shown that patients with hyperammonemia do not necessarily have HE, and not all patients with HE show significantly elevated blood ammonia which requires us to distinguish HE from other diseases [30]. Therefore, the theory of ammonia toxicity alone cannot well explain the pathogenesis of HE, and it should be along with other hypotheses such as inflammatory response, oxidation, and nitrification stress, amino acid metabolism imbalance, neurotransmitter imbalance, and manganese toxicity. Consequently, the clinical value of assessing blood ammonia concentration in HE classification and MHE diagnosis remains unclear. Lactulose is widely used as a clinical treatment for MHE, as it promotes the metabolism of ammonia, by reducing the intestinal absorption leading to an overall reduction in circulating ammonia [31]. In the present study, we treated MHE patients with lactulose for 2 months, resulting in a decline in ammonia levels (from 63.45 ± 21.33 to 43.36 ± 10.63, $P = 0.004$), indicating that lactulose is an effective treatment for MHE via the compounds ability to reduce ammonia.

Current literatures demonstrated a good understanding of cerebral hemodynamics, cerebral metabolism, and cerebral autoregulation function in acute/fulminant hepatic failure, whilst their role in HE and chronic liver disease/cirrhosis remains poorly understood. Felipo et al. found that determining noninvasive brain blood flow using arterial spin labeling (ASL) could detect MHE earlier than Psychometric Hepatic Encephalopathy Score (PHES) [32] indicating there are early changes to cerebral hemodynamics in the preliminary stages of HE. In the present study, prior to treatment, we observed no differences in V_p ($P = 0.356$) of right MCA, while significant differences were evident in V_m, V_d, PI, and RI ($P < 0.05$). Furthermore, our results demonstrate that more serious HE was associated with decreased cerebral blood flow velocity, particularly mean velocity and end diastolic velocity. Simultaneously, PI and RI paralleled the severity of HE. As PI reflects the compliance and elasticity of the cerebral vasculature and RI reflects diastolic, systolic, and resistant status of the cerebral vasculature this result suggests that systolic and diastolic cerebral autoregulation is impaired, as PI and RI increased in cirrhotic patients with HE and cerebral hemodynamics was related to severity of HE, consistent with results from previous studies [33, 34].

Many studies have established that cerebral blood flow, cerebral autoregulation, and cerebral edema are improved in acute/fulminant hepatic failure through a series of active treatments [35–37]. However, to date little is known about the changes of cerebral hemodynamics in cirrhotic patients with MHE after treatment. Lactulose can reduce the impact of ammonia on cerebral blood flow and brain function by reducing ammonia and as confirmed in our study may therefore improve cerebral hemodynamics in patients with HE. Following two months of treatment with lactulose, V_d increased (from 27.55 ± 6.27 to 34.09 ± 7.38, $P = 0.007$), whilst PI (from 1.06 ± 0.09 to 0.93 ± 0.12, $P = 0.008$) and RI (from 0.69 ± 0.06 to 0.63 ± 0.06, $P = 0.019$) declined. In addition, the treatment did not significantly alter V_p and V_m ($P = 0.185$, $P = 0.143$). As such, we demonstrate that lactulose treatment not only does improve cerebral blood flow and cerebral autoregulation in acute/fulminant hepatic failure, but also has potential for use in patients with MHE. Furthermore, it was an effective method for disease surveillance, efficacy evaluation by detection, and monitoring of TCD.

Cognition is the mental action and process of acquiring and understanding of knowledge, with the basis of the normal functioning of cerebral cortex. Consequently, any factors including ammonia which cause abnormity in brain function and structure may lead to declining cognitive function. Our study found that, in patients with MHE, there was positive correlation between ammonia and PI, RI, and also NCT-A ($P < 0.001$). In contrast, there was negative correlation between ammonia and V_d and DST ($P < 0.001$). Similarly, there was negative correlation between V_d and NCT-A and positive correlation between V_d and DST ($P < 0.05$), which was opposite to PI and RI ($P < 0.05$). This indicated that there were tight correlations among ammonia, reduced cerebral blood flow velocity, impaired systolic and diastolic cerebral autoregulation, and declining cognitive function in patients with MHE.

However, TCD application is still associated with some issues such as the impact of different operators and lack of uniform criteria about normal and abnormal values. The failure rate of TCD is 2.7% to 5% in older patients, who often have thickening of the skull, arterial tortuosity, and arterial shift [7]. The present study addressed changes in cerebral

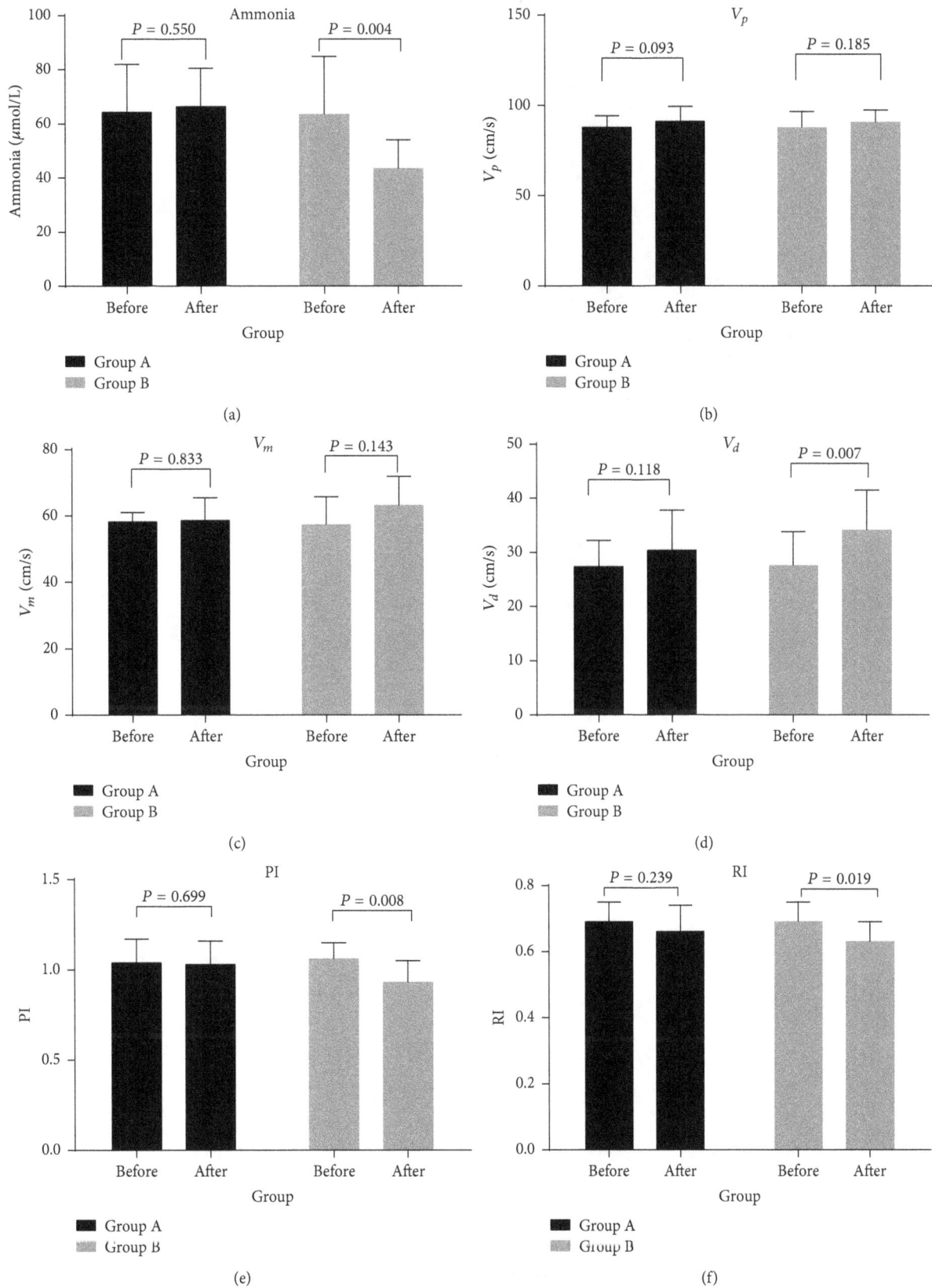

FIGURE 2: *Comparison of ammonia and TCD before and after treatment in groups A and B.* It includes the subfigures (a, b, c, d, e, and f). Subfigure (a) is comparison of ammonia. Subfigure (b) is comparison of V_p. Subfigure (c) is comparison of V_m. Subfigure (d) is comparison of V_d. Subfigure (e) is comparison of PI. Subfigure (f) is comparison of RI. Group A is the control group; group B is the treated group. The data were compared using t-test. $P < 0.05$ means significant differences in an index among groups.

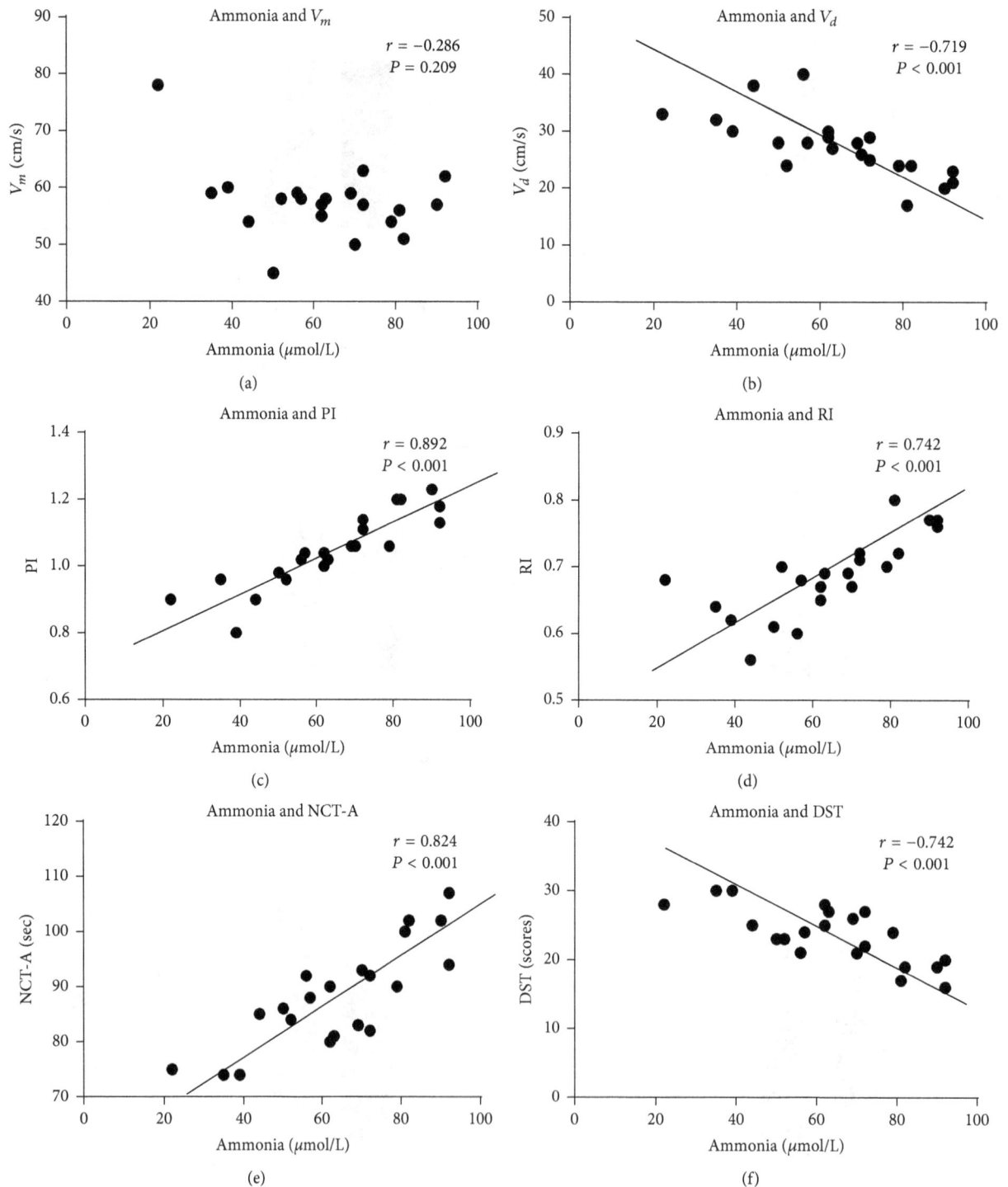

FIGURE 3: *Correlation between ammonia and cerebral hemodynamics (V_m, V_d, PI, and RI) and declining cognitive function (NCT-A and DST) in patients with MHE*. It includes the subfigures (a, b, c, d, e, and f). Subfigure (a) is correlation between ammonia and V_m. Subfigure (b) is correlation between ammonia and V_d. Subfigure (c) is correlation between ammonia and PI. Subfigure (d) is correlation between ammonia and RI. Subfigure (e) is correlation between ammonia and NCT-A. Subfigure (f) is correlation between ammonia and DST. Correlation was analyzed by Pearson's correlation coefficient. $P < 0.05$ means significant differences in correlation between two indexes.

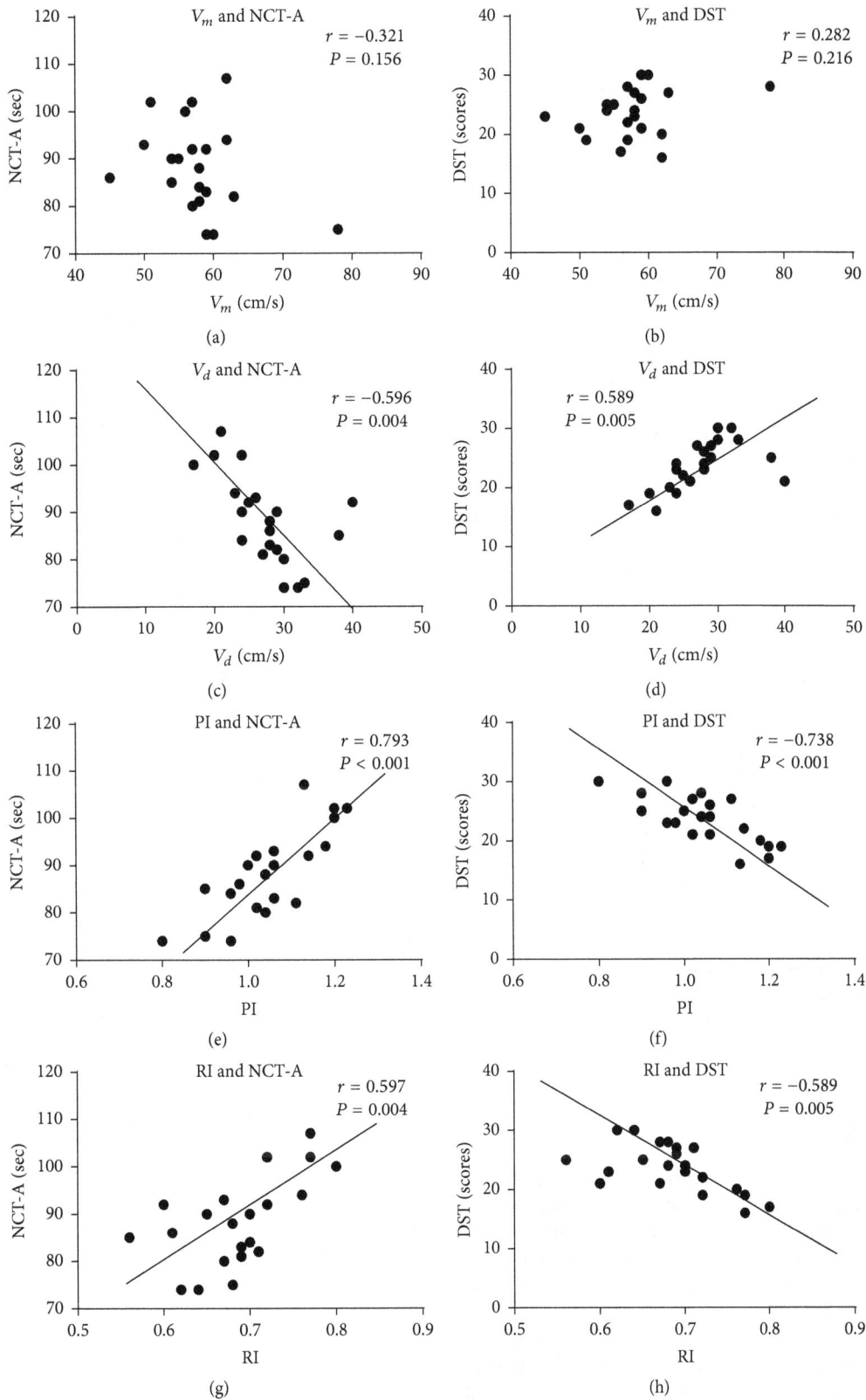

FIGURE 4: *Correlation between cerebral hemodynamics (V_m, V_d, PI, and RI) and declining cognitive function (NCT-A and DST) in patients with MHE.* It includes the subfigures (a, b, c, d, e, f, g, and h). Subfigure (a) is correlation between V_m and NCT-A. Subfigure (b) is correlation between V_m and DST. Subfigure (c) is correlation between V_d and NCT-A. Subfigure (d) is correlation between V_d and DST. Subfigure (e) is correlation between PI and NCT-A. Subfigure (f) is correlation between PI and DST. Subfigure (g) is correlation between RI and NCT-A. Subfigure (h) is correlation between RI and DST. Correlation was analyzed by Pearson's correlation coefficient. $P < 0.05$ means significant differences in correlation between two indexes.

hemodynamics in patients with HE as well as its role in monitoring severity of HE and efficacy assessment. Future studies will need to further explore the critical value for diagnosis and classification. Although this study reports some important findings in the improvement of cerebral hemodynamics after 2 months of treatment, further long-term follow-up of such patients is required to better understand these findings.

The incidence of MHE in cirrhotic patients has been reported to be from 30% to 84% according to foreign data [38–40] while it is between 29.2% and 57.1% in China [1] and 22.8% in the present study. These differences may be due to the lack of uniform diagnostic criteria of MHE, the different operators, sample size, and individual and regional differences. It has been reported by Groeneweg et al. that cirrhotic patients of Child-Pugh A had a low prevalence (15%) of MHE, while MHE was present in half of the patients with advanced cirrhosis (B/C) [41]. Our study confirmed there was a significant difference in the prevalence of MHE amongst these groups, with the lowest incidence observed in Child-Pugh A (19%); MHE had a higher incidence in Child-Pugh B (38.1%) and C (42.9%) groups. Accordingly, patients' liver function should be taken into account in the diagnosis of MHE and more attention directed to cirrhotic patients without OHE clinically, especially in patients with Child-Pugh B and Child-Pugh C.

Patients with MHE do not demonstrate any overt clinical symptoms of HE but do exhibit mild cognitive and psychomotor deficits [42]. It has been previously reported that the majority of patients with MHE have changes in memory, reaction, attention, and behavior, which may impact their work and personal life to different degrees. Approximately 60% of patients with MHE have been found to be unfit for work and approximately 50% unfit to drive [43]. However, due to the subtle nature of MHE symptoms, preventative and treatment strategies are difficult to implement. Therefore, a better understanding of MHE pathology may lead to improvements in early diagnosis, treatment, and disease surveillance to significantly improve the quality of life of MHE patients.

5. Conclusion

Our study reports that, in patients with HE, ammonia, PI, and RI increased and cerebral blood flow velocity slowed down. At the same time, ammonia, PI, and RI paralleled the severity of HE, which indicated reduced cerebral blood flow and impairment of systolic and diastolic cerebral autoregulation in patients with HE. There were tight correlations among ammonia, reduced cerebral blood flow velocity, impaired systolic and diastolic cerebral autoregulation, and declining cognitive function in patients with MHE. After treatment with lactulose, ammonia level, PI, and RI decreased significantly while V_d increased. A better understanding of these parameters in the context of HE may provide an important basis for disease surveillance and the development of new treatment strategies to improve cerebral hemodynamics. The results of this study highlight the importance of correct diagnosis, monitoring, and treatment of patients with HE, particularly MHE.

Consent

This research was conducted with the human subjects' understanding and consent.

Disclosure

The content of the study will not cause harm or risk to the patients. The analysis will try to maximize the protection of the rights and privacy of the patients.

Competing Interests

The authors declare that there is no conflict of interests regarding the publication of this paper.

Authors' Contributions

Yuqing Zhou, Qian Dong, and Rong Zhang contributed equally to this work and share first authorship.

Acknowledgments

The authors would like to sincerely thank Dr. Chuanyong Guo, Dr. Yingqun Zhou, and all doctors from Second Ward of Department of Gastroenterology in Shanghai Tenth People's Hospital, for assistance with data collection and insightful discussions throughout the development, conduct, and analysis of this study. This study was supported by National Nature Science Foundation of China (81670472; 81500466).

References

[1] Chinese Society of Gastroenterology, Chinese Society of Hepatology, and Chinese Medical Association, "Consensus on the diagnosis and treatment of hepatic encephalopathy in China (Chongqing, 2013)," *Chinese Journal of Hepatology*, vol. 21, pp. 641–651, 2013 (Chinese).

[2] J. Fichet, E. Mercier, O. Genée et al., "Prognosis and 1-year mortality of intensive care unit patients with severe hepatic encephalopathy," *Journal of Critical Care*, vol. 24, no. 3, pp. 364–370, 2009.

[3] M. M. Lauridsen, P. Jepsen, and H. Vilstrup, "Critical flicker frequency and continuous reaction times for the diagnosis of minimal hepatic encephalopathy. A comparative study of 154 patients with liver disease," *Metabolic Brain Disease*, vol. 26, no. 2, pp. 135–139, 2011.

[4] K. D. Mullen and R. K. Prakash, "Management of covert hepatic encephalopathy," *Clinics in Liver Disease*, vol. 16, no. 1, pp. 91–93, 2012.

[5] P. Amodio, S. Montagnese, A. Gatta, and M. Y. Morgan, "Characteristics of minimal hepatic encephalopathy," *Metabolic Brain Disease*, vol. 19, no. 3-4, pp. 253–267, 2004.

[6] J. S. Bajaj, "Review article: the modern management of hepatic encephalopathy," *Alimentary Pharmacology and Therapeutics*, vol. 31, no. 5, pp. 537–547, 2010.

[7] P. Neu, P. Schlattmann, A. Schilling, and A. Hartmann, "Cerebrovascular reactivity in major depression: a pilot study," *Psychosomatic Medicine*, vol. 66, no. 1, pp. 6–8, 2004.

[8] C. Montoliu, B. Piedrafita, M. A. Serra et al., "IL-6 and IL-18 in blood may discriminate cirrhotic patients with and without minimal hepatic encephalopathy," *Journal of Clinical Gastroenterology*, vol. 43, no. 3, pp. 272–279, 2009.

[9] Chinese Society of Hepatology, Chinese Society of Infectious Diseases, and Chinese Medical Association, "The guideline of prevention and treatment for chronic hepatitis B(2010 version)," *Chinese Journal of Hepatology*, vol. 19, pp. 13–24, 2011 (Chinese).

[10] K. V. Rama Rao, A. R. Jayakumar, and M. D. Norenberg, "Ammonia neurotoxicity: role of the mitochondrial permeability transition," *Metabolic Brain Disease*, vol. 18, no. 2, pp. 113–127, 2003.

[11] P. Ferenci, A. Lockwood, K. Mullen, R. Tarter, K. Weissenborn, and A. T. Blei, "Hepatic encephalopathy—definition, nomenclature, diagnosis, and quantification: final report of the Working party at the 11th world congresses of gastroenterology, vienna, 1998," *Hepatology*, vol. 35, no. 3, pp. 716–721, 2002.

[12] A. J. L. Cooper and F. Plum, "Biochemistry and physiology of brain ammonia," *Physiological Reviews*, vol. 67, no. 2, pp. 440–519, 1987.

[13] T. R. Elliott, B. Hudspith, C. Karaiskos, N. Rayment, and J. D. Sanderson, "Prolonged survival of E coli but not *Staphylococcus aureus* in monocytes from patients with Crohn's disease," *Gut*, vol. 60, no. 1, pp. A61–A62, 2011.

[14] D. Häussinger and F. Schliess, "Pathogenetic mechanisms of hepatic encephalopathy," *Gut*, vol. 57, no. 8, pp. 1156–1165, 2008.

[15] D. Häussinger, "Low grade cerebral edema and the pathogenesis of hepatic encephalopathy in cirrhosis," *Hepatology*, vol. 43, no. 6, pp. 1187–1190, 2006.

[16] J. Córdoba, F. Sanpedro, J. Alonso, and A. Rovira, "^{1}H magnetic resonance in the study of hepatic encephalopathy in humans," *Metabolic Brain Disease*, vol. 17, no. 4, pp. 415–429, 2002.

[17] D. L. Shawcross, S. Balata, S. W. M. Olde Damink et al., "Low myo-inositol and high glutamine levels in brain are associated with neuropsychological deterioration after induced hyperammonemia," *American Journal of Physiology—Gastrointestinal and Liver Physiology*, vol. 287, no. 3, pp. G503–G509, 2004.

[18] C. Rose, W. Kresse, and H. Kettenmann, "Acute insult of ammonia leads to calcium-dependent glutamate release from cultured astrocytes, an effect of pH," *The Journal of Biological Chemistry*, vol. 280, no. 22, pp. 20937–20944, 2005.

[19] R. Rodrigo, O. Cauli, J. Boix, N. ElMlili, A. Agusti, and V. Felipo, "Role of NMDA receptors in acute liver failure and ammonia toxicity: therapeutical implications," *Neurochemistry International*, vol. 55, no. 1-3, pp. 113–118, 2009.

[20] H. Mardini and C. Record, "Pathogenesis of hepatic encephalopathy: lessons from nitrogen challenges in man," *Metabolic Brain Disease*, vol. 28, no. 2, pp. 201–207, 2013.

[21] R. F. Butterworth, "Pathophysiology of hepatic encephalopathy: the concept of synergism," *Hepatology Research*, vol. 38, supplement 1, pp. S116–S121, 2008.

[22] J. B. Gregorios, L. W. Mozes, and M. D. Norenberg, "Morphologic effects of ammonia on primary astrocyte cultures. II. Electron microscopic studies," *Journal of Neuropathology and Experimental Neurology*, vol. 44, no. 4, pp. 404–414, 1985.

[23] R. K. Dhiman and Y. K. Chawla, "Minimal hepatic encephalopathy," *Indian Journal of Gastroenterology*, vol. 28, no. 1, pp. 5–16, 2009.

[24] A. S. Seyan, R. D. Hughes, and D. L. Shawcross, "Changing face of hepatic encephalopathy: role of inflammation and oxidative stress," *World Journal of Gastroenterology*, vol. 16, no. 27, pp. 3347–3357, 2010.

[25] M. D. Norenberg, K. V. Rama Rao, and A. R. Jayakumar, "Signaling factors in the mechanism of ammonia neurotoxicity," *Metabolic Brain Disease*, vol. 24, no. 1, pp. 103–117, 2009.

[26] K. S. Panickar, A. R. Jayakumar, K. V. R. Rao, and M. D. Norenberg, "Ammonia-induced activation of p53 in cultured astrocytes: role in cell swelling and glutamate uptake," *Neurochemistry International*, vol. 55, no. 1-3, pp. 98–105, 2009.

[27] A. Chastre, W. Jiang, P. Desjardins, and R. F. Butterworth, "Ammonia and proinflammatory cytokines modify expression of genes coding for astrocytic proteins implicated in brain edema in acute liver failure," *Metabolic Brain Disease*, vol. 25, no. 1, pp. 17–21, 2010.

[28] A. T. Blei and J. Córdoba, "Hepatic encephalopathy," *American Journal of Gastroenterology*, vol. 96, no. 7, pp. 1968–1976, 2001.

[29] J. P. Ong, A. Aggarwal, D. Krieger et al., "Correlation between ammonia levels and the severity of hepatic encephalopathy," *The American Journal of Medicine*, vol. 114, no. 3, pp. 188–193, 2003.

[30] M. A. Bragagnolo Jr., V. Teodoro, L. M. Lucchesi, T. C. D. R. Ribeiro, S. Tufik, and M. Kondo, "Minimal hepatic encephalopathy detection by neuropsychological and neurophysiological methods and the role of ammonia for its diagnosis," *Arquivos de Gastroenterologia*, vol. 46, no. 1, pp. 43–49, 2009.

[31] Q. Jiang, X.-H. Jiang, M.-H. Zheng, and Y.-P. Chen, "L-Ornithine-L-aspartate in the management of hepatic encephalopathy: a meta-analysis," *Journal of Gastroenterology & Hepatology*, vol. 24, no. 1, pp. 9–14, 2009.

[32] V. Felipo, A. Urios, C. Giménez-Garzó et al., "Non invasive blood flow measurement in cerebellum detects minimal hepatic encephalopathy earlier than psychometric tests," *World Journal of Gastroenterology*, vol. 20, no. 33, pp. 11815–11825, 2014.

[33] R. U. Macías-Rodríguez, A. Duarte-Rojo, C. Cantú-Brito et al., "Cerebral haemodynamics in cirrhotic patients with hepatic encephalopathy," *Liver International*, vol. 35, no. 2, pp. 344–352, 2015.

[34] M. Kawakami, M. Koda, Y. Murawaki, H. Kawasaki, and S. Ikawa, "Cerebral vascular resistance assessed by transcranial color Doppler ultrasonography in patients with chronic liver diseases," *Journal of Gastroenterology and Hepatology*, vol. 16, no. 8, pp. 890–897, 2001.

[35] M. Raghavan and P. E. Marik, "Therapy of intracranial hypertension in patients with fulminant hepatic failure," *Neurocritical Care*, vol. 4, no. 2, pp. 179–189, 2006.

[36] K.-W. Huang, A. Chao, N.-K. Chou, and W.-J. Ko, "Hepatic encephalopathy and cerebral blood flow improved by liver dialysis treatment," *International Journal of Artificial Organs*, vol. 26, no. 2, pp. 149–151, 2003.

[37] L. E. Schmidt, L. B. Svendsen, V. R. Sørensen, B. A. Hansen, and F. S. Larsen, "Cerebral blood flow velocity increases during a single treatment with the molecular adsorbents recirculating system in patients with acute on chronic liver failure," *Liver Transplantation*, vol. 7, no. 8, pp. 709–712, 2001.

[38] I. J. C. Hartmann, M. Groeneweg, J. C. Quero et al., "The prognostic significance of subclinical hepatic encephalopathy," *American Journal of Gastroenterology*, vol. 95, no. 8, pp. 2029–2034, 2000.

[39] A. Das, R. K. Dhiman, V. A. Saraswat, M. Verma, and S. R. Naik, "Prevalence and natural history of subclinical hepatic

encephalopathy in cirrhosis," *Journal of Gastroenterology and Hepatology*, vol. 16, no. 5, pp. 531–535, 2001.

[40] A. Gupta, R. K. Dhiman, S. Kumari et al., "Role of small intestinal bacterial overgrowth and delayed gastrointestinal transit time in cirrhotic patients with minimal hepatic encephalopathy," *Journal of Hepatology*, vol. 53, no. 5, pp. 849–855, 2010.

[41] M. Groeneweg, W. Moerland, J. C. Quero, W. C. J. Hop, P. F. Krabbe, and S. W. Schalm, "Screening of subclinical hepatic encephalopathy," *Journal of Hepatology*, vol. 32, no. 5, pp. 748–753, 2000.

[42] C. Wein, H. Koch, B. Popp, G. Oehler, and P. Schauder, "Minimal hepatic encephalopathy impairs fitness to drive," *Hepatology*, vol. 39, no. 3, pp. 739–745, 2004.

[43] K. Weissenborn, "The clinical relevance of minimal hepatic encephalopathy—a critical look," *Digestive Diseases*, vol. 33, no. 4, pp. 555–561, 2015.

22

Transanal Irrigation for Refractory Chronic Idiopathic Constipation: Patients Perceive a Safe and Effective Therapy

Kevin J. Etherson,[1] **Ian Minty,**[2] **Iain M. Bain,**[1] **Jeremy Cundall,**[1] **and Yan Yiannakou**[1]

[1]*Department of Colorectal Surgery, County Durham and Darlington NHS Foundation Trust, Durham, UK*
[2]*Department of Radiology, County Durham and Darlington NHS Foundation Trust, Durham, UK*

Correspondence should be addressed to Kevin J. Etherson; kevinetherson@doctors.net.uk

Academic Editor: Branka Filipović

Background. Transanal irrigation (TAI) can successfully treat neurogenic bowel dysfunction (NBD), but patient perception of its use in chronic idiopathic constipation (CIC) is unknown. *Objective.* To evaluate patient perceptions of the efficacy and safety of TAI for CIC and whether there are predictive factors of perceived treatment response. *Methods.* Prospective data collection of baseline physiology and symptom severity; retrospective evaluation of efficacy and safety perceptions using a snapshot survey. All patients fulfilling the Rome III criteria for functional constipation with chronic idiopathic aetiology were included. The main outcome measure was the duration of patients' usage of TAI. *Results.* 102 patients reported 21,476 irrigations over 119 patient years, with a mean duration of therapy use of 60.5 weeks [SD 73.2 : SE 7.3]. Overall symptom improvement included general well-being (65%), rectal clearance (63%), bloating (49%), abdominal pain (48%), and bowel frequency (42%). 68 patients (67%) were "moderately better" or "very much better" on a satisfaction question. Reported complications were minor. No correlation was demonstrated between duration of therapy use and baseline measures. *Conclusion.* A significant proportion of CIC sufferers use TAI as a long-term or bridging therapy and perceive it as safe. This therapy demands a prospective investigation of efficacy and safety.

1. Introduction

Chronic idiopathic constipation (CIC) is characterised by multiple symptoms and classified according to the Rome III criteria [1], with a half of patients typically suffering for 5 or more years [2]. CIC causes a significant reduction in health related quality of life (HRQOL) compared to the general population [3] in the community, HRQOL can be worse than inflammatory bowel disease in those attending secondary care [4], and the burden on healthcare resources is widely recognised [4–6]. Roughly 50% of patients are refractory to laxatives and lifestyle measures [7] and are often referred to secondary care where they have investigations including tests of transit and functional defecation disorder (FDD). A proportion of these cases are also refractory to drug therapy and biofeedback [8] and require further invasive therapy. Transanal irrigation (TAI, also commonly known as "rectal irrigation") is a possible treatment for these patients.

TAI is a type of colonic irrigation which is self-administered by the patient at home after adequate training in the technique and which differs from commercialised colonic irrigation (hydrotherapy) only in the volume and length of time the water is left in situ. It typically involves transanal insertion of a rectal catheter or cone in order to instil lukewarm water retrograde into the colon. This is achieved through various commercially available irrigation systems which have either hand controlled or mechanical pumps, in a volume ranging from 500 mL to 1000 mL depending on patients' experience and tolerance. This is then drained naturally after a few minutes and can result in a satisfactory bowel movement.

The published literature provides very little evidence of efficacy in the CIC group and mostly reports effect in patients suffering faecal incontinence or constipation secondary to neurogenic bowel dysfunction (NBD) [9]. A systematic review of TAI studies reported successful treatment of constipation in 117/259 cases (45%) [10]. Of these 259 patients only 2 cohorts had a significant proportion with CIC in the mixed aetiology [11, 12] with numbers of 79 and 37 patients, respectively, and the remaining 143 patients mostly suffered neurogenic aetiology. The procedure has been extensively reported as simple to perform and relatively safe [11], with the estimated risk of the most serious complication (TAI induced colonic perforation) being less than 0.0002% per irrigation [9]. In 2013 an expert consensus review has specifically stated that there is an urgent need to evaluate effectiveness in the other conditions where TAI is an emerging treatment and if there are any physiological predictors of long-term response [9].

Patients who suffer from CIC are clearly a separate and distinctly different group of patients; the aetiology of the condition is completely unknown; there is evidence of its marked prevalence (14%) and chronicity [13] and subsequent detrimental effect on quality of life [4]. In this paper we aim to present retrospective evidence of the efficacy and safety of TAI in the largest reported cohort of tertiary care patients receiving this therapy for refractory CIC and use the prospective database these patients are enrolled on to identify any baseline predictors of efficacy.

2. Materials and Methods

Patients for this study were treated at the Durham Constipation Clinic (DCC), a tertiary referral centre in the North East of England receiving around 150 new patient referrals each year and with around 850 patients under follow-up. All patients prospectively give informed consent for enrolment onto an ethically approved database. This includes data of symptom and severity measures, physiological tests (transit, proctography, and physiology), and scores of symptom severity using the validated PAC-SYM [14] questionnaire.

The DCC team are experienced in using TAI as a minimally invasive technique for treating CIC after failed medical and behavioural therapies. Patients are selected for one of 3 differing forms of irrigation equipment based on patient choice and the ability of patients to manage the differing practical aspects of each type. Peristeen™ (Coloplast A/S®, Denmark), Qufora™ (MBH International A/S®, Denmark), and the Irrimatic pump™ (B. Braun Melsungen AG®, Germany) systems are all used, with the vast majority given the Peristeen™ system.

A service evaluation was designed to gain patient perspective on TAI as a treatment specific to refractory CIC. Patients under active clinic follow-up were identified through the prospective database and included if they fulfilled the Rome III criteria for functional constipation, had past or present treatment with TAI, and received TAI specifically for refractory CIC (failed all medical and behavioural therapies). Patients were excluded for any secondary causes of constipation (e.g., neurological or opioid use) or concomitant faecal incontinence. Evaluation of patients was not at specific timepoints after commencement of therapy but was a snapshot of all patients who had used the therapy in our service within the preceding 12 months.

A 12-question form was designed for self-completion in clinic or via telephone interview by a team member. The form asked patients to indicate therapy commencement/cessation and total use, how they perceived response to the treatment, the number of irrigations performed on average each week, whether it improved particular CIC symptoms (stating yes or no if TAI improved), how satisfied they were with the therapy, and any adverse events or complications they encountered. Data was collected from February to June 2012. The duration of therapy was calculated from both participants answers on the actual length of time they had used it (to the nearest week) and notes entries on when it was started by the specialist nurse. The duration of therapy use was considered the main outcome measure as a surrogate marker of efficacy. The total number of irrigations for each person was calculated by participants reporting their frequency of use, which was then extrapolated over the therapy duration.

The prospective database of DCC patients' baseline assessments was used to identify baseline predictors of long-term TAI efficacy. Patients who had completed the service evaluation had their baseline data checked on the database and these were extracted and included in the analysis if present and consistent with investigation prior to commencing TAI. PAC-SYM score, transit study time, isotope proctogram, and barium proctogram results were included as relevant indicators of symptom severity and physiological profile of constipation. Transit time was calculated according to the day 4 time on the Metcalf protocol [15], and PAC-SYM mean item score as a validated outcome measure of symptom severity in CIC [14]. Proctograms were checked by team members and used to classify patients as having a functional defecation disorder (FDD) according to the Rome 3 criteria [1], by consensus opinion of 3 consultants. Where patients had both isotope and barium proctograms the measured evacuation percentage of the isotope proctogram was considered superior to the barium proctogram in classifying FDD. Data was analysed in SPSS in order to create a Kaplan-Meier survival curve of continuing use of TAI. The endpoint on the curve is defined as the duration of use until cessation of TAI due to lack of efficacy. Patients are censored on the curve where they continue with the therapy at their current duration of usage. Possible correlations between therapy duration and baseline measures were explored using scatter plots and Pearson's correlation. A Student's t-test was performed to assess for significant differences in length of therapy use between patients classified as FDD or non-FDD.

3. Results and Discussion

3.1. Results. 148 people were identified (via database and specialist nurse records) and contacted, and 102 completed the service evaluation (69%) with consent for survey and demographic data analysis (Figure 1). Table 1 demonstrates the demographics of the cohort. 53% of participants were currently still using TAI at data collection (Table 2), with a combined total of 21,476 irrigations reported over nearly 119 years of therapy use. Patients used TAI on average once every second day.

Participants reported "yes" or "no" if they believed that particular symptoms of CIC had been improved by TAI use (Table 3), with >42% reporting improvement in 4 of the 6

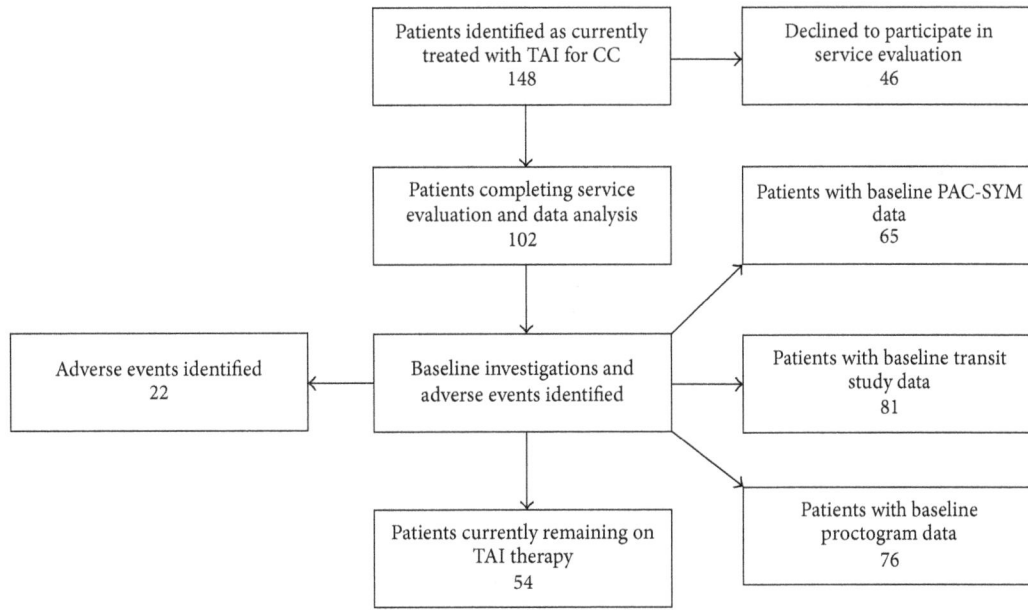

FIGURE 1: Patient flow.

TABLE 1: Baseline *demographics*.

Number of patients	102
Median age in years [range]	45 [25–84]
Number of females [%]	95 [93%]
Number of males [%]	7 [7%]
Mean duration of CIC in years [SD : SE]	21.8 [16.9 : 1.7]

SD = standard deviation, SE = standard error.

TABLE 2: Transanal irrigation *(TAI) therapy use*.

Presently still using TAI	54 [53%]
Completely stopped TAI	48 [47%]
Combined length of therapy weeks [years]	6,175 [118.8]
Mean length of therapy use in weeks [SD : SE]	60.5 [73.2 : 7.3]
Median length of therapy use in weeks [range]	30.15 [1–468]
Combined irrigations	21,476
Mean irrigations/week [SD : SE]	3.7 [2.6 : 0.26]

SD = standard deviation, SE = standard error.

TABLE 3: Symptom improvement and overall satisfaction with transanal irrigation (TAI).

Symptoms improved	
Bowel frequency	43 (42%)
Clearance of rectum	64 (63%)
Abdominal pain	49 (48%)
Bloating	50 (49%)
General well-being	66 (65%)
Awareness of urge	25 (25%)
Spontaneous complete bowel movements (SCBMs)	22 (22%)
Overall satisfaction	
No better	34 (33%)
Moderately better	40 (39%)
Very much better	28 (28%)

fields and >22% in all fields. Overall satisfaction with TAI (as a therapy) was reported by 67% of respondents as either moderately or very much better.

In the Kaplan-Meier survival curve (Figure 2) it should be noted that 40 patients reached the endpoint with 62 (60.8%) censored at their current duration of use of TAI. The curve demonstrates that a significant proportion of the cohort continue with the therapy, although most are censored at their current duration of use within 2 years. Table 4 outlines the baseline data collected from the prospective database on patient colonic transit times, PAC-SYM score, and categorisation of FDD through either isotope or barium proctogram (or both). A Pearson's correlation analysis did not demonstrate significant correlations in the duration of TAI use with any

baseline demographics: age [$N = 102, r = 0.018, P = 0.86$], duration of CIC symptoms [$N = 102, r = 0.033, P = 0.74$], and frequency of TAI use [$N = 102, r = -0.07, P = 0.48$]. Similarly the baseline symptom severity and transit times did not demonstrate any correlation: mean item PAC-SYM [$N = 65, r = -0.19, P = 0.13$] and transit time [$N = 81, r = -0.073, P = 0.52$]. Figure 3 is a boxplot comparing the TAI therapy use of patients classified from baseline proctograms as having a FDD [$N = 40$, mean use = 45 weeks, SD = 49.5] and no FDD [$N = 36$, mean use = 59 weeks, SD = 60.7], with no significant difference in TAI therapy use (Student's t-test for equality of means) detected between these groups [$P = 0.29$].

Adverse events reported (Table 5) were relatively minor given the frequency and total duration of use, although 1 in 5 patients experienced one or more. Device and equipment problems were most frequently reported and minor medical complications such as rectal bleeding were easily managed by

TABLE 4: Baseline investigations on prospective database (cohort).

Investigation	N	Result
Transit study mean time (hours) [SD : SE]	81	60.9 [15.6 : 1.7]
PAC-SYM mean total score [SD : SE]	65	2.23 [0.76 : 0.09]
Baseline isotope & barium proctograms classified to FDD or no	76	FDD 40
FDD by consensus of consultant coauthors		None 36

Standard deviation (SD), standard error (SE), functional defecation disorder (FDD).

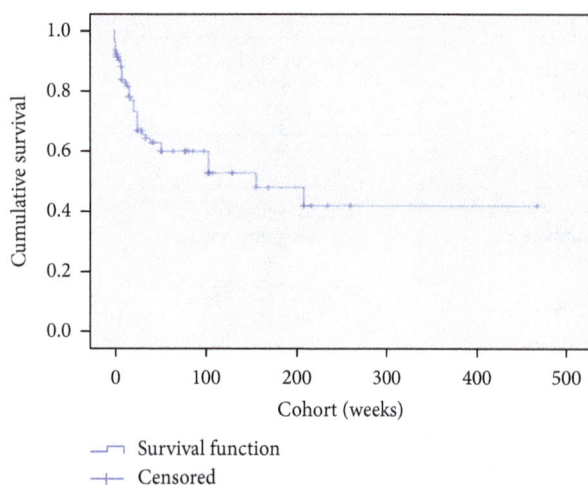

FIGURE 2: Kaplan-Meier survival of transanal irrigation. In this survival curve the endpoint was defined as patients' discontinuing TAI therapy due to perceived ineffectiveness. 40 patients reached the endpoint with 62 (60.0%) censored at their current duration of use of TAI. The curve demonstrates that a significant proportion of the cohort continue with the therapy.

patients. A small proportion (2%) attributed new anal fissures to TAI usage. This series does not report any rectal or colonic perforations, and the unit has not experienced any of these major complications to date.

3.2. Discussion. Investigators across Europe have been reporting for 10 years that TAI is a beneficial treatment for patients suffering faecal incontinence and constipation due to a range of aetiologies [10–12, 16–18]. Our cohort is the largest reported who suffer specifically from CIC, with demonstrable chronicity (mean 21.8 years), symptom severity (mean item total PAC-SYM 2.23), and slow transit (mean 60.9 hrs), with a proportion suffering from FDD (53%).

The results in this cohort demonstrate that around 60% of patients with CIC use TAI for an extended period of time (1-2 years or more) and feel their symptoms are significantly improved. As this was a retrospective snapshot of outcomes, satisfaction rates at specific time intervals cannot be determined. However the duration of TAI therapy use is a justified outcome measure as this is a procedure which requires commitment and time (unlike drug treatments) and patients tend to discontinue ineffective treatments early. Duration of TAI therapy use is therefore a reasonable surrogate marker for efficacy.

TABLE 5: Adverse events (AEs).

All AEs	22/102 (21.6%)
TAI devices	
Bursting balloons	10 (9.8%)
Catheters splitting	3 (2.9%)
Medical problems	
Rectal bleeding	6 (5.9%)
Painful irrigations	3 (2.9%)
Painful haemorrhoids	2 (2.0%)
New anal fissure	2 (2%)
Perforation	0 (0%)

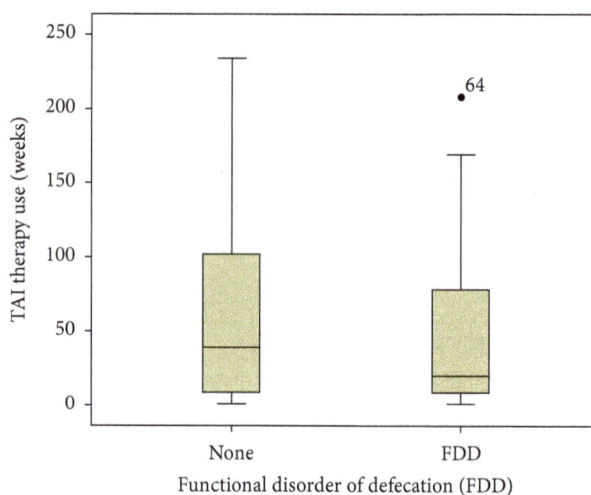

FIGURE 3: This boxplot compares the reported TAE therapy duration (*y*-axis, weeks) of patients classified from baseline proctograms as having a functional defecation disorder (FDD) [$N = 40$, mean use = 45 weeks, SD = 49.5] and no FDD [$N = 36$, mean use = 59 weeks, SD = 60.7], with no significant difference detected between these groups [$P = 0.29$].

The most severe symptoms of CIC (abdominal pain, bloating, incomplete emptying [of rectum], and bowel frequency) improved in over 42% of patients. Remarkably awareness of urge and spontaneous complete bowel movements occurred in a quarter and a fifth, respectively. No correlation was demonstrated between duration of TAI therapy use and patient age or duration of CIC, suggesting that the treatment can be just as effective in a patient who has suffered for 20 years as in someone with a six-month history. There was also no correlation between therapy duration and baseline transit time or presence of FDD suggesting that, on present evidence, the treatment can be offered to patients with any type of constipation. It might be a therapy that could be offered to community-assessed patients with only the treatment refractory referred for detailed investigations. A very slight negative correlation exists between baseline PAC-SYM severity and duration of therapy use: this does not reach statistical significance and merely reflects that patients with more severe symptoms fail treatments faster, which is hardly surprising.

There were no serious complications recorded despite over 20,000 irrigations used by this cohort. Indeed TAI has been used in our service for 7 years and the cohort studied probably represents less than a third of the total number of patients treated. We have not encountered any cases of rectal perforation or other serious complications in this time, though these problems have been reported and remain an unlikely possibility. A small proportion of patients developed new anal fissures during therapy but without a control group it is difficult to know if this is treatment related.

The exact mechanism through which TAI causes a bowel motion is unclear, although it is postulated to be due to stimulation or initiation of peristaltic waves through either stretching and/or warming the colon, and scintigraphic assessment has previously demonstrated washout to the splenic flexure [19]. This may explain the marked effects on chronic symptom improvements reported in our cohort. The spontaneous bowel movements between irrigations that occurred in a fifth of cases may suggest that the treatment has effects that go beyond a simple washout. One possible mechanism could be the initiation of a normal rectal urge to defecate, which is lost or diminished in around two-thirds of patients with chronic constipation [20] and may be due to raised sensorimotor thresholds [21]. An alternative hypothesis relates to the release of 5HT when colonic muscle is distended, thus increasing peristalsis [22].

Overall, a significant proportion of patients in this cohort are globally satisfied with the therapy, reporting marked symptom improvements and minimal complications. International expert consensus on the treatment algorithms of CIC in both Europe and the US has failed to adequately recognise the value and position of this treatment [23, 24].

4. Conclusions

Our results are retrospective, uncontrolled, and possibly affected by reporting bias as patients were interviewed by clinic staff and as such should be treated with caution. A prospective controlled multicentre study is therefore required together with assessments of cost-effectiveness and qualitative studies of the experience of the procedure.

These results do add weight to a body of evidence that TAI is an effective and safe minimally invasive treatment for CIC, either definitively in some or as a bridge to other treatments. For now, the medical ethos of "first do no harm" and common sense dictate that it should be considered as an option on the CIC treatment algorithm before any form of invasive abdominal surgery.

Abbreviations

TAI: Transanal irrigation
CIC: Chronic idiopathic constipation
NBD: Neurogenic bowel dysfunction
FDD: Functional defecation disorder
DCC: Durham Constipation Clinic
HRQOL: Health related quality of life
PAC-SYM: Patient assessment of constipation symptoms.

Disclosure

This manuscript has been presented as two separate conference presentations:

(1) Association of Surgeons of Great Britain and Ireland 90th International Surgical congress, Harrowgate, North Yorkshire, UK, 30/04/2014–02/05/2014.

(2) Tripartite Colorectal Meeting 2014, Birmingham, UK, 30/06/2014–03/07/2014.

Competing Interests

The authors declare that they have no competing interests.

Authors' Contributions

Kevin J. Etherson and Yan Yiannakou made substantial contributions to conception and design and were responsible for acquisition of data. Kevin J. Etherson, Yan Yiannakou, Ian Minty, Iain M. Bain, and Jeremy Cundall were responsible for analysis and interpretation of data, drafting manuscript and revising it critically for important intellectual content, and final approval of manuscript version to be published.

Acknowledgments

Yan Yiannakou has received an educational grant from Coloplast A/S. The authors thank Deborah Rowley-Conwy and Anne Kelly for help with data collection and Professor Charles Knowles for proofreading the manuscript and providing reliable scholarly advice.

References

[1] D. A. Drossman, E. Corazziari, and M. Delvaux, *Rome III: The Functional Gastrointestinal Disorders*, Degnon Associates, McLean, Va, USA, 3rd edition, 2006.

[2] W. F. Stewart, J. N. Liberman, R. S. Sandler et al., "Epidemiology of constipation (EPOC) study in the United States: relation of clinical subtypes to sociodemographic features," *American Journal of Gastroenterology*, vol. 94, no. 12, pp. 3530–3540, 1999.

[3] E. J. Irvine, S. Ferrazzi, P. Pare, W. G. Thompson, and L. Rance, "Health-related quality of life in functional GI disorders: focus on constipation and resource utilization," *The American Journal of Gastroenterology*, vol. 97, no. 8, pp. 1986–1993, 2002.

[4] J. Belsey, S. Greenfield, D. Candy, and M. Geraint, "Systematic review: impact of constipation on quality of life in adults and children," *Alimentary Pharmacology and Therapeutics*, vol. 31, no. 9, pp. 938–949, 2010.

[5] K. Walsh, S. R. McWilliams, M. M. Maher, and E. M. Quigley, "The spectrum of functional gastrointestinal disorders in a tertiary referral clinic in Ireland," *Irish Journal of Medical Science*, vol. 181, no. 1, pp. 81–86, 2012.

[6] K. A. Nyrop, O. S. Palsson, R. L. Levy et al., "Costs of health care for irritable bowel syndrome, chronic constipation, functional diarrhoea and functional abdominal pain," *Alimentary Pharmacology and Therapeutics*, vol. 26, no. 2, pp. 237–248, 2007.

[7] A. Wald, C. Scarpignato, S. Mueller-Lissner et al., "A multinational survey of prevalence and patterns of laxative use among adults with self-defined constipation," *Alimentary Pharmacology and Therapeutics*, vol. 28, no. 7, pp. 917–930, 2008.

[8] U. Khan, D. Dubois, F. Schenck et al., "Patient satisfaction with current management strategies in chronic constipation," *Gut*, vol. 60, article A160, 2011.

[9] A. V. Emmanuel, K. Krogh, G. Bazzocchi et al., "Consensus review of best practice of transanal irrigation in adults," *Spinal Cord*, vol. 51, no. 10, pp. 732–738, 2013.

[10] P. Christensen and K. Krogh, "Transanal irrigation for disordered defecation: a systematic review," *Scandinavian Journal of Gastroenterology*, vol. 45, no. 5, pp. 517–527, 2010.

[11] P. Christensen, K. Krogh, S. Buntzen, F. Payandeh, and S. Laurberg, "Long-term outcome and safety of transanal irrigation for constipation and fecal incontinence," *Diseases of the Colon and Rectum*, vol. 52, no. 2, pp. 286–292, 2009.

[12] M. P. Gosselink, M. Darby, D. D. E. Zimmerman et al., "Long-term follow-up of retrograde colonic irrigation for defaecation disturbances," *Colorectal Disease*, vol. 7, no. 1, pp. 65–69, 2005.

[13] D. A. Drossman, Z. Li, E. Andruzzi et al., "U. S. Householder survey of functional gastrointestinal disorders," *Digestive Diseases and Sciences*, vol. 38, no. 9, pp. 1569–1580, 1993.

[14] L. Frank, L. Kleinman, C. Farup, L. Taylor, and P. Miner Jr., "Psychometric validation of a constipation symptom assessment questionnaire," *Scandinavian Journal of Gastroenterology*, vol. 34, no. 9, pp. 870–877, 1999.

[15] A. M. Metcalf, S. F. Phillips, A. R. Zinsmeister, R. L. MacCarty, R. W. Beart, and B. G. Wolff, "Simplified assessment of segmental colonic transit," *Gastroenterology*, vol. 92, no. 1, pp. 40–47, 1987.

[16] P. Christensen, J. Andreasen, and L. Ehlers, "Cost-effectiveness of transanal irrigation versus conservative bowel management for spinal cord injury patients," *Spinal Cord*, vol. 47, no. 2, pp. 138–143, 2009.

[17] P. Christensen, G. Bazzocchi, M. Coggrave et al., "A randomized, controlled trial of transanal irrigation versus conservative bowel management in spinal cord-injured patients," *Gastroenterology*, vol. 131, no. 3, pp. 738–747, 2006.

[18] A. M. Tod, E. Stringer, C. Levery, J. Dean, and J. Brown, "Rectal irrigation in the management of functional bowel disorders: a review," *British Journal of Nursing*, vol. 16, no. 14, pp. 858–864, 2007.

[19] P. Christensen, N. Olsen, K. Krogh, T. Bacher, and S. Laurberg, "Scintigraphic assessment of retrograde colonic washout in fecal incontinence and constipation," *Diseases of the Colon and Rectum*, vol. 46, no. 1, pp. 68–76, 2003.

[20] F. Harraf, M. Schmulson, L. Saba et al., "Subtypes of constipation predominant irritable bowel syndrome based on rectal perception," *Gut*, vol. 43, no. 3, pp. 388–394, 1998.

[21] J. M. Remes-Troche, S. De-Ocampo, J. Valestin, and S. S. C. Rao, "Rectoanal reflexes and sensorimotor response in rectal hyposensitivity," *Diseases of the Colon and Rectum*, vol. 53, no. 7, pp. 1047–1054, 2010.

[22] N. J. Spencer, S. J. Nicholas, L. Robinson et al., "Mechanisms underlying distension-evoked peristalsis in guinea pig distal colon: is there a role for enterochromaffin cells?" *American Journal of Physiology—Gastrointestinal and Liver Physiology*, vol. 301, no. 3, pp. G519–G527, 2011.

[23] A. E. Bharucha, J. H. Pemberton, and G. R. Locke III, "American gastroenterological association technical review on constipation," *Gastroenterology*, vol. 144, no. 1, pp. 218–238, 2013.

[24] J. Tack, S. Müller-Lissner, V. Stanghellini et al., "Diagnosis and treatment of chronic constipation—a European perspective," *Neurogastroenterology and Motility*, vol. 23, no. 8, pp. 697–710, 2011.

23

Face-to-Face Cognitive-Behavioral Therapy for Irritable Bowel Syndrome: The Effects on Gastrointestinal and Psychiatric Symptoms

Hanna Edebol-Carlman,[1] Brjánn Ljótsson,[2] Steven J. Linton,[3] Katja Boersma,[3] Martien Schrooten,[3] Dirk Repsilber,[1] and Robert J. Brummer[1]

[1]*Nutrition-Gut-Brain Interactions Research Centre, Örebro University, 701 82 Örebro, Sweden*
[2]*Department of Clinical Neuroscience, Division of Psychiatry, Karolinska Institutet, Stockholm, Sweden*
[3]*Center for Health and Medical Psychology (CHAMP), School of Law, Psychology and Social Work,
Örebro University, Örebro, Sweden*

Correspondence should be addressed to Hanna Edebol-Carlman; hanna.edebol-carlman@oru.se

Academic Editor: Tamar Ringel-Kulka

Irritable bowel syndrome (IBS) is a gastrointestinal disorder linked to disturbances in the gut-brain axis. Visceral hypersensitivity and pain are hallmarks of IBS and linked to the physiological and psychological burden and to the nonadaptive coping with stress. Cognitive-behavioral therapy (CBT) for IBS has proven effective in reducing gastrointestinal and psychiatric symptoms in IBS by means of coping with stress. The present pilot study evaluated for the first time whether CBT for IBS affected visceral sensitivity and pain. Individual CBT was performed for 12 weeks in 18 subjects with IBS and evaluated in terms of visceral sensitivity and pain during rectal distensions using the barostat method and self-rated visceral sensitivity and gastrointestinal and psychiatric symptoms. Visceral discomfort, urge, and pain induced by the barostat were not affected by CBT but were stable across the study. However, the level of self-rated visceral sensitivity and gastrointestinal and psychiatric symptoms decreased after the intervention. Central working mechanisms and increased ability to cope with IBS-symptoms are suggested to play a key role in the alleviation of IBS symptoms produced by CBT.

1. Background

Irritable bowel syndrome (IBS) is a common multifactorial functional gastrointestinal disorder with a point prevalence of 11% in the adult western population [1]. Clinical symptoms include visceral hypersensitivity, abdominal pain, discomfort, altered gastrointestinal motility, and secretion as described in the Rome criteria [2]. Its pathophysiology is not fully understood but a multicomponent conceptual model involving physiological, affective, cognitive, and behavioral factors has been postulated [3]. Visceral hypersensitivity is a key hallmark of IBS that involves pain originating from the intestinal organs and is poorly understood in terms of its etiology and management or treatment. It is enhanced by stress, anticipation, and inflammatory factors as implicated in preclinical and clinical studies in the context of for example,

gender, gut microbiota, immune functioning in IBS [4], and neonates maternally separated [5]. Visceral sensitivity can be pharmacologically and psychologically manipulated as was done in a study of hypnotherapy for IBS in which normalized levels of visceral sensitivity, GI, and psychological symptoms were reported [6]. Rectal thresholds can be adversely affected by acute and psychological stress and cognition influences pain perception shown by pain-rating scores higher during attention towards aversive stimuli than during distraction task in healthy volunteers [7]. Cognitions involving catastrophizing, rumination, and maladaptive coping are examples of cognitive-affective factors that play a role in the exacerbation of stress and IBS symptoms [8].

Visceral sensitivity is a robust hallmark of IBS. Previous studies, selecting the visceral stimuli of a barostat as a stressful trigger to assess visceral hypersensitivity in IBS, report increased attention via dorsal anterior cingulate cortex (ACC) towards pain sensation in IBS versus healthy controls [9], as well as impaired inhibitory control of rectal pain in emotional-sensory regulatory areas including amygdala, insula, and thalamus, as well as primary and secondary sensory cortex [10]. Acute tryptophan depletion in healthy volunteers during rectal stimuli to induce IBS-like processing of stressful pain altered hormonal response and decreased negative amygdaloid feedback to, for example, ACC, which yielded hypervigilance and amplified pain scores [11–13]. Autonomous nervous system reactivity during barostat assessment is also typically presented in IBS and provides further evidence that rectal hypersensitivity is not only a gastrointestinal symptom of IBS but also a reliable indicator of IBS-related cognitive impairment including abnormal processing of rectal pain and response to stress [14].

Cognitive-behavioral therapy (CBT) for IBS emphasizes cognitive, emotional, and behavioral strategies to better cope with physiological and psychological stressors. Previous studies report on the effectiveness of CBT for IBS in terms of improved gastrointestinal symptoms, quality of life, and the role of stress management as key mechanisms to regulate IBS pathophysiology [15–21]. The treatment, delivered over the Internet, showed promising results regarding gastrointestinal and psychological symptoms associated with IBS, as well as quality of life [15–21]. Our first study of CBT for IBS in a face-to-face format [22] reported improved gastrointestinal and psychological function, as well as improved quality of life in the majority of the subjects. However, there has not yet been a study on the actual visceral sensitivity and pain during an ecologically valid condition. Because we included measures of visceral sensitivity and pain during rectal stimulation in the study above (22) using the barostat method, this paper explores bidirectional gut-brain interactions by means of a top-down (i.e., brain initiated) intervention in subjects with IBS.

Aim. The aim of the present pilot study was to elucidate whether or not a cognitive-behavioral intervention for IBS affects (1) visceral sensitivity and pain during rectal stimuli using the barostat method in subjects with IBS and (2) self-rated visceral sensitivity and fear and worry about symptoms, as well as gastrointestinal symptoms in patients with IBS. Specifically, we asked whether face-to-face CBT for IBS affects

(1) visceral pain, discomfort, and/or urge in subjects with IBS during rectal distensions at the pressure of 20, 30, 40, and 50 mmHg, respectively,

(2) the continuous tolerable pressure (mmHg) at 20, 40, 60, and 80% of the estimated maximum of the highest visual analogue score, respectively, in subjects with IBS,

(3) self-rated visceral sensitivity and gastrointestinal and psychiatric symptoms in subjects with IBS.

2. Methods

2.1. Design. The study included 18 subjects with IBS whose ratings of visceral pain, urge, and discomfort as well as the

induced visceral pressure (mmHg) during rectal distensions with the barostat method were measured four weeks before the CBT intervention (t1, $n = 8$) and/or just before the CBT intervention (t2, $N = 15$) as well as after the intervention (t3, $N = 15$). In addition, subjects self-rated visceral sensitivity, symptoms of depression and anxiety, and gastrointestinal complaints of IBS were measured four weeks before ($n = 13$), just before ($N = 18$), and after the intervention ($N = 18$). Dependent variables were visceral sensitivity during rectal distensions (ratings of pain, urge, and discomfort using 100 mm VAS scales at the pressure of 20, 30, 40, and 50 mmHg), the continuous and maximal tolerable pressure (mmHg at 20, 40, 60, and 80% of the estimated maximum of the highest VAS score), and self-rated visceral sensitivity and gastrointestinal and psychiatric symptoms (visceral sensitivity index (VSI), gastrointestinal symptoms rating scale (GSRS), and Hospital Anxiety and Depression Scale (HADS)).

2.2. Subjects. A total of 18 subjects (14 females and 4 men; mean age = 35, SD = 13.31) suffering from IBS symptoms for one to five ($n = 6$) or more than five ($n = 12$) years prior to inclusion and having been diagnosed with constipation ($n = 5$), diarrhea ($n = 9$), and unspecified ($n = 3$) or mixed ($n = 1$) type IBS at a gastroenterological clinic according to Rome III criteria were included [23]. All subjects were eligible for an IBS diagnosis according to Rome III self-ratings at the time of inclusion; none had other gastrointestinal or psychiatric disorders, but chronic medical disorders included polycystic ovary syndrome ($n = 1$) and asthma ($n = 1$).

Current medications for IBS included loperamide and/or sterculia gum ($n = 7$) and alternative treatments included probiotics (at any time, $n = 9$; regular use, $n = 6$). Social status was either married ($n = 3$), shared household ($n = 6$), or single household ($n = 9$). Ten participants had completed high school and the rest had graduated from college. Three persons were on sick leave because of IBS.

Criteria for participation included (1) fulfilling Rome III diagnostic criteria for IBS and pain/discomfort frequency at least 2 days a week in the last 12 weeks, (2) having VAS score of global assessment of abdominal pain and discomfort equal to or >35 mm, (3) age being between 18 and 65 years, and (4) signing informed consent. Criteria for exclusion were (1) concurrent or recent treatment with drugs affecting intestinal function or mood, for example, antidepressants, (2) concurrent or recent (<2 weeks) use of nutritional supplements or herb products affecting intestinal function or mood (e.g., aloe vera, St. John's Wort), (3) depression or suicide tendencies according to Montgomery Åsberg Depression Rating Scale-Short (MADRS-S) screen [24] and/or clinical judgment, (4) abuse of alcohol or drugs according to Alcohol Use Disorder Identification Test screen [25] and/or clinical judgment, and (5) ongoing titration of psychopharmacological treatment.

2.3. The CBT Intervention. After a baseline, participants were introduced to their CBT therapist and the intervention was performed individually with 12 weekly one-hour sessions. During the whole study period, participants filled out weekly ratings about their gastrointestinal and psychological health using the online dedicated web portal [26]. Participants also filled out paper and pencil diaries consisting of five questions about their gut health using a five-point response scale [22].

Six clinical psychologists and two last-term psychology students at the Center for Health and Medical Psychology, CHAMP, at Örebro University, familiar with conducting CBT, were trained to conduct the CBT intervention. Supervision was provided by experienced psychologists (coauthors Brjánn Ljótsson and Steven J. Linton). Twelve participants performed a four-week baseline and six participants started treatment directly within a week from the first barostat assessment. The intervention was based on techniques and a manual developed and tested previously [18, 19]. The main modules of the manual consisted of exposure and mindfulness components. The total treatment entailed 12 sessions of therapy provided on an individual basis and guided by the manual. Thirteen participants participated in one session per week and the remaining five participants participated in the same therapy distributed over six weeks because of time constraints.

2.4. Rectal Pain Induction with the Barostat Method.

To reduce the influence of a adipose tissue mass and abdominal wall tone during the barostat assessment, subjects fasted 12 hours prior to assessment and were placed in the left lateral decubitus position; the rectal probe was lubricated and placed 10–15 cm into the rectum. The probe consists of a 700 mL polyethylene bag secured on a rectal catheter (external diameter = 18 French). Rectal distensions were applied with a barostat (Electronic barostat, distender series II; G & J Electronic Inc., Toronto, Ontario, Canada) according to our previous study [11]. The barostat protocol consists of intermittent semi-random staircase distensions of 60 seconds' duration (15, 10, 25, and 20 mmHg, etc.) separated by an interval of 30 seconds of baseline pressure. The end point to stop the series of distensions is the perceptual threshold for maximal tolerable pain, discomfort, and/or urge or if the safety value of the maximal volume of 600 mL is exceeded. During each distension (after 13 seconds of distensions), subjects are asked to report their perception of pain, discomfort, and urge, respectively, using 100 mm VAS scales (no pain/discomfort/urge maximal tolerable pain/discomfort/urge). The barostat protocol has previously been approved by EPN (Etikprövningsnämnden, Ethical Review Board, Drn 2010-261, 2010-08-11, Dnr 2010-282, 2010-08-25) and described in detail [27].

2.5. Measurement of Symptoms with Rating Scales

2.5.1. Gastrointestinal Symptoms Rating Scale (GSRS).

This is a 15-item clinical rating scale for gastrointestinal symptoms scored on a 7-point Likert scale in which 1 represents no symptoms and 7 the highest level of symptoms. The reliability and validity of the GSRS are well documented [28]. Interrater reliability is excellent and ranges from 0.86 to 0.90 for the separate items and from 0.92 to 0.94 for different gastrointestinal syndromes [28].

2.5.2. Visceral Sensitivity Index (VSI).

This 15-item self-report questionnaire [29] measures gastrointestinal symptoms in IBS including unique aspects of anxiety related to gastrointestinal sensations, fear and hypervigilance that accompany misappraisals of GI-specific sensations, and discomfort. Items cover symptomatic areas like pain, diarrhea, constipation, bloating, or sense of urgency and are rated on 6-point scale ranging from strongly disagree (0) to strongly agree (5). VSI demonstrates excellent reliability (Cronbach's alpha = 0.93) as well as good content, convergent (0.61–0.66, $p <$ 0.001), divergent, and predictive validity [29].

2.5.3. Hospital Anxiety and Depression Scale (HADS).

This clinical scale [30] is a widely used and well-validated 14-item self-rating questionnaire that taps symptoms of depression and anxiety with seven questions, respectively. The instrument was originally developed to detect anxious and depressive symptoms in patients with physical health disorders. In a systematic overview of the HADS literature [31], correlations between the subscales varied from 0.40 to 0.74, Cronbach's alpha for the anxious subscale varied from 0.68 to 0.93, and the depressive subscale varied from 0.67 to 0.90. In most studies, an optimal balance between sensitivity and specificity (i.e., 0.80 for both) was achieved when the cut-off was set at ≥8 points on both subscales. HADS has been found to perform well in terms of evaluating and indicating cases of anxiety disorders and depression in somatic, psychiatric, and primary care patients [31].

2.6. Statistical Analyses.

The slopes of a fitted linear function of the estimated VAS scores for pain, discomfort, and urge, respectively, at the fixed pressures of 20, 30, 40, 50, and 60 mmHg as well as the maximum tolerable pressure, that is, the highest visceral pressure that each subject could tolerate, were calculated and the fitted slopes were analyzed with paired samples t-tests ($ps < 0.05$).

The pressure (mmHg) of the barostat was measured but in order to achieve better comparability across subjects it was normalized based on 20, 40, 60, and 80% of the largest fitted VAS score using fits of logistic functions with intercept (see below). To characterize a subject's VAS score-pressure-curve, normalized pressures are reported for the above quantiles of the largest fitted VAS score value. The resulting normalized pressures were compared with paired samples t-tests ($ps <$ 0.05) before and after CBT therapy. The function for the fitting of the observed scores was score $= K/(1 + e^{\wedge}(r * (x - d))) - K/(1 + e^{\wedge}(-r * d))$, with measured pressure x and parameters K (limit of the logistic function), d (shift with respect to pressure), and r (slope of the logistic function). The second term of the fitted function represents the fitted score at zero pressure, forcing a zero intercept for better comparability. The fit was obtained using the Levenberg-Marquardt algorithm, as implemented in R-package nlsLM [32, 33]. The formula for the pressure at 80%-of-max-VAS score estimate was $x.80 = \log(K/(0.8 * \text{max.score} + K/(1 + e^{\wedge}(-r * d))) - 1)/r + d$, with "max.score" being the largest fitted VAS score value. Normalized pressures for 20, 40, and 60% of max-VAS scores were calculated accordingly.

The total score for the visceral sensitivity index (VSI), the Gastrointestinal Symptoms Ratings Scale (GSRS), and the Hospital Anxiety and Depression Scale (HADS) as well as the subscores for anxiety and depression on the HADS was analyzed with paired samples t-tests and for the skewed data according to the Shapiro-Wilk test of normality, the Wilcoxon signed ranks test was applied ($p < 0.05$). Because several t-tests were made, significance levels were adjusted with a Bonferroni correction. Effect sizes are reported in terms of Cohen's d for paired comparisons. In case of a significant difference between t1 and t2 (four weeks and directly before CBT; $n = 12$) for a certain dependent variable, as assessed with paired samples t-tests, the difference between t2 and t3 for that dependent variable was examined with an ANCOVA ($n = 12$), controlling for the (centered) difference between t1 and t2. The comparison of t2 and t3 was also assessed for all variables with paired samples t-tests and skewed data was analyzed with the nonparametric Wilcoxon signed rank test.

The statistical power was calculated post hoc using the g*power software [34] based on a two-way paired samples t-test with an achieved effect size of around 0.48, an alpha level of 0.05, and a total sample size of 18. The power of the study was around 0.45, which is lower than previous studies on the efficacy of CBT for IBS [18, 35]. In order to achieve a power of 0.80 for the ANS measurement, a total sample size of at least 38 participants (SD = 1) would have been required which was not feasible for the present study.

2.7. Ethics. The study was approved by the ethical board EPN in Uppsala (Drn 2013/275) and conducted according to good clinical practice and the ethics of the Helsinki declaration [36].

3. Results

3.1. Sample Characteristics. Two of the original 20 subjects included in the study terminated their participation because of personal reasons and because of a lack of motivation for performing the exposure therapy, respectively. For the barostat analysis, data from three subjects could not be analyzed because of technical limitations during the barostat assessment; this left a total of 15 participants for the barostat analysis. A total of 12 participants at t1 and 18 participants at t2 and t3 were left for the analyses of the rating scales.

3.2. Discomfort, Pain, and Urge at the Pressure of 20, 30, 40, and 50 mmHg. Paired samples t-tests were conducted to compare the estimated ratings of discomfort, pain, and urge, respectively, at the pressure of 20, 30, 40, and 50 mmHg before and after CBT (t2-t3) as well as for the two rectal assessments performed before the intervention (t1-t2). None of the comparisons yielded significant results. For means and standard deviations, see Table 1. For a graphical presentation of the estimated visceral pain, see Figure 1.

3.3. Pressure at 20, 40, 60, and 80% of the Highest VAS Ratings. Paired t-tests were conducted to compare the estimated ratings of discomfort, pain, and urge, respectively, at 20, 40, 60, and 80% of the highest VAS rating before and after CBT (t2-t3) as well as for the two rectal assessments performed before the intervention (t1-t2). None of the comparisons yielded a significant difference. For means and standard

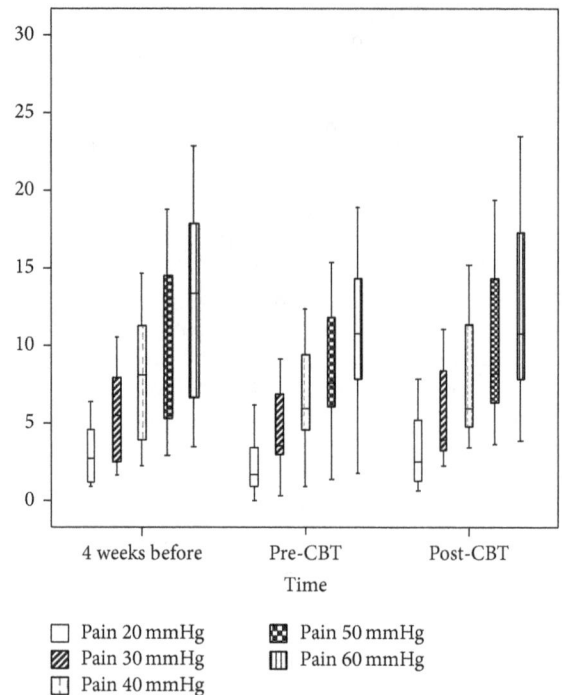

FIGURE 1: The estimated visceral pain based on ratings made by subjects with IBS at the rectal pressure of 20, 30, 40, 50, and 60 mmHg, respectively, four weeks before CBT, before, and after CBT. The pressure was induced by a barostat device.

deviations, see Table 2. For a graphical presentation of the pressure (mmHg) at 20, 40, 60, 80, and 100% of the maximal tolerable rectal pain, see Figure 2.

3.4. Maximal Tolerable Pressure. The participants' maximum tolerable pressures were calculated and compared before and after CBT (t2-t3). On average, participants maximum tolerable pressure did not improve after (M = 42.55, SD = 10.69) as compared to before (M = 42.05, SD = 11.76, $t(14)$ = -0.174, $p = 0.864$) the intervention. A paired samples t-test was conducted for the maximal tolerable pressure for the two rectal assessments performed before the intervention (t1-t2). On average, participants' maximal tolerable pressure did not differ at t1 (M = 42.44, SD = 8.62) compared to t2 (M = 37.59, SD = 7.94, $t(7) = 0.996$, $p = 0.352$). Figure 2 presents a graphical presentation of the maximal tolerable rectal pain.

3.5. Self-Rated Symptoms. Participants visceral sensitivity decreased after as compared to before the intervention ($t(17)$ = -5.980, $p = 0.000$) but did not differ at t1 compared to t2 ($t(12) = 1.945$, $p = 0.076$), although there was a trend towards lower scores at t2. Gastrointestinal symptoms decreased after as compared to before the intervention ($t(16) = -3.606$, $p = 0.002$) but did not differ at t1 compared to t2 ($t(12) = 0.559$, $p = 0.587$). The hospital anxiety and depression total score decreased after the intervention as compared to before the intervention ($t(17) = -2.224$, $p = 0.040$) but did not differ for t1 and t2 ($t(11) = -1.00$, $p = 0.339$). Anxiety subscores did not decrease after as compared to before the intervention

TABLE 1: Descriptive data for dependent variables.

(a)

mmHg	Pain, 4 weeks before		Pain, pre-CBT		Pain, post-CBT	
	M	SD	M	SD	M	SD
20	3.00	2.05	2.61	2.31	3.29	2.38
30	5.44	3.23	4.96	3.27	5.57	3.13
40	7.89	4.45	7.33	4.36	7.84	3.97
50	10.33	5.68	9.70	5.51	10.12	4.87

(b)

mmHg	Discomfort, 4 weeks before		Discomfort, pre-CBT		Discomfort, post-CBT	
	M	SD	M	SD	M	SD
20	3.83	1.67	3.48	2.16	4.31	2.35
30	6.66	2.15	6.63	4.16	6.74	2.78
40	10.03	2.52	8.53	4.16	9.29	3.35
50	12.34	3.21	11.06	5.39	11.60	4.23

(c)

mmHg	Urge, 4 weeks before		Urge, pre-CBT		Urge, post-CBT	
	M	SD	M	SD	M	SD
20	4.39	1.68	3.96	2.41	4.35	2.31
30	7.18	2.34	6.37	3.50	6.69	2.46
40	9.97	3.08	9.02	2.89	9.02	2.89
50	12.76	3.84	11.19	6.16	11.35	3.50

Note. Means (M) and standard deviations (SD) for dependent variables of visceral pain, discomfort, and urge in subjects with IBS during rectal distensions at the pressure of 20, 30, 40, and 50 mmHg collected four weeks before, just before (pre-CBT), and after CBT (post-CBT). N for the 4 weeks before measurement = 7; N for the pre- and post-CBT measurement = 14.

$(t(17) = 1.393$, $p = 0.181)$ and did not differ for t1 and t2 $(t(11) = 0.312$, $p = 0.761)$. Depression subscores decreased after as compared to before the intervention $(t(17) = -3.073$, $p = 0.007)$ but did not differ for t1 and t2 $(t(11) = -1.688$, $p = 0.119)$. For means and standard deviations, see Table 3.

4. Discussion

The present pilot study investigated for the first time whether or not induced rectal pain and hypersensitivity can be modulated in IBS by means of CBT. The study also evaluated whether CBT affected self-rated visceral sensitivity and gastrointestinal and psychiatric symptoms in subjects with IBS. Our results show that visceral pain, discomfort, and urge during rectal distensions were not affected by the CBT treatment. Likewise, the continuous and the maximal tolerable rectal pressure were not affected by CBT. Moreover, there was no change in visceral sensitivity and rectal pain across the entire study. However, self-rated visceral sensitivity, gastrointestinal symptoms, and psychiatric symptoms of anxiety and depression did significantly decrease after CBT.

CBT for IBS did not seem to affect either the physiological perception or the intensity of visceral sensitivity and pain. The finding is consistent with earlier studies on IBS [37] suggesting high levels of stress and difficulties coping with

anxiety and ANS activity in general and during physically and psychologically stressful situations in particular. Despite the fact that CBT improves gastrointestinal, visceral, and psychiatric symptoms according to the present and a previous study [22], it does not seem to affect the physiological perception and intensity of visceral pain during rectal distensions, which suggests more of central coping mechanisms related to IBS rather than physically altered functions regarding the disorder.

CBT seems to affect how participants cope with IBS, which in turn leads to reduced visceral sensitivity and gastrointestinal symptoms. In line with previous studies on CBT for IBS [22], the present study suggests that the intervention involves central mechanisms of coping rather than physiological visceral-afferent alterations of the gut. One plausible explanation of the CBT effect seen in the present study sample [22] and in other groups with IBS [15–21, 38] is suggested to be related to increased abilities to cope with IBS signs and symptoms which reduces manifestations of these symptoms [18, 19]. Several mediational analyses have also suggested that the effect of exposure-based CBT on IBS symptom is mediated through reduced symptom fear [20, 39, 40]. However, these meditational analyses have all been based on self-reported measures. The present study used for the first time the barostat technique to assess a biological

TABLE 2: Descriptive data for dependent variables.

(a)

%	Pain, 4 weeks before		Pain, pre-CBT		Pain, post-CBT	
	M	SD	M	SD	M	SD
20	19.40	10.77	20.54	11.86	17.69	10.18
40	24.95	9.42	25.32	11.86	23.39	11.07
60	28.08	11.57	29.49	8.86	28.08	11.57
80	34.23	8.75	33.46	11.55	28.70	12.08

(b)

%	Discomfort, 4 weeks before		Discomfort, pre-CBT		Discomfort, post-CBT	
	M	SD	M	SD	M	SD
20	16.50	4.96	17.28	9.07	15.85	9.12
40	22.55	6.70	22.39	10.16	20.91	10.15
60	27.43	8.03	21.19	6.64	25.12	10.95
80	32.68	8.98	31.41	11.77	29.83	11.68

(c)

%	Urge, 4 weeks before		Urge, pre-CBT		Urge, post-CBT	
	M	SD	M	SD	M	SD
20	13.39	3.22	13.78	6.96	14.65	8.62
40	19.54	5.02	19.03	9.12	19.69	10.03
60	23.37	11.02	24.74	6.85	23.91	11.11
80	30.51	8.47	28.12	12.86	28.70	12.08

Note. Means (M), and standard deviations (SD) for dependent variables, that is, the estimated pressure (mmHg) at 20, 40, 60, and 80% of the maximum ratings with regard to discomfort, pain, and urge, respectively, during the barostat assessment collected four weeks before (−4 weeks), just before (pre-CBT), and after CBT (12 weeks after CBT). N for the 4 weeks before measurement = 7; N for the pre- and post-CBT measurement = 15.

TABLE 3: Descriptive statistics for questionnaire data.

	−4 w			Day 0			Week 12		
	M	SD	95% CI	M	SD	95% CI	M	SD	95% CI
VSI	43.92	14.14	38.25, 53.91	41.06	17.21	31.35, 47.32	21.28[**]	14.74	14.42, 26.41
GSRS	40.23	12.98	34.50, 49.50	37.83	14.67	31.04, 50.30	29.82[**]	13.82	22.52, 41.32
HADS-T	14.00	5.66	10.41, 17.59	14.22	5.75	11.34, 18.16	11.39[*]	6.39	7.96, 15.54
HADS-D	3.83	2.79	2.06, 5.61	4.5	2.81	2.91, 6.59	2.83[**]	2.55	1.33, 4.67
HADS-A	10.17	3.30	8.07, 12.26	9.72	3.68	7.85, 12.15	8.56	4.19	6.36, 11.14

Note. Means (M), medians (Mdn), standard deviations (SD), and 95% confidence intervals (CI) for dependent variables of visceral sensitivity index (VSI), Gastrointestinal Symptoms Rating Scale (GSRS), and hospital anxiety and depression symptom scale (total, anxiety, and depression) in subjects with IBS collected four weeks before (−4 weeks), just before (day 0), and after cognitive behavioral therapy (CBT) (12 weeks). [*]$p < 0.05$, [**]$p < 0.01$.

marker of visceral pain and indicated that CBT effects arise primarily via psychological coping of IBS symptoms rather than visceral-afferent signaling of decreased symptoms.

The present study suggests that the effect of CBT upon IBS symptoms is initiated by improved psychological coping of IBS rather than an altered visceral-afferent physiological functioning, tolerance, and/or ability to perceive rectal pain, discomfort, urge, and pressure. In fact, the ability of the subjects to experience visceral pain and the intolerance of visceral pain seem to have remained constant, in contrast to the overall symptoms of IBS and associated impairments. Finally, improving IBS symptoms seem to be possible by means of altering psychological functioning related to the

experience and coping of IBS symptoms, rather than altering IBS symptoms themselves.

4.1. Limitations. This study has some methodological confinements. First, post hoc calculations of the statistical power suggest only moderate power (0.45). Further, the effect sizes for many of the comparisons are limited to low to moderate effects. Taken together, these limitations reduce our ability to draw firm conclusions. Although we found a significant effect of CBT on IBS symptomatology in another report with these same participants, our sample size may be too small for physiological measures, for example, barostat assessment of visceral pain. Second, the lack of a control group raises

Face-to-Face Cognitive-Behavioral Therapy for Irritable Bowel Syndrome: The Effects on Gastrointestinal...

207

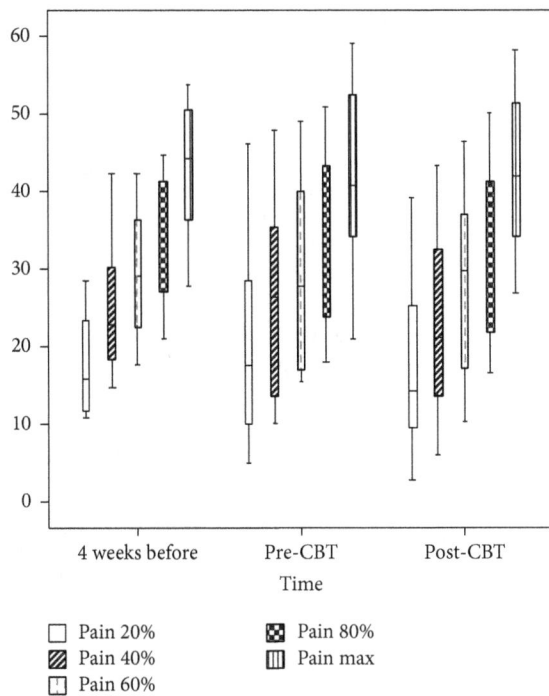

FIGURE 2: The actual pressure (mmHg) to the rectum at 20, 40, 60, 80, and 100% of the maximal tolerable rectal pain according to ratings made by subjects with IBS four weeks before CBT, before, and after CBT. The pressure was induced by a barostat device.

questions as to whether the results of the present study were affected by psychological mechanisms not related to the intervention. Also, the selection of participants was not based on barostat data but only on self-ratings and clinical judgment, and thus the lack of a control group makes the presence of visceral hypersensitivity difficult to verify. Third, the evaluation took place immediately after finalizing the intervention and with no follow-up measurement and, thus, a more gradual effect on the intestinal visceral mechanisms may have been overlooked. Taken together, future research will need to test further the effects of CBT in randomized studies with larger samples.

5. Conclusions

The present study investigated for the first time whether CBT for IBS alters visceral sensitivity, pain, and the maximal tolerable pressure during rectal stimuli using the barostat method. While we did not find significant changes in the barostat measurements, the level of self-rated visceral sensitivity and gastrointestinal and psychiatric symptoms did decrease after the intervention. Changes in central working mechanisms and increased ability to cope with IBS symptoms are suggested to play a key role in the alleviation of IBS symptoms produced by CBT. More studies exploring the effect of CBT upon IBS in terms of biological markers and visceral pain during rectal distensions are needed.

Abbreviations

ACC: Anterior cingulate cortex
ANS: Autonomous nervous system
CBT: Cognitive-behavioral therapy
GI: Gastrointestinal
GSRS: Gastrointestinal Symptoms Ratings Scale
HADS: Hospital Anxiety and Depression Scale
IBS: Irritable bowel syndrome
VAS: Visual Analogue Scale
VSI: Visceral sensitivity index.

Ethical Approval

The study was approved by the regional ethical board Etik-prövningsnämnden (http://www.epn.se/start/) in Uppsala (number of the application: 2013/275) and conducted according to good clinical practice and the ethics of the Helsinki declaration [36].

Competing Interests

The authors declare that they have no competing interests.

Authors' Contributions

Hanna Edebol-Carlman facilitated the study design, collection, analysis, and interpretation of data and wrote the draft of the manuscript and approved the final version of the manuscript. Brjánn Ljótsson facilitated the study design, developed the intervention, facilitated data collection, critically revised the manuscript, contributed with important intellectual content, and approved the final version of the manuscript. Steven J. Linton facilitated the study design, facilitated the intervention and data collection, critically revised the manuscript, contributed with important intellectual content, and approved the final version of the manuscript. Katja Boersma facilitated the study design, facilitated the intervention and data collection, critically revised the manuscript, contributed with important intellectual content, and approved the final version of the manuscript. Martien Schrooten facilitated analysis of data, critically revised the manuscript, contributed with important intellectual content, and approved the final version of the manuscript. Dirk Repsilber facilitated analysis of data, critically revised the manuscript, contributed with important intellectual content, and approved the final version of the manuscript. Robert J. Brummer facilitated design and funding of the study, facilitated collection and analysis of the data, critically revised the manuscript, contributed with important intellectual content, and approved the final version of the manuscript.

Acknowledgments

The authors would like to thank all of the participants and the CBT therapists of the present study. The authors would also like to thank the Endoscopy Department at the University Hospital in Örebro, Sweden, for their helpful facilitation during data collection. The authors wish to thank

Sam Jundler, president at G&J Electronics, Canada, for his technical expertise during data acquisition.

References

[1] E. M. Quigley, H. Abdel-Hamid, G. Barbara et al., "A global perspective on irritable bowel syndrome: a consensus statement of the World Gastroenterology Organisation Summit Task Force on irritable bowel syndrome," *Journal of Clinical Gastroenterology*, vol. 46, no. 5, pp. 356–366, 2012.

[2] W. G. Thompson, G. L. Longstreth, D. A. Drossman et al., "Functional bowel disorders," in *Rome II: The Functional Gastrointestinal Disorders. Diagnosis, Pathophysiology and Treatment. A Multinational Consensus*, D. A. Drossman, E. Corazziari, N. J. Talley et al., Eds., Allen Press Inc, Lawrence, Kan, USA, 2000.

[3] P. P. J. van der Veek, E. Dusseldorp, Y. R. van Rood, and A. A. M. Masclee, "Testing a biobehavioral model of irritable bowel syndrome," *European Journal of Gastroenterology & Hepatology*, vol. 22, no. 4, pp. 412–419, 2010.

[4] R. D. Moloney, S. M. O'Mahony, T. G. Dinan, and J. F. Cryan, "Stress-induced visceral pain: toward animal models of irritable-bowel syndrome and associated comorbidities," *Frontiers in Psychiatry*, vol. 6, article no. 15, 2015.

[5] S. Elsenbruch, "Abdominal pain in Irritable Bowel Syndrome: a review of putative psychological, neural and neuro-immune mechanisms," *Brain, Behavior, and Immunity*, vol. 25, no. 3, pp. 386–394, 2011.

[6] R. Lea, L. A. Houghton, E. L. Calvert et al., "Gut-focused hypnotherapy normalizes disordered rectal sensitivity in patients with irritable bowel syndrome," *Alimentary Pharmacology and Therapeutics*, vol. 17, no. 5, pp. 635–642, 2003.

[7] P. Dunckley, Q. Aziz, R. G. Wise, J. Brooks, I. Tracey, and L. Chang, "Attentional modulation of visceral and somatic pain," *Neurogastroenterology and Motility*, vol. 19, no. 7, pp. 569–577, 2007.

[8] W. Deechakawan, K. C. Cain, M. E. Jarrett, R. L. Burr, and M. M. Heitkemper, "Effect of self-management intervention on cortisol and daily stress levels in irritable bowel syndrome," *Biological Research for Nursing*, vol. 15, no. 1, pp. 26–36, 2013.

[9] B. D. Naliboff, S. W. G. Derbyshire, J. Munakata et al., "Cerebral activation in patients with irritable bowel syndrome and control subjects during rectosigmoid stimulation," *Psychosomatic Medicine*, vol. 63, no. 3, pp. 365–375, 2001.

[10] C. H. Wilder-Smith, D. Schindler, K. Lovblad, S. M. Redmond, and A. Nirkko, "Brain functional magnetic resonance imaging of rectal pain and activation of endogenous inhibitory mechanisms in irritable bowel syndrome patient subgroups and healthy controls," *Gut*, vol. 53, no. 11, pp. 1595–1601, 2004.

[11] T. O. C. Kilkens, A. Honig, M. A. Van Nieuwenhoven, W. J. Riedel, and R.-J. M. Brummer, "Acute tryptophan depletion affects brain-gut responses in irritable bowel syndrome patients and controls," *Gut*, vol. 53, no. 12, pp. 1794–1800, 2004.

[12] T. O. C. Kilkens, A. Honig, D. Fekkes, and R.-J. M. Brummer, "The effects of an acute serotonergic challenge on brain-gut responses in irritable bowel syndrome patients and controls," *Alimentary Pharmacology and Therapeutics*, vol. 22, no. 9, pp. 865–874, 2005.

[13] J. S. Labus, E. A. Mayer, J. Jarcho et al., "Acute tryptophan depletion alters the effective connectivity of emotional arousal circuitry during visceral stimuli in healthy women," *Gut*, vol. 60, no. 9, pp. 1196–1203, 2011.

[14] K. Tillisch, E. A. Mayer, J. S. Labus, J. Stains, L. Chang, and B. D. Naliboff, "Sex specific alterations in autonomic function among patients with irritable bowel syndrome," *Gut*, vol. 54, no. 10, pp. 1396–1401, 2005.

[15] B. Ljótsson, S. Andréewitch, E. Hedman, G. Rück, G. Andersson, and N. Lindefors, "Exposure and mindfulness based therapy for irritable bowel syndrome—an open pilot study," *Journal of Behavior Therapy and Experimental Psychiatry*, vol. 41, no. 3, pp. 185–190, 2010.

[16] B. Ljótsson, L. Falk, A. W. Vesterlund et al., "Internet-delivered exposure and mindfulness based therapy for irritable bowel syndrome—a randomized controlled trial," *Behaviour Research and Therapy*, vol. 48, no. 6, pp. 531–539, 2010.

[17] B. Ljótsson, E. Hedman, P. Lindfors et al., "Long-term follow-up of internet-delivered exposure and mindfulness based treatment for irritable bowel syndrome," *Behaviour Research and Therapy*, vol. 49, no. 1, pp. 58–61, 2011.

[18] B. Ljótsson, E. Hedman, E. Andersson et al., "Internet-delivered exposure-based treatment vs. stress management for irritable bowel syndrome: a randomized trial," *The American Journal of Gastroenterology*, vol. 106, no. 8, pp. 1481–1491, 2011.

[19] B. Ljótsson, G. Andersson, E. Andersson et al., "Acceptability, effectiveness, and cost-effectiveness of internet-based exposure treatment for irritable bowel syndrome in a clinical sample: a randomized controlled trial," *BMC Gastroenterology*, vol. 11, article 110, 2011.

[20] B. Ljótsson, H. Hesser, E. Andersson et al., "Mechanisms of change in an exposure-based treatment for irritable bowel syndrome," *Journal of Consulting and Clinical Psychology*, vol. 81, no. 6, pp. 1113–1126, 2013.

[21] B. Ljótsson, H. Hesser, E. Andersson et al., "Provoking symptoms to relieve symptoms: a randomized controlled dismantling study of exposure therapy in irritable bowel syndrome," *Behaviour Research and Therapy*, vol. 55, no. 1, pp. 27–39, 2014.

[22] K. Boersma, B. Ljótsson, H. Edebol-Carlman, M. Schrooten, S. J. Linton, and R. J. Brummer, "Exposure-based cognitive behavioral therapy for irritable bowel syndrome. A single-case experimental design across 13 subjects," *Cognitive Behaviour Therapy*, vol. 45, no. 6, pp. 415–430, 2016.

[23] G. F. Longstreth, W. G. Thompson, W. D. Chey, L. A. Houghton, F. Mearin, and R. C. Spiller, "Functional bowel disorders," *Gastroenterology*, vol. 130, no. 5, pp. 1480–1491, 2006.

[24] P. Svanborg and M. Asberg, "A new self-rating scale for depression and anxiety states based on the comprehensive psychopathological rating scale," *Acta Psychiatrica Scandinavica*, vol. 89, no. 1, pp. 21–28, 1994.

[25] J. B. Saunders, O. G. Aasland, T. F. Babor, J. R. De La Fuente, and M. Grant, "Development of the alcohol use disorders identification test (AUDIT): WHO collaborative project on early detection of persons with harmful alcohol consumption—II," *Addiction*, vol. 88, no. 6, pp. 791–804, 1993.

[26] B. Ljotsson, 2013, http://www.webskattning.se/ibsorebro.

[27] S. A. L. W. Vanhoutvin, F. J. Troost, T. O. C. Kilkens et al., "Alternative procedure to shorten rectal barostat procedure for the assessment of rectal compliance and visceral perception: a feasibility study," *Journal of Gastroenterology*, vol. 47, no. 8, pp. 896–903, 2012.

[28] J. Svedlund, I. Sjödin, and G. Dotevall, "GSRS-A clinical rating scale for gastrointestinal symptoms in patients with irritable bowel syndrome and peptic ulcer disease," *Digestive Diseases and Sciences*, vol. 33, no. 2, pp. 129–134, 1988.

[29] J. S. Labus, R. Bolus, L. Chang et al., "The Visceral Sensitivity Index: development and validation of a gastrointestinal symptom-specific anxiety scale," *Alimentary Pharmacology and Therapeutics*, vol. 20, no. 1, pp. 89–97, 2004.

[30] A. S. Zigmond and R. P. Snaith, "The hospital anxiety and depression scale," *Acta Psychiatrica Scandinavica*, vol. 67, no. 6, pp. 361–370, 1983.

[31] I. Bjelland, A. A. Dahl, T. T. Haug, and D. Neckelmann, "The validity of the Hospital Anxiety and Depression Scale: an updated literature review," *Journal of Psychosomatic Research*, vol. 52, no. 2, pp. 69–77, 2002.

[32] R Core Team, *R: A Language and Environment for Statistical Computing*, R Foundation for Statistical Computing, Vienna, Austria, 2015, http://www.R-project.org/.

[33] T. V. Elzhov, K. M. Mullen, A.-N. Spiess, and B. Bolker, "minpack.lm: R interface to the Levenberg-Marquardt nonlinear least-squares algorithm found in MINPACK, plus support for bounds," R package version 1.1-8, 2013, https://cran.r-project.org/package=minpack.lm.

[34] F. Faul, E. Erdfelder, A.-G. Lang, and A. Buchner, "G*Power 3: a flexible statistical power analysis program for the social, behavioral, and biomedical sciences," *Behavior Research Methods*, vol. 39, no. 2, pp. 175–191, 2007.

[35] I. L. Zijdenbos, N. J. de Wit, G. J. van der Heijden, G. Rubin, and A. O. Quartero, "Psychological treatments for the management of irritable bowel syndrome," *Cochrane Database of Systematic Reviews*, no. 1, Article ID CD006442, 2009.

[36] D. Human, "Declaration of Helsinki," *Lance*, vol. 353, pp. 1418–1419, 1974.

[37] N. Mazurak, N. Seredyuk, H. Sauer, M. Teufel, and P. Enck, "Heart rate variability in the irritable bowel syndrome: a review of the literature," *Neurogastroenterology and Motility*, vol. 24, no. 3, pp. 206–216, 2012.

[38] L. Li, L. Xiong, S. Zhang, Q. Yu, and M. Chen, "Cognitive-behavioral therapy for irritable bowel syndrome: a meta-analysis," *Journal of Psychosomatic Research*, vol. 77, no. 1, pp. 1–12, 2014.

[39] Q.-L. Tang, G.-Y. Lin, and M.-Q. Zhang, "Cognitive-behavioral therapy for the management of irritable bowel syndrome," *World Journal of Gastroenterology*, vol. 19, no. 46, pp. 8605–8610, 2013.

[40] J. M. Lackner, J. Jaccard, S. S. Krasner, L. A. Katz, G. D. Gudleski, and E. B. Blanchard, "How does cognitive behavior therapy for irritable bowel syndrome work? A mediational analysis of a randomized clinical trial," *Gastroenterology*, vol. 133, no. 2, pp. 433–444, 2007.

Permissions

List of Contributors

Takaharu Matsunaga, Shinichi Hashimoto, Ryo Kawasato, Tomohiro Shirasawa, Atsushi Goto, Taro Takami, Takeshi Okamoto and Isao Sakaida
Department of Gastroenterology and Hepatology, Yamaguchi University Graduate School of Medicine, 1-1-1 Minami Kogushi, Ube, Yamaguchi 755-8505, Japan

Naoki Yamamoto
Department of Gastroenterology and Hepatology, Yamaguchi University Graduate School of Medicine, 1-1-1 Minami Kogushi, Ube, Yamaguchi 755-8505, Japan
Yamaguchi University Health Administration Center, 1677-1 Yoshida, Yamaguchi, Yamaguchi 753-8511, Japan

Koichi Fujisawa
Department of Gastroenterology and Hepatology, Yamaguchi University Graduate School of Medicine, 1-1-1 Minami Kogushi, Ube, Yamaguchi 755-8505, Japan
Center of Research and Education for Regenerative Medicine, Yamaguchi University Graduate School of Medicine, 1-1-1 Minami Kogushi, Ube, Yamaguchi 755-8505, Japan

Jun Nishikawa
Department of Gastroenterology and Hepatology, Yamaguchi University Graduate School of Medicine, 1-1-1 Minami Kogushi, Ube, Yamaguchi 755-8505, Japan
Department of Laboratory Science, Yamaguchi University Graduate School of Medicine, 1-1-1 Minami Kogushi, Ube, Yamaguchi 755-8505, Japan

Martin Hübner, Hugo Teixeira Farinha, Fabian Grass, Dieter Hahnloser and Nicolas Demartines
Department of Visceral Surgery, University Hospital of Lausanne (CHUV), Lausanne, Switzerland

Anita Wolfer
Department of Medical Oncology, University Hospital of Lausanne (CHUV), Lausanne, Switzerland

Patrice Mathevet
Department of Gynecology, University Hospital of Lausanne (CHUV), Lausanne, Switzerland

ReneWarschkow
Department of Surgery, Cantonal Hospital of St. Gallen, 9007 St. Gallen, Switzerland
Institute of Medical Biometry and Informatics, University of Heidelberg, 69120 Heidelberg, Germany

SabrinaM. Ebinger
Department of Surgery, Cantonal Hospital of St. Gallen, 9007 St. Gallen, Switzerland
Department of Surgery, Hospital ofThun, 3600Thun, Switzerland

Walter Brunner and BrunoM. Schmied
Department of Surgery, Cantonal Hospital of St. Gallen, 9007 St. Gallen, Switzerland

Lukas Marti
Department of Surgery, Cantonal Hospital of St. Gallen, 9007 St. Gallen, Switzerland
Department of Surgery, Universit'atsmedizin Mannheim, Medical Faculty Mannheim, University of Heidelberg, 68167 Mannheim, Germany

Fumio Omata and Tsuguya Fukui
Department of Internal Medicine, St. Luke's International Hospital, Chuo-Ku, Japan
Center for Clinical Epidemiology, St. Luke's International University, Chuo-Ku, Japan

Takuro Shimbo
Ohta Nishinouchi Hospital, Koriyama, Japan

Sachiko Ohde and Gautam A. Deshpande
Center for Clinical Epidemiology, St. Luke's International University, Chuo-Ku, Japan

Lin Jia
Department of Medical Oncology, The Affiliated Hospital of Hebei University, Baoding 071000, China

Shuguang Ren and JianhuaWu
Department of Animal Center,The Fourth Hospital, Hebei Medical University, Shijiazhuang 050017, China

Tao Li
Department of Epidemiology and Health Statistics, School of Public Health, Hebei Medical University, Shijiazhuang 050011, China

JianingWu and Yan Zhang
Hebei Province China-Japan Friendship Center for Cancer Detection, Shijiazhuang 050017, China

Xinliang Zhout
Department of Medical Oncology,The Fourth Hospital, Hebei Medical University, Shijiazhuang 050017, China

Wei Liu
Department of Palliative Care Center, Beijing Cancer Hospital, Beijing 100000, China

Long-Hai Cui, Sang-Yong Son, Ho-Jung Shin, Cheulsu Byun, Hoon Hur,
Sang-Uk Han and Yong Kwan Cho
Department of Surgery, Ajou University School of Medicine, Suwon, Republic of Korea

Wei-chun Zhao, Yan-shan Xu, Yan Guo, Dan-yi Wang and Gui-binMeng
College of Life Sciences, Zhejiang Chinese Medical University, Hangzhou 310053, China

Gang Chen
Department of Chemistry, Simon Fraser University, Burnaby, BC, Canada V5A 1S6

Chenyu Li, Aixia Gong, Jingwen Zhang, Linmei Ge, Nan Xia, Jing Leng, Mei Li and Yanjie Liu
Department of Digestive Endoscopy,The First Affiliated Hospital of Dalian Medical University, Dalian, Liaoning 116000, China

Zhijun Duan
Department of Gastroenterology,The First Affiliated Hospital of Dalian Medical University, Dalian, Liaoning 116000, China

Runhua Chen
Department of Gastroenterology, Dongfang Hospital, Beijing University of Chinese Medicine, Beijing, China

Han Deng
Postgraduate College, Dalian Medical University, Dalian, China

Xia Ding
Department of Hospital Administration, Beijing University of Chinese Medicine, Beijing, China

Chune Xie
Department of Personnel, Dongfang Hospital, Beijing University of Chinese Medicine, Beijing, China

WeiWang
Department of Cardiology,Wangjing Hospital, China Academy of Chinese Medical Sciences, Beijing, China

Qian Shen
Department of Massage and Physiotherapy, Dongfang Hospital, Beijing University of Chinese Medicine, Beijing, China

Zhikun Liu, Feng Gao and Zhou Shao
Division of Hepatobiliary and Pancreatic Surgery, First Affiliated Hospital, Zhejiang University School of Medicine, Hangzhou, China
Key Lab of Combined Multi-Organ Transplantation, Ministry of Public Health, Hangzhou, China

Haiyang Xie and Lin Zhou
Key Lab of Combined Multi-Organ Transplantation, Ministry of Public Health, Hangzhou, China
Collaborative Innovation Center for Diagnosis and Treatment of Infectious Diseases, Hangzhou, China

Xiao Xu and Shusen Zheng
Division of Hepatobiliary and Pancreatic Surgery, First Affiliated Hospital, Zhejiang University School of Medicine, Hangzhou, China
Key Lab of Combined Multi-Organ Transplantation, Ministry of Public Health, Hangzhou, China
Collaborative Innovation Center for Diagnosis and Treatment of Infectious Diseases, Hangzhou, China

Jennifer M. Weiss
Division of Gastroenterology and Hepatology, University of Wisconsin School of Medicine and Public Health, Madison, WI, USA
Department of Medicine, University ofWisconsin School of Medicine and Public Health, Madison, WI, USA
University of Wisconsin Carbone Cancer Center, Madison, WI, USA

Perry J. Pickhardt and David H. Kim
Department of Radiology, University of Wisconsin School of Medicine and Public Health, Madison, WI, USA

Jessica R. Schumacher
Department of Surgery, University of Wisconsin School of Medicine and Public Health, Madison, WI, USA

Aaron Potvien
Department of Population Health Sciences, University of Wisconsin School of Medicine and Public Health, Madison, WI, USA

Patrick R. Pfau
Division of Gastroenterology and Hepatology, University of Wisconsin School of Medicine and Public Health, Madison, WI, USA
Department of Medicine, University of Wisconsin School of Medicine and Public

Elizabeth A. Jacobs
Department of Medicine, University of Wisconsin School of Medicine and Public

Maureen A. Smith
University of Wisconsin Carbone Cancer Center, Madison, WI, USA
Department of Surgery, University ofWisconsin School of Medicine and Public Health, Madison,WI, USA
Department of Population Health Sciences, University ofWisconsin School of Medicine and Public Health, Madison,WI, USA
Department of Family Medicine, University ofWisconsin School of Medicine and Public Health, Madison, WI, USA

Muyun Liu, Tian Xia, Di Zhang, Lianghao Hu, Zhuan Liao, Chang Sun and Zhaoshen Li
Department of Gastroenterology, Changhai Hospital, Second Military Medical University, Shanghai, China

BrunoMärkl, Simon Franz and Tina Schaller
Institute of Pathology, Klinikum Augsburg, Augsburg, Germany

Jochen Hardt and Reinhard Hoffmann
Institute of Laboratory Medicine and Microbiology, Klinikum Augsburg, Augsburg, Germany

Gerhard Schenkirsch
Clinical and Population-Based Cancer Registry Augsburg, Augsburg, Germany

Bernadette Kriening and Stefan Rüth
Department of Visceral Surgery, Klinikum Augsburg, Augsburg, Germany

Kang Nyeong Lee and Oh Young Lee
Department of Internal Medicine, Hanyang University College of Medicine, Seoul, Republic of Korea

Hassan K. Dakik
Duke Gastroenterology Division, Duke University Hospital, Durham, NC, USA

F. Douglas Srygley
Austin Gastroenterology, Austin, TX, USA

Shih-Ting Chiu and Shein-Chung Chow
Duke Biostatistics Division, Duke University Hospital, Durham, NC, USA

Deborah A. Fisher
Duke Gastroenterology Division, Duke University Hospital, Durham, NC, USA
Durham VA Health Services Research and Development Center, Durham, NC, USA

Yoichiro Okubo, Tomoyuki Yokose, Emi Yoshioka, Masaki Suzuki, Kota Washimi, Kae Kawachi and Yoichi Kameda
Department of Pathology, Kanagawa Cancer Center, 2-3-2 Nakao, Asahi-Ku, Yokohama, Kanagawa 241-8515, Japan

OsamuMotohashi
Department of Gastroenterology, Kanagawa Cancer Center, 2-3-2 Nakao, Asahi-Ku, Yokohama, Kanagawa 241-8515, Japan

YoheiMiyagi
Molecular Pathology and Genetics Division, Kanagawa Cancer Center Research Institute, 2-3-2 Nakao, Asahi-Ku, Yokohama, Kanagawa 241-8515, Japan

Madoka Nito
Department ofThoracic Surgery, Kanagawa Cancer Center, 2-3-2 Nakao, Asahi-Ku, Yokohama, Kanagawa 241-8515, Japan

Tetsuo Nemoto and Kazutoshi Shibuya
Department of Surgical Pathology, Toho University School of Medicine, 6-11-1 Omori-Nishi, Ota-Ku, Tokyo 143-8541, Japan

Ou Cai and Shiyun Tan
Department of Gastroenterology, Renmin Hospital of Wuhan University, Wuhan, Hubei, China

F. Scaldaferri, M. Pizzoferrato, L. R. Lopetuso, T. Musca, F. Ingravalle,
L. L. Sicignano, E. Gaetani, C. Graziani, V. Petito, G. Cammarota and A. Gasbarrin
Gastroenterology Division, Catholic University of Sacred Heart, Rome, Italy

M. Mentella, G. Miggiano and M. C. Mele
Nutrition Team, Catholic University of Sacred Heart, Rome, Italy

E. Marzetti, A. Martone and F. Landi
Gerontology Division, Catholic University of Sacred Heart, Rome, Italy

Hao Wu
Qilu Hospital, Shandong University, Ji'nan, Shandong 250012, China
Department of Gastroenterology, The Second Affiliated Hospital, Wenzhou Medical University, Wenzhou, China

Liang Sun, Dao-po Lin, Xiao-xiao Shao and Sheng-long Xia
Department of Gastroenterology, The Second Affiliated Hospital, Wenzhou Medical University, Wenzhou, China

Ming Lv
Qilu Hospital, Shandong University, Ji'nan, Shandong 250012, China

Mengjie Jiang, Xiaofen Li, Hanguang Hu, Xianyun Ye, Ying Cao,
and Ying Yuan
Department of Medical Oncology, The Second Affiliated Hospital, Zhejiang University School of Medicine, Hangzhou, Zhejiang Province, China

Yinuo Tan
Department of Surgical Oncology, The Second Affiliated Hospital, Zhejiang University School of Medicine, Hangzhou, Zhejiang Province, China

Jianfei Fu
Cancer Institute (Key Laboratory of Cancer Prevention and Intervention, Chinese National Ministry of Education; Key Laboratory of Molecular Biology in Medical Sciences, Zhejiang Province, China),The Second Affiliated Hospital, Zhejiang University School of Medicine, Hangzhou, Zhejiang Province, China
Department of Oncology, Jinhua Central Hospital (Jinhua Hospital of Zhejiang University School of Medicine), Jinhua, Zhejiang Province, China

Jinghong Xu
Department of Pathology, The Second Affiliated Hospital, Zhejiang University School of Medicine, Hangzhou, Zhejiang Province, China

Yuqing Zhou, Shunfeng Zhou, Linqiang Li, Keran Cheng and Rui Kong
Department of Gastroenterology, Shanghai Tenth People's Hospital, School of Medicine, Tongji University, Shanghai 200072, China
The School of Medicine of Soochow University, Suzhou 215006, China

Qian Dong
The Shanghai Tenth Hospital, School of Clinical Medicine of Nanjing Medical University, Shanghai 200072, China

Rong Zhang, Qiang Yu and Shizan Xu
Department of Gastroenterology, Shanghai Tenth People's Hospital, School of Medicine, Tongji University, Shanghai 200072, China
The Shanghai Tenth Hospital, School of Clinical Medicine of Nanjing Medical University, Shanghai 200072, China

Jingjing Li, Sainan Li, Jiao Feng, LiweiWu, Tong Liu, Xiya Lu, Kan Chen, Yujing Xia, Jie Lu, Yingqun Zhou and Chuanyong Guo
Department of Gastroenterology, Shanghai Tenth People's Hospital, School of Medicine, Tongji University, Shanghai 200072, China

Kevin J. Etherson, Iain M. Bain, Jeremy Cundall and Yan Yiannakou
Department of Colorectal Surgery, County Durham and Darlington NHS Foundation Trust, Durham, UK

IanMinty
Department of Radiology, County Durham and Darlington NHS Foundation Trust, Durham, UK

Hanna Edebol-Carlman, Dirk Repsilber, and Robert J. Brummer
Nutrition-Gut-Brain Interactions Research Centre, Örebro University, 701 82 Örebro, Sweden

Brjánn Ljótsson
Department of Clinical Neuroscience, Division of Psychiatry, Karolinska Institutet, Stockholm, Sweden

Steven J. Linton, Katja Boersma and Martien Schrooten
Center for Health and Medical Psychology (CHAMP), School of Law, Psychology and Social Work, Örebro University, Örebro, Sweden

Index

www.ingramcontent.com/pod-product-compliance
Lightning Source LLC
Chambersburg PA
CBHW080629200326
41458CB00013B/4563